LIBYA

EGYPT

NORTH AFRICA

0 200 400 600 MILES

0 200 400 600 KILOMETERS

Medicinal Plants
of
North Africa

BOOKS BY LOUTFY BOULOS

COMMON WEEDS IN EGYPT (1967)

STREET TREES IN EGYPT (1968; 2nd ed. 1979)

SUPPLEMENTARY NOTES TO STUDENTS' FLORA OF EGYPT, SECOND EDITION (1974)

FIREWOOD CROPS (1980)

BOOKS ILLUSTRATED BY MAGDY EL-GOHARY

COMMON WEEDS IN EGYPT (1967)

STREET TREES IN EGYPT (1968; 2nd ed. 1979)

STUDENTS' FLORA OF EGYPT, SECOND EDITION (1974)

FLORA OF EGYPT, AMARANTHACEAE (1981)

MEDICINAL PLANTS of NORTH AFRICA

Loutfy Boulos
Illustrated by Magdy El-Gohary

Reference Publications, Inc.

This is a book in the series "Medicinal Plants of the World."

Published 1983

Printed in the United States of America

Library of Congress Cataloging in Publication Data

Boulos, Loutfy.
Medicinal plants of North Africa.

(Medicinal plants of the world; no. 3)
Bibliography: p.
Includes index.
1. Medicinal plants—Africa, North. 2. Materia medica, Vegetable—Africa, North. 3. Folk medicine—Africa, North. I. Title. II. Series.
QK99.A43B68 1982 581.6'34'0961 82-20412
ISBA 0-917256-16-6

Library of Congress Catalog Card Number: 82-20412
International Standard Book Number: 0-917256-16-6

Reference Publications, Inc.
218 St. Clair River Drive, Box 344
Algonac, Michigan 48001

This work is dedicated to
the memory of my teachers

Louis Emberger (1897-1969)
Vivi Täckholm (1898-1978)
Charles Sauvage (1909-1980)

who devoted most of their lifework
to study the plants of North Africa.

Acknowledgements

I wish to thank Professor Edward S. Ayensu, Director, Office of Biological Conservation, Smithsonian Institution, Washington, D.C., for introducing me to Mr. Keith Irvine, President, Reference Publications, who kindly asked me to undertake this work.

I am most grateful to Professor Mohamed Kamel, Director, National Research Center, Dokki, Cairo, for his encouragement and help, to Mr. Magdy El-Gohary for his great skill and patience in drawing the plates, and to Dr. Robert DeFilipps, Smithsonian Institution, for his careful reading of the manuscript. Thanks are also due to Professor M. Nabil El-Hadidi, Cairo University Herbarium, for the facilities and help during the preparation of the work. Dr. Raymond M. Harley, Royal Botanic Gardens, Kew, England, kindly determined the *Mentha* species. Dr. E. Le Floc'h, Centre d'Etudes Phytosociologiques et Ecologiques Louis Emberger, Montpellier, France, generously supplied numerous publications on the subject during the preparation of the work and during my visit to Montpellier in 1981.

During my visit to Rabat, Morocco, in 1980, Dr. José Lewalle, Mr. Francis Collin, Dr. Abdelhamid Daoudi and Mr. Mohamed Atbibi kindly helped me to obtain material, information, literature, and to determine some specimens. Madame Nicole Bounaga and Mr. Faid Abdelkader kindly allowed me to work in the Library of the Botany Department, University of Algiers, during my visit in 1980. I am also grateful to Dr. Sidky T. Boulos for his kind hospitality and help during my stay in Algiers.

The indexes were compiled at the Computer Department, National Research Center, Cairo, Egypt, through the courtesy of Dr. Nadia Hegazi and her colleagues.

Dr. Adel K. El-Duweini, National Information Center, Cairo, (NIDOC), kindly supplied several items of literature.

To my friends and colleagues who helped in many different ways throughout the preparation of this book, I owe a word of thanks. None are mentioned by name, but my gratitude goes to them all.

I also wish to thank my sister and my brother-in-law, Soad and Ahdy Mansour, of Cleveland, Ohio, for their kind hospitality during my stay with them in the spring of 1983.

I am indebted to my wife, Soad, for her tolerance and support, especially during the last four years, when this work was being prepared.

LOUTFY BOULOS

Foreword

This volume—the third in the series "Medicinal Plants of the World"—is yet another manifestation of the deliberate effort by modern scientists to find useful medicinal agents in the plant kingdom. Prehistoric man began to use plants to battle diseases, induce hallucinogenic experiences, and to ward off evil spirits. These uses of plants continue to be witnessed throughout the world, especially in developing nations where over eighty percent of the population relies on herbal treatments as their major health delivery system.

Plants represent a fantastic source of chemical compounds, ranging in complexity from those which are simple but potentially toxic, to complicated derivatives. The systematic isolation and identification of these compounds is essential if we are to help the search for new useful drugs. Unfortunately the impressive variety of plants being used in different parts of the world has not been subjected to careful study. One of the main objectives of this volume and those in the series is to assemble, in one place, basic information on the plant species used frequently in folk medicine, for the guidance of plant chemists and pharmacologists desiring to investigate the chemical constituents and to determine the efficacy of these plant resources. The volumes will also help modern medical practitioners to learn enough about herbal medicine so that they can communicate more knowledgeably with traditional healers with whom the World Health Organization is currently seeking collaboration.

The advent of western medicine diminished the importance of herbal remedies especially since scientific discoveries showed how fatal the indiscriminate use of plants could be. Various studies have shown that plant principles which produce medicinal effects usually are also poisonous. In small quantities they may only stimulate and produce beneficial effects; but in large doses they begin to produce stronger physiological reactions that can prove to be quite lethal. For example, hypertension or high blood pressure, which is a common fatal disorder, is currently controlled by the alkaloid reserpine found in *Rauwolfia serpentina,* a species which features prominently in Asiatic folklore and is currently grown in many parts of the world. This plant, if misused, can destroy stores of the neurotransmitter noradrenaline in the brain and can lead to suicidal depression. It is therefore important that as herbal medicine assumes new importance in health delivery systems in developing countries, every effort should be made to ensure that avoidable catastrophes are totally eliminated. This can only be achieved when herbalists receive the confidence of plant scientists and medical doctors in their own societies.

I am extremely grateful to my friend and colleague Dr. Loutfy Boulos for accepting my request to contribute this volume covering North Africa—an area for which he is regarded worldwide as the foremost systematic botanist. By combing the local drug emporiums of Cairo, Algiers and several other North African cities and villages, he has given us a unique insight into the preparations used in this part of the Arabic-speaking world, where intensified multi-purpose utilization of individual medicinal species has evolved over centuries of trial and error by both stationary and nomadic cultures. One notes with interest that some of the plants used by the desert nomadic tribes to cure ailments of their camels, the mainstay of their economy and society, are also used effectively to cure human disorders. Researchers will be intrigued by the numerous human abortifacients, aphrodisiacs, and female weight-inducing drugs, even some Saharan war poisons of decades not far gone, which on the whole present a great potential of species for further chemical inventory.

Dr. Boulos is to be congratulated for the remarkable exhibition of his knowledge of medicinal plants of North Africa and for his understanding of the need to make such knowledge available to a wide audience.

EDWARD S. AYENSU

Introduction

The use of herbs for therapeutic purposes in North Africa dates back to immemorial times. In desert countries, like the greater part of our area, where people live in communities far away from each other, the inhabitants used to be short of, or almost deprived of proper medical care. Naturally, a group of local prescribers have to fill the gap using folk medicine formulae, based on crude materials from their local environment. Indigenous and naturalized plants, their infusions, decoctions, powders, juices, etc., constitute the backbone of their medicinal activities. In North Africa, plants were traditionally prescribed and used for generations and probably for centuries with slight or almost no change, and with strong belief, leading in most cases to satisfactory results. If the patient is not cured or little progress is noted, then the reason is attributed to other unseen factors such as evil eye or heaven's curse, while the medicinal herbs have always been considered as good and effective drugs.

The aim of this book, as one of a series of books on medicinal plants covering different parts of the world, is to bridge the gap between folk and modern medicine, and to introduce, in our case, the medicinal plants of North Africa and their uses, a tradition experienced by many generations of the indigenous people, yet unknown to most of us. Many herbalists, scientists and travellers, during different ages, old and recent, have studied some of these plants and recorded their uses, yet the modern literature covering this subject, especially for some parts of the world like the tropics and arid regions, has been insufficient to revive these traditions.

In order to bring back to life the use of these plants, I may quote here the following words from a recent publication (1980) of "The Beneficial Plant Research Association," a non-profit scientific and educational corporation formed in 1979 in Carmel Valley, California, to investigate and promote the use of plants to improve human life. "A special concern of the Association is to make available natural pharmaceuticals that are effective but less dangerous than many of the potent synthetic drugs now in common use. In the past century, interest in botanical drugs has waxed and waned. In general, however, their use has steadily decreased in medical practice. Presently, there is a resurgence of interest in these traditional medicines, stimulated by growing awareness of the dangers of the overuse of synthetics. Adverse drug reactions are today the leading iatrogenic (physician-caused) illness. Moreover, the inflated prices of synthetic pharmaceutical drugs contribute heavily to escalating medical costs. Synthetic chemicals certainly have their place in treatment, but physicians and patients should have the option of choosing the milder, natural forms of medicines when appropriate."

I have kept an interest in the subject during my numerous field trips to different areas in Egypt and the neighboring countries for botanical investigations since I was a student in Cairo University in 1952. Specimens and information were collected during my five years' assignment (1966-1971) with the University of Libya, and published in an article (1970) on the "Medicinal herbs in Libya." In 1968 I visited Tunisia and collected some 500 species of its flora. In September 1980 I paid a visit both to Morocco and Algeria, exclusively to collect drugs and some basic information on the medicinal plants of these interesting regions of North Africa. Especially interesting were the "souks" or local markets where the medicinal herbs were sold, and the drug seller would prescribe to the buyer how to use the drug and when it should be taken, together with the appropriate dose. In October 1981, I also spent a few weeks in Montpellier where I was introduced to some of the literature covering the subject of North Africa.

This work deals with 369 species of vascular plants, alphabetically arranged according to the 97 families to which they belong. The species are indigenous, naturalized or cultivated in North Africa; also included are some drugs which are traditionally used by the people and which constitute a part of the folk medicine in the area. For every species the scientific name is given and whenever appropriate the synonym or synonyms which are to be expected in the literature due to the latest changes in the botanical nomenclature. The distribution of the plant only within North Africa is given. If the species is spontaneous (wild) and known from all the five countries of North Africa from east to west: Egypt, Libya, Tunisia, Algeria and Morocco, then the phrase "Egypt to Morocco" is given; otherwise, the country or countries from which the species is known is stated. If the species is naturalized, cultivated or imported as a drug, this is also mentioned. If only one country is mentioned for the distribution of the species, this does not mean that it is not known from other parts of the world, e.g., *Blepharis ciliaris,* Egypt, is also known from other countries of the Middle East; *Origanum compactum,* Morocco, is also known from Spain. For species only known from our area, the term "endemic" is added, e.g., *Thymus broussonettii* is endemic to Morocco, *Arbutus pavari,* endemic to Libya and *Cedrus atlantica* endemic to Algeria and Morocco.

The vernacular names are given in Arabic, Berber, English and French, whenever available. The Arabic names usually vary according to their origin, often with different orthographic versions which are often listed for the same name, otherwise the most common version is mentioned. "Berber" refers to the different local languages used by various tribes in villages or in the desert regions of the Sahara, Atlas Mountains, etc.

The drawings cover 107 species in 103 plates. Some groups, such as all the *Mentha* species and most of the cultivated species of Umbelliferae, are drawn in order to help the users of the book to identify their specimens, which are often difficult to separate. For species marked with an asterisk (*)the reader is advised to consult the section on Notes and Explanations for synonyms and names of other taxa included within the species. A medicinal index and a glossary of medical terms are included.

LOUTFY BOULOS

Contents

Dedication 3
Acknowledgements 5
Foreword by Edward S. Ayensu 6
Introduction by the Author 8

MEDICINAL PLANTS OF NORTH AFRICA

Acanthaceae 23
Acanthus mollis L. 23
Blepharis ciliaris (L.) B.L. Burtt 23
Adiantaceae 23
Adiantum capillus-veneris L. 23
Alismataceae 23
Alisma plantago-aquatica L. 23
Alliaceae 23
Allium cepa L. 23
Allium sativum L. 23
Amaryllidaceae 25
Narcissus tazetta L. 25
Anacardiaceae 25
Rhus tripartita (Ucria) Grande 25
Apocynaceae 25
Nerium oleander L. 25
Araceae 25
Arisarum vulgare Targ.-Tozz. 25
Arum italicum Miller 27
Eminium spiculatum (Blume) Kuntze 27
Araliaceae 27
Hedera helix L. 27
Asclepiadaceae 27
Calotropis procera (Ait.) Ait. fil. 27
Leptadenia pyrotechnica (Forssk.) Decne 27
Pergularia tomentosa L. 32
Periploca laevigata Ait. 32
Solenostemma arghel (Del.) Hayne 32
Aspidiaceae 32
Dryopteris filix-mas (L.) Schott 32
Aspleniaceae 32
Asplenium adiantum-nigrum L. 32
Asplenium trichomanes L. 32
Ceterach officinarum DC. 32
Phyllitis scolopendrium (L.) Newman 35
Balanitaceae 35
Balanites aegyptiaca (L.) Del. 35
Berberidaceae 35

Berberis hispanica Boiss. & Reuter 35
Boraginaceae 35
Alkanna tinctoria (L.) Tausch 35
Anchusa azurea Miller 35
Borago officinalis L. 37
Cynoglossum officinale L. 37
Echium plantagineum L. 37
Heliotropium bacciferum Forssk. 37
Moltkiopsis ciliata (Forssk.) Johnst. 37
Buxaceae 37
Buxus sempervirens L. 37
Cactaceae 40
Opuntia ficus-indica (L.) Miller 40
Cannabidaceae 40
Cannabis sativa L. 40
Capparaceae 40
Capparis decidua (Forssk.) Edgew. 40
Capparis spinosa L. 40
Maerua crassifolia Forssk. 42
Caprifoliaceae 42
Sambucus ebulus L. 42
Sambucus nigra L. 42
Caryophyllaceae 42
Corrigiola telephiifolia Pourret 42
Herniaria hirsuta L. 45
Paronychia arabica (L.) DC. 45
Paronychia argentea Lam. 45
Spergularia media (L.) C. Presl 45
Spergularia rubra (L.) J. & C. Presl 45
Stellaria media (L.) Vill. 45
Vaccaria pyramidata Medicus 45
Chenopodiaceae 45
Atriplex halimus L. 45
Chenopodium ambrosioides L. 46
Chenopodium vulvaria L. 46
Cornulaca monacantha Del. 46
Haloxylon scoparium Pomel 46
Cistaceae 46
Cistus albidus L. 46
Cistus ladanifer L. 46
Cistus monspeliensis L. 52
Cleomaceae 52
Cleome amblyocarpa Barr. & Murb. 52
Compositae 52
Achillea fragrantissima (Forssk.) Sch. Bip. 52
Achillea santolina L. 52
Ageratum conyzoides L. 52
Ambrosia maritima L. 52
Anacyclus pyrethrum (L.) Link 52

Anthemis pseudocotula Boiss. 54
Artemisia absinthium L. 54
Artemisia arborescens L. 54
Artemisia atlantica Coss. & Dur. 57
Artemisia campestris L. 57
Artemisia herba-alba Asso 57
Artemisia judaica L. 57
Atractylis gummifera L. 57
Calendula officinalis L. 60
Centaurea acaulis L. 60
Centaurea alexandrina Del. 60
Centaurea calcitrapa L. 60
Chamaemelum nobile (L.) All. 60
Chamomilla recutita (L.) Rauschert 60
Chrysanthemum coronarium L. 61
Cichorium intybus L. 61
Conyza bonariensis (L.) Cronq. 61
Cotula cinerea Del. 61
Cotula coronopifolia L. 61
Cynara cardunculus L. 61
Cynara humilis L. 64
Cynara scolymus L. 64
Echinops spinosus L. 64
Eclipta prostrata (L.) L. 64
Eupatorium cannabinum L. 64
Helianthus annuus L. 64
Inula viscosa (L.) Ait. 64
Lactuca sativa L. 67
Lactuca serriola L. 67
Lactuca virosa L. 67
Otanthus maritimus (L.) Hoffmanns. & Link 67
Pulicaria crispa (Forssk.) Benth. ex Oliver 67
Pulicaria incisa (Lam.) DC. 67
Santolina chamaecyparissus L. 67
Senecio anteuphorbium L. 68
Senecio vulgaris L. 68
Silybum marianum (L.) Gaertner 68

Convolvulaceae 68
Convolvlus althaeoides L. 68
Convolvulus arvensis L. 68
Convolvulus hystrix Vahl 68
Cressa cretica L. 68
Cuscuta epithymum (L.) L. 70
Cuscuta planiflora Ten. 70

Coriariaceae 70
Coriaria myrtifolia L. 70

Cruciferae 70
Alliaria petiolata (Bieb.) Cavara & Grande 70
Anastatica hierochuntica L. 70
Brassica nigra (L.) Koch 70
Capsella bursa-pastoris (L.) Medicus 71

Eruca sativa Miller 71
Lepidium sativum L. 71
Lobularia maritima (L.) Desv. 71
Nasturtium officinale R. Br. 71
Raphanus sativus L. 73
Sinapis alba L. 73
Sisymbrium officinale (L.) Scop. 73
Zilla spinosa (L.) Prantl 73
Cucurbitaceae 73
Bryonia dioica Jacq. 73
Citrullus colocynthis (L.) Schrader 73
Cucumis melo L. 75
Cucurbita pepo L. 75
Ecballium elaterium (L.) A. Rich. 75
Lagenaria siceraria (Molina) Standley 75
Luffa cylindrica (L.) M. Roem. 79
Cupressaceae 79
Cupressus sempervirens L. 79
Juniperus communis L. 79
Juniperus oxycedrus L. 79
Juniperus phoenicea L. 79
Juniperus thurifera L. 80
Tetraclinis articulata (Vahl) Masters 80
Cynomoriaceae 80
Cynomorium coccineum L. 80
Cyperaceae 80
Cyperus esculentus L. 80
Cyperus papyrus L. 82
Cyperus rotundus L. 82
Dioscoreaceae 82
Tamus communis L. 82
Ephedraceae 82
Ephedra alata Decne. 82
Ericaceae 82
Arbutus pavari Pamp. 82
Euphorbiaceae 83
Euphorbia balsamifera Ait. var. *sepium* N.E. Br. 83
Euphorbia echinus Hook. fil. & Coss. 83
Euphorbia falcata L. 83
Euphorbia granulata Forssk. 83
Euphorbia helioscopia L. 83
Euphorbia lathyrus L. 83
Euphorbia peplis L. 83
Euphorbia resenifera Berg. 83
Mercurialis annua L. 86
Ricinus communis L. 86
Fagaceae 86
Quercus coccifera L. 86
Fumariaceae 89

Fumaria judaica Boiss. 89
Fumaria officinalis L. 89
Fumaria parviflora Lam. 89
Gentianaceae 89
Centaurium erythraea Rafn 89
Centaurium spicatum (L.) Fritsch 89
Geraniaceae 92
Erodium cicutarium (L.) L'Hérit. 92
Geranium robertianum L. 92
Globulariaceae 92
Globularia alypum L. 92
Gramineae 92
Avena sativa L. 92
Cymbopogon proximus (Hochst. ex A. Rich.) Stapf 92
Cymbopogon schoenanthus (L.) Spreng. 94
Cynodon dactylon (L.) Pers. 94
Eleusine indica (L.) Gaertner 94
Elymus repens (L.) Gould 94
Imperata cylindrica (L.) Beauv. 94
Lolium perenne L. 94
Lolium temulentum L. 96
Panicum turgidum Forssk. 96
Phragmites australis (Cav.) Trin. ex Steud. 96
Stipagrostis pungens (Desf.) de Winter 96
Zea mays L. 96
Guttiferae 96
Hypericum perforatum L. 96
Iridaceae 97
Crocus sativus L. 97
Iris foetidissima L. 97
Iris germanica L. 97
Iris pseudacorus L. 97
Juglandaceae 98
Juglans regia L. 98
Juncaceae 98
Juncus acutus L. 98
Juncus maritimus Lam. 98
Labiatae 98
Ajuga iva (L.) Schreber 98
Ballota nigra L. 101
Lavandula angustifolia Miller 101
Lavandula dentata L. 101
Lavandula multifida L. 101
Lavandula stoechas L 101
Lycopus europaeus L. 101
Marrubium vulgare L. 101
Melissa officinalis L. 104
Mentha longifolia (L.) Huds. subsp. *typhoides* (Briq.) R. Harley 104
Mentha pulegium L. 104
Mentha spicata L. 104

Mentha suaveolens Ehrh. 109
Mentha x *villosa* Huds. 109
Ocimum basilicum L. 109
Origanum compactum Benth. 109
Origanum majorana L. 109
Origanum vulgare L. subsp. *glandulosum* (Desf.) Ietswaart 109
Otostegia fruticosa (Forssk.) Schweinf. ex Penzig 110
Rosmarinus officinalis L. 110
Salvia fruticosa Miller 110
Salvia officinalis L. 110
Salvia sclarea L. 110
Stachys officinalis (L.) Trev. 112
Teucrium chamaedrys L. 112
Teucrium polium L. 112
Thymus algeriensis Boiss. & Reut. 112
Thymus broussonettii Boiss. 112
Thymus capitatus (L.) Hoffmanns. & Link 112

Lauraceae 116
Laurus nobilis L. 116

Leguminosae 116
Acacia albida Del. 116
Acacia nilotica (L.) Willd. ex Del. 116
Acacia raddiana Savi 116
Acacia seyal Del. 116
Alhagi graecorum Boiss. 119
Anagyris foetida L. 119
Anthyllis vulneraria L. 119
Cassia italica (Miller) F.W. Andr. 119
Cassia senna L. 119
Ceratonia siliqua L. 119
Cicer arietinum L. 123
Colutea arborescens L. 123
Coronilla scorpioides (L.) Koch 123
Crotalaria aegyptiaca Benth. 123
Glycyrrhiza foetida Desf. 123
Glycyrrhiza glabra L. 123
Lupinus albus L. 123
Melilotus indica (L). All. 126
Ononis spinosa L. 126
Ononis tournefortii Cosson 126
Psoralea plicata Del. 126
Retama raetam (Forssk.) Webb 126
Spartium junceum L. 126
Tamarindus indica L. 126
Trigonella foenum-graecum L. 128
Vicia faba L. 128
Vicia sativa L. 128

Liliaceae 128
Aloe perryi Baker 128
Androcymbium gramineum (Cav.) McBride 128
Asparagus stipularis Forssk. 130

Asphodelus aestivus Brot. 130
Colchicum autumnale L. 130
Urginea maritima (L.) Baker 130
Linaceae 131
Linum usitatissimum L. 131
Loranthaceae 131
Viscum cruciatum Sieber ex Boiss. 131
Lythraceae 131
Lawsonia inermis L. 131
Lythrum salicaria L. 131
Malvaceae 134
Althaea officinalis L. 134
Malva parviflora L. 134
Malva sylvestris L. 134
Moraceae 134
Ficus carica L. 134
Morus alba L. 135
Myristicaceae 135
Myristica fragrans Houtt. 135
Myrtaceae 135
Eucalyptus globulus Labill. 135
Myrtus communis L. 135
Syzygium aromaticum (L.) Merr. 137
Nyctaginaceae 137
Boerhavia repens L. 137
Oleaceae 137
Fraxinus angustifolia Vahl 137
Olea europaea L. 137

Orchidaceae 138
Aceras anthropophorum (L.) Ait. fil. 138
Orobanchaceae 138
Cistanche phelypaea (L.) Coutinho 138
Paeoniaceae 138
Paeonia coriacea Boiss. 138
Palmae 138
Hyphaene thebaica (L.) Mart. 138
Phoenix dactylifera L. 140
Papaveraceae 140
Papaver dubium L. 140
Papaver rhoeas L. 140
Papaver somniferum L. 140
Pedaliaceae 142
Sesamum indicum L. 142
Pinaceae 142
Cedrus atlantica (Endl.) Carrière 142
Pinus halepenis Miller 142
Piperaceae 142

Piper cubeba L. fil. 142
Piper nigrum L. 142
Pistaciaceae 145
Pistacia atlantica Desf. 145
Pistacia lentiscus L. 145
Plantaginaceae 145
Plantago afra L. 145
Plantago coronopus L. 146
Plantago major L. 146
Plumbaginaceae 146
Plumbago europaea L. 146
Polygonaceae 146
Polygonum aviculare L. 146
Polygonum maritimum L. 146
Rumex vesicarius L. 149
Polypodiaceae 149
Polypodium vulgare L. 149
Portulacaceae 149
Portulaca oleracea L. 149
Punicaceae 149
Punica granatum L. 149
Ranunculaceae 150
Adonis aestivalis L. 150
Adonis annua L. 150
Clematis flammula L. 150
Delphinium staphisagria L. 150
Nigella sativa L. 150
Ranunculus macrophyllus Desf. 151
Ranunculus sceleratus L. 151
Resedaceae 151
Reseda luteola L. 151
Rhamnaceae 151
Rhamnus alaternus L. 151
Ziziphus lotus (L.) Lam. 151
Ziziphus spina-christi (L.) Willd. 153
Ziziphus zizyphus (L.) Meikle 153
Rosaceae 153
Agrimonia eupatoria L. 153
Crataegus monogyna Jacq. 153
Fragaria vesca L. 153
Geum urbanum L. 153
Potentilla reptans L. 154
Rosa canina L. 154
Rosa damascena Miller 154
Rubus ulmifolius Schott 154
Rubiaceae 154
Galium odoratum (L.) Scop. 154
Rubia peregrina L. 154
Rubia tinctorum L. 155

Ruscaceae 155
Ruscus aculeatus L. 155

Rutaceae 155
Citrus aurantium L. 155
Haplophyllum tuberculatum (Forssk.) A. Juss. 155
Ruta chalepensis L. 158
Ruta montana (L.) L. 158

Salicaceae 158
Populus nigra L. 158
Salix alba L. 158

Salvadoraceae 158
Salvadora persica L. 158

Sapotaceae 162
Argania spinosa (L.) Skeels 162

Scrophulariaceae 162
Verbascum sinuatum L. 162

Smilacaceae 162
Smilax aspera L. 162

Solanaceae 162
Atropa bella-donna L. 162
Capsicum annuum L. 164
Capsicum frutescens L. 164
Datura stramonium L. 164
Hyoscyamus albus L. 164
Hyoscyamus faleslez Coss. 167
Hyoscyamus muticus L. 167
Lycium intricatum Boiss. 167
Mandragora autumnalis Bertol. 167
Nicotiana rustica L. 167
Physalis alkekengi L. 168
Solanum dulcamara L. 168
Solanum nigrum L. 168
Withania somnifera (L.) Dunal 168

Tamaricaceae 172
Tamarix aphylla L. 172

Thymelaeaceae 172
Daphne gnidium L. 172
Thymelaea hirsuta (L.) Endl. 172

Typhaceae 172
Typha domingensis (Pers.) Steud. 172

Ulmaceae 172
Ulmus campestris L. 172

Umbelliferae 175
Ammi majus L. 175
Ammi visnaga L. 175
Ammodaucus leucotrichus Coss. & Dur. 175
Ammoides pusilla (Brot.) Breistr. 175
Anethum graveolens L. 175

Apium graveolens L. 175
Carum carvi L. 180
Conium maculatum L. 180
Coriandrum sativum L. 180
Crithmum maritimum L. 183
Cuminum cyminum L. 183
Daucus carota L. var. *boissieri* Wittm. 183
Eryngium campestre L. 183
Eryngium ilicifolium Lam. 183
Ferula communis L. 183
Foeniculum vulgare Miller 187
Petroselinum crispum (Miller) A. W. Hill 187
Pimpinella anisum L. 187
Pituranthos tortuosus (Desf.) Benth. & Hook. fil. 187
Thapsia garganica L. 187
Urticaceae 191
Urtica pilulifera L. 191
Urtica urens L. 191
Verbenaceae 191
Aloysia triphylla (L'Hérit.) Britt. 191
Verbena officinalis L. 191
Vitex agnus-castus L. 193
Violaceae 193
Viola odorata L. 193
Viola tricolor L. 193
Zingiberaceae 193
Alpinia officinarum Hance 193
Curcuma zedoaria (Christm.) Roscoe 193
Zingiber officinale Roscoe 193
Zygophyllaceae 195
Peganum harmala L. 195
Tribulus terrestris L. 195
Zygophyllum coccineum L. 195
Zygophyllum gaetulum Emberger & Maire 197

Notes and Explanations 198
Glossary 201
Bibliography 210
Indexes 215
1. Medicinal Index
2. Common Names Index
3. Index to Species

Medicinal Plants of North Africa

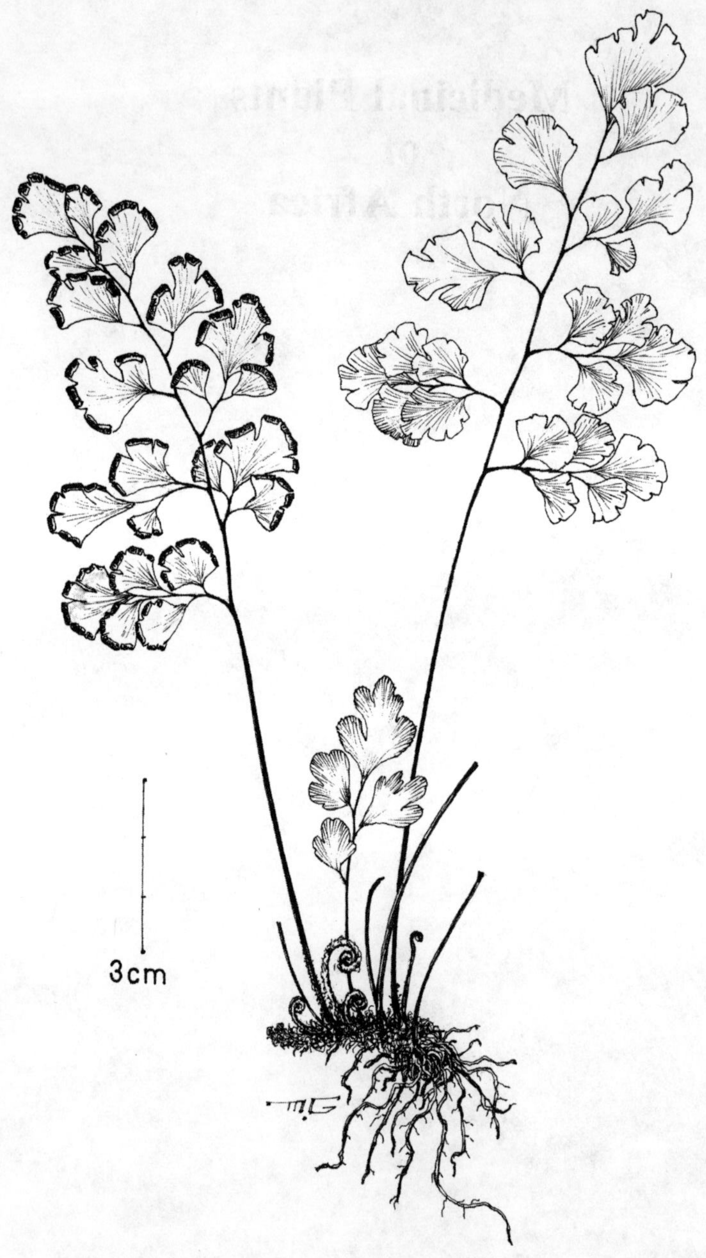

Adiantum capillus-veneris

Acanthaceae

Acanthus mollis L. *Area:* Tunisia to Morocco.
Names: Arabic: Bakhbakh, Sabounia, Selikh, Shouk el-yahoudi (66). Berber: Tasmas, Tafrira (66); Zeku (26). English: Bear's breech (4, 24); Branke ursine (4). French: Acanthe molle, Branc ursine (4, 24).
Uses: Plant vulnerary. Infusion of root and leaves emollient. *Ref:* 23, 24, 26, 42

***Blepharis ciliaris** (L.) B.L. Burtt *Area:* Egypt.
Names: Arabic: Shawk ed-dab'a, Shawk ed-dib (58); Shawk ed-dabb, Zughaf, Shuqaf (4). French: Blépharie (4).
Uses: Charcoal from roots ground into a powder used as "kohl" (eye powder) for feeble sight, probably against cataract (Bedouins, Egypt). Seeds for wound healing, anti-inflammatory, antihemorrhoidal, keratolytic and emollient. *Ref:* 2

Adiantaceae

***Adiantum capillus-veneris** L. *Area:* Egypt to Morocco.
Names: Arabic: Kuzbarat el-bir (17, 62); Saq el-akhal (62); Sha'ar el-khanzir, Sha'ar el-ard (4, 17); Sha'ar el-ghul (17, 42, 62). Berber: Guengit, Rajraf (62). English: Maidenhair, Venus's hair (4). French: Capillaire de Montpellier (23); Adiante, Capillaire (4).
Uses: Fronds expectorant, emollient. Concentrated decoctions as emmenagogue; infusion for all chest diseases: colds, bronchitis, asthma; obstructions of liver and spleen, to provoke perspiring urine. *Ref:* 17, 23, 42

Alismataceae

Alisma plantago-aquatica L. *Area:* Egypt to Morocco.
Names: Arabic: Seif el-maa, Semouma, Massas (13, 23, 62); Mizmar er-rai (4, 13, 62); Ouden el-'anz (13, 62). English: Water plantain (4). French: Plantain d'eau (13, 23, 24, 62); Flûteau (62, 23); Alisma plantain (23); Alisme (4).
Uses: Dried rhizome is diuretic, astringent, galactogogue, antiscorbutic, depurative, used for epilepsy and rabies. *Ref:* 13, 23, 24

Alliaceae

***Allium cepa** L. *Area:* Commonly cultivated in North Africa.
Names: Arabic: Bassal, Besla (62). Berber: Zalim, Baslim, Lebsal, Tibsal (62); Azalim, Azlim (5). English: Onion (4). French: Oignon (4).
Uses: Bulbs are diuretic, hypoglycemic, antiscorbutic, antidiabetic, bacteriostatic, antibiotic, intestinal disinfectant in homeopathy. Dried powder of onion mixed with honey is locally applied to eyes for protection against cataract; when salt and wine are added to the mixture, it becomes effective against dog bites. *Ref:* 5, 24, 37, 42

Allium sativum L. *Area:* Commonly cultivated in North Africa.
Names: Arabic: Thoum, Toum (4, 62). Berber: Tiskert, Tissert (5). English: Garlic (4). French: Ail cultivé (4); Ail commum (45).

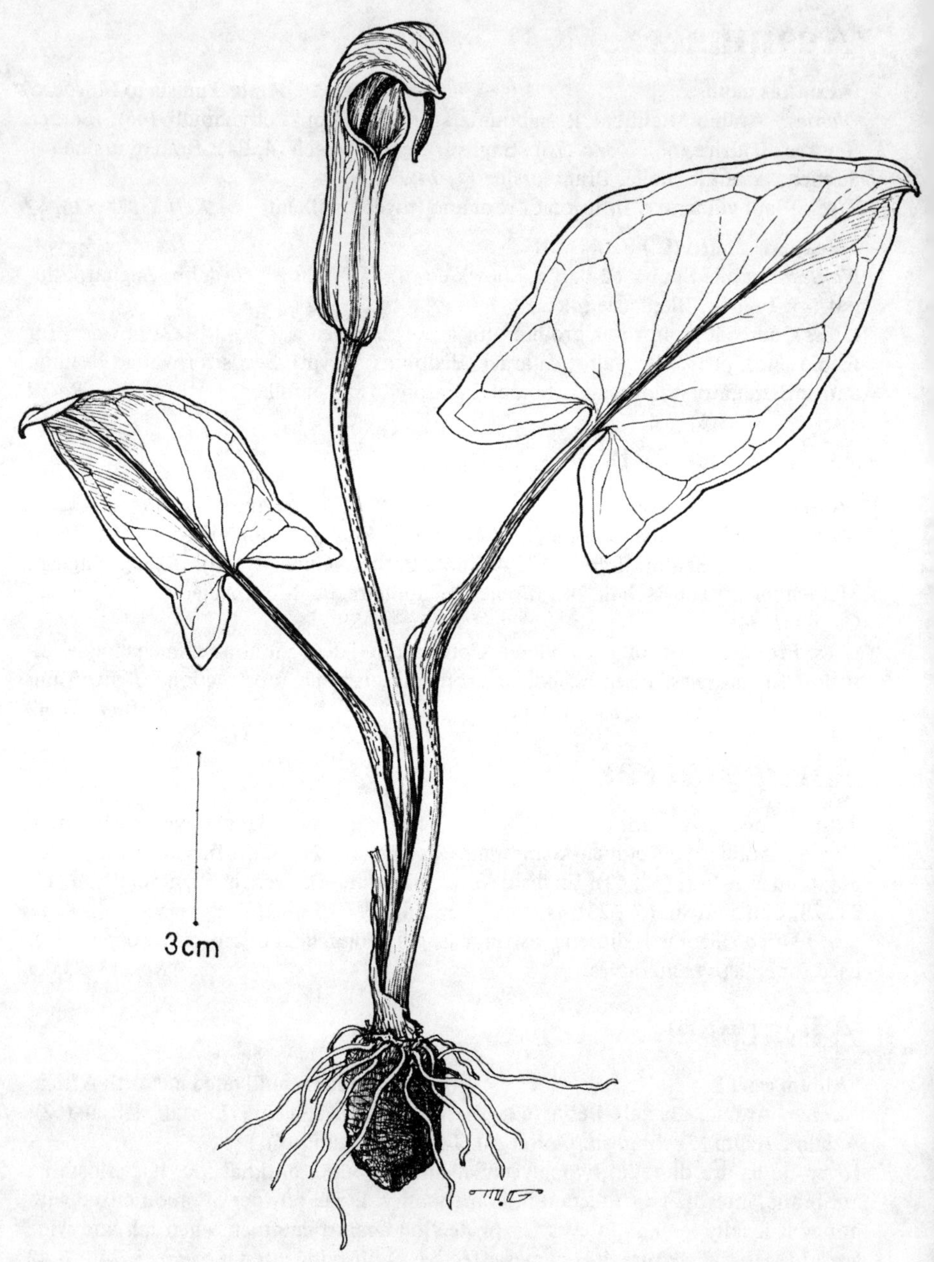

Arisarum vulgare

Uses: Bulbs are powerful antidote for poisons of all kinds, antibacterial, stimulant, vermifuge, hypotensive, chologogue, expectorant, digestive, anthelmintic, depurative, tonic, general antiseptic; for dysentery, typhoid, plague, intestinal worms, suppository for hemorrhoids, tuberculosis, cough, colds. Drops of hot fat previously cooked with sliced garlic useful in treating otitis, also used in veterinary medicine for multiple purposes *Ref.* 5. 24. 45. 46

Amaryllidaceae

Narcissus tazetta L. *Area:* Egypt to Morocco.
Names: Arabic: Nardjes (42, 62); Nargis (58); Behar, Khenounat En-Nebi, Teif ed-dib, Berengat, Nowar zouawa, 'Ain serdouk (62). Berber: Tikheloulin En-Nebi (62). English: French daffodil (4). French: Narcisse (42); Narcisse tazette (4).
Uses: Crushed fresh bulbs mixed with honey are applied in form of cataplasm on burns to soothe pain and avoid suppuration. Dried bulbs ground and ingested for poisoning and ill health. *Ref:* 42

Anacardiaceae

Rhus tripartita (Ucria) Grande *Area:* Egypt to Morocco.
Names: Arabic: Gdari (5); 'Ern (58, 62); 'Oronfel, Za'rour (58); Leqq (62). Berber: Addou, Tadoumkheit, Tahammak (62). English: Lac sumach (4). French: Sumac vernis (4).
Uses: Infusion of fruits and leaves recommended for gastric and intestinal ailments. *Ref:* 5

Apocynaceae

Nerium oleander L. *Area:* Libya to Morocco. Cultivated in Egypt.
Names: Arabic: Defla (5, 13, 42, 62); Ward el-homar (4). Berber: Alili (13, 42, 62); Anini, Ariri (13, 62). English: Oleander (4). French: Laurier-rose (4, 5, 13, 62); Oleandre (4).
Uses: Plant poisonous and not used orally. Infusion of plant abortive. Macerated leaves for itch and fall of hair; fresh leaves applied to tumors; lotion or soap made by mixing wood ash with olive oil used for itch. Decoction of leaves and bark antisyphilitic; leaves general paralyzing and toxic agent by contact or ingestion, hence used as insecticide. Decoction of plant antipoison; decoction of leaves used as a gargle to strengthen teeth and gum and as nose drops for children (Algiers drug market); extracts of plant show cardiotonic activity; pounded dry leaves for ulcers in animals. Infusion of flowers febrifuge. *Ref:* 2, 5, 13, 42

Araceae

Arisarum vulgare Targ.-Tozz. *Area:* Egypt to Morocco.
Names: Arabic: Niriche, Reiniche (58, 62); Snei'ah, Loof (58); Ouden el-fil (26, 62); Hiermi, Begouga, Sebhora, Irni (26). Berber: Tiougda (26, 62); Abbouk, Idjened (62); Taourza (26). English: Friar's cow (4). French: Gouët à capuchon (4).

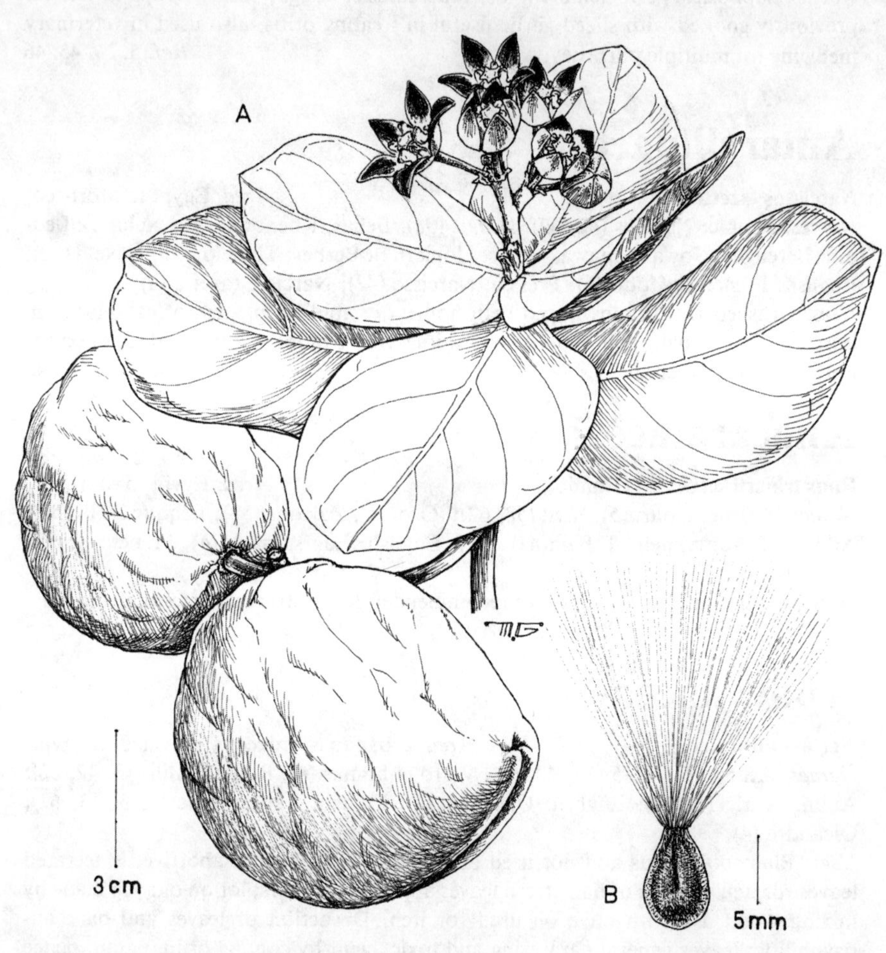

Calotropis procera
A. flowering and fruiting branch
B. seed, enlarged

Uses: Although young corms are edible, raw plants are considered dangerous and poisonous by locals in Egypt, and used for committing suicide. Corms contain glucosides, edible without danger if well cooked, emetic-cathartic. *Ref:* 5

Arum italicum Miller *Area:* Libya to Morocco.
Names: Arabic: Dharirah, Luf ga'd (4); Begouga, Bou qesas, Qesas el-lesan, Ouden el-fil (13, 62). Berber: Abqouq, Tikelmout, Germi, Airni (13, 62). English: Large cuckoo-pint, Italian arum (4). French: Gouët d'Italie (4, 13); Arum d'Italie (24).
Uses: Corms rich in amidon and contain a very irritant saponin, purgative, hydragogue, emetic-cathartic, resolvent, expectorant for chronic conditions of respiratory organs. *Ref:* 24, 42

Eminium spiculatum (Blume) Kuntze *Area:* Egypt.
Names: Arabic: Erqeita, Arqat, Loof (58).
Uses: Considered by locals in Egypt a dangerous, poisonous plant, used for committing suicide. Juice hypotensive; alcoholic extract hypertensive; aqueous extract devoid of toxicity. Purified alcoholic extract of corms contains glycosides. *Ref:* 19

Araliaceae

Hedera helix L. *Area:* Libya to Morocco. Cultivated in Egypt.
Names: Arabic: Qessous, Habl el-masakin (4, 13, 42, 62); Lablab kebir (4); Leblab, Beglet el-berba (62). Berber: Afal (13, 42, 62); Barga, Koubbar, Azemnoun, Tassouflal (13, 62). English: Common ivy (4); Ivy (24); English ivy. French: Lierre (4, 13, 37, 62); Lierre grimpant (4, 24).
Uses: Leaves emmenagogue, antispasmodic, used for cancerous growths, dysmenorrhea, wound ulcers, boils, burns, corns and various skin diseases. Fruits emetocathartic, sudorific, febrifuge. *Ref:* 24, 37, 41

Asclepiadaceae

Calotropis procera (Ait.) Ait. fil. *Area:* Egypt, Libya, Algeria, Morocco.
Names: Arabic: 'Oshar (4, 5, 7, 8, 57, 58, 62); Baranbakh (8, 13, 62); Krenka (13, 62). Berber: Torcha (5, 13, 62); Tourza, Ngeyi (13). English: Apple of Sodom (8); French cotton, Mudar plant (4). French: Calotrope, Arbre à soie, Fafetone (4); Pomme de Sodome (13).
Uses: Decoction of bark and latex used in veterinary medicine, anti-leprosy, for scabies. Powdered dried leaves vermifuge in small doses; dry leaves smoked as cigarettes for asthma; latex causes serious inflammations and may lead to blindness if it gets into the eyes. Cataplasm of fresh leaves for sunstroke, latex for scabies of camels and goats; latex applied on teeth to loosen them, also for toothache (Bedouins, Egypt). Leaf extracts cardiotonic. Root emetic, expectorant; root bark for dysentery, elephantiasis, syphilitic ulcers, stomachic, diaphoretic.
Ref: 2, 5, 8, 49, 57

Leptadenia pyrotechnica (Forssk.) Decne *Area:* Egypt to Morocco.
Names: Arabic: Markh (58, 62); Assabay (5, 62); Kalenba (62). Berber: Titarek (5, 62); Kizzen, Kanouri (62).
Uses: Branches diuretic; infusion of branches used for retention of urine and to help

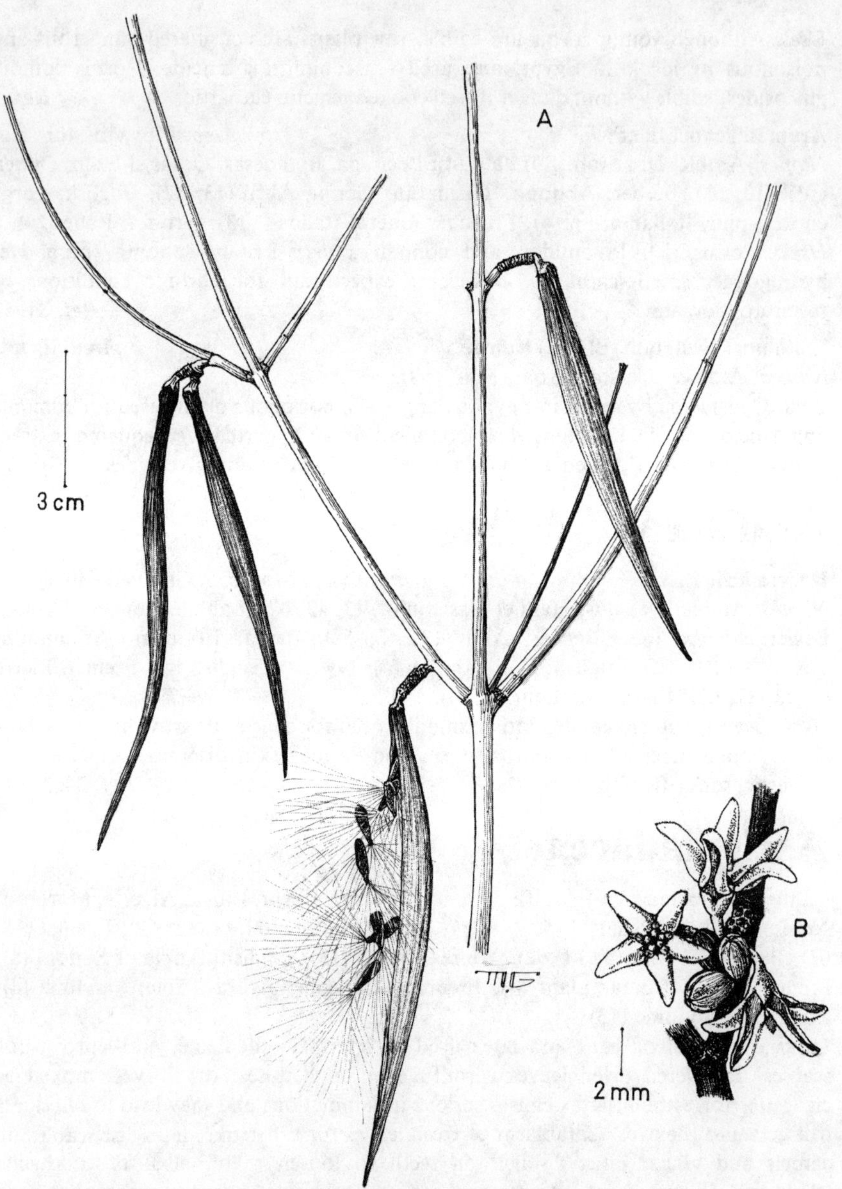

Leptadenia pyrotechnica
A. fruiting branch
B. flowers in a cluster, enlarged

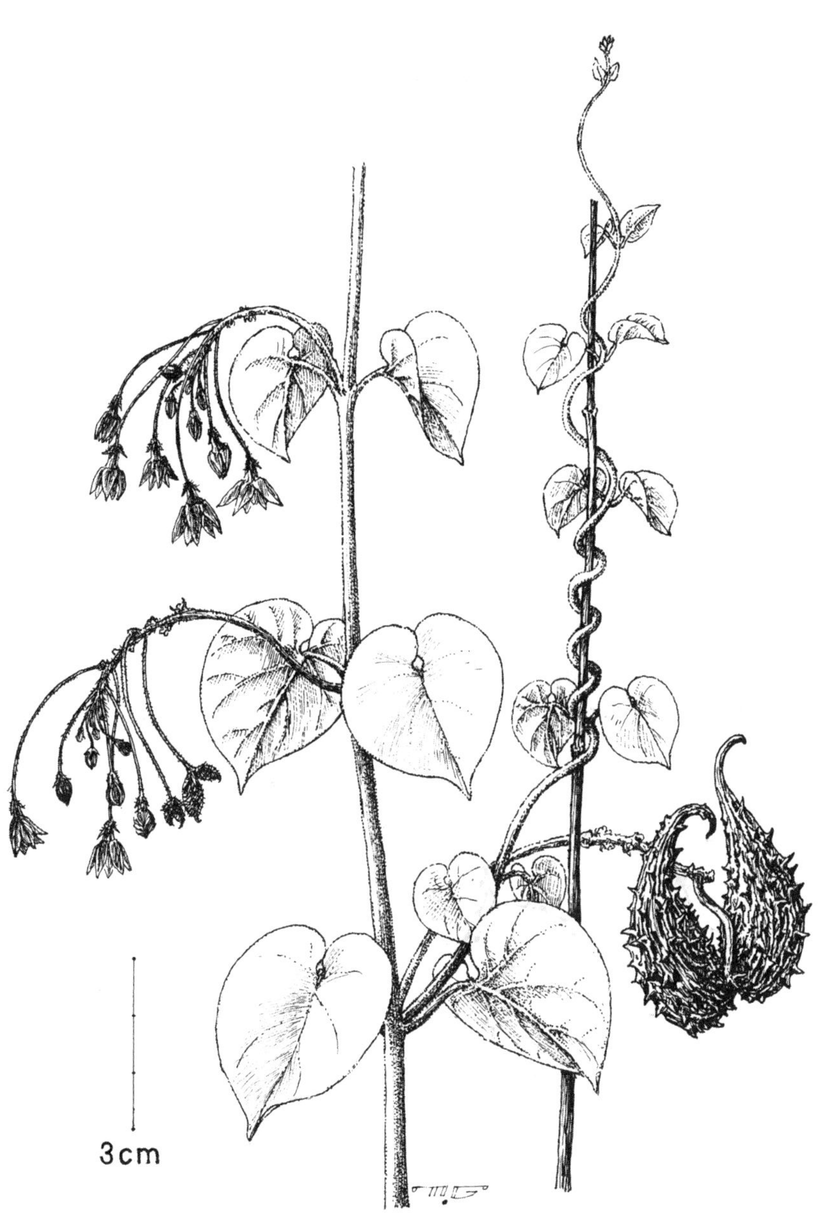

Pergularia tomentosa

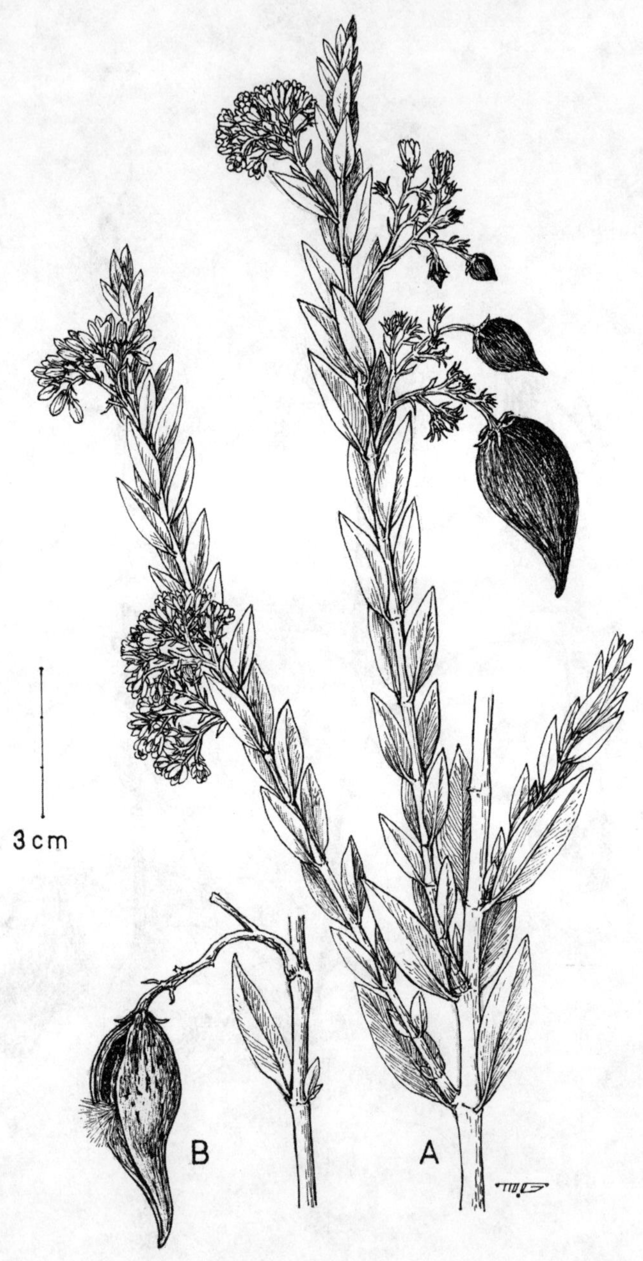

Solenostemma arghel
A. flowering and fruiting branch
B. opened fruit with seeds

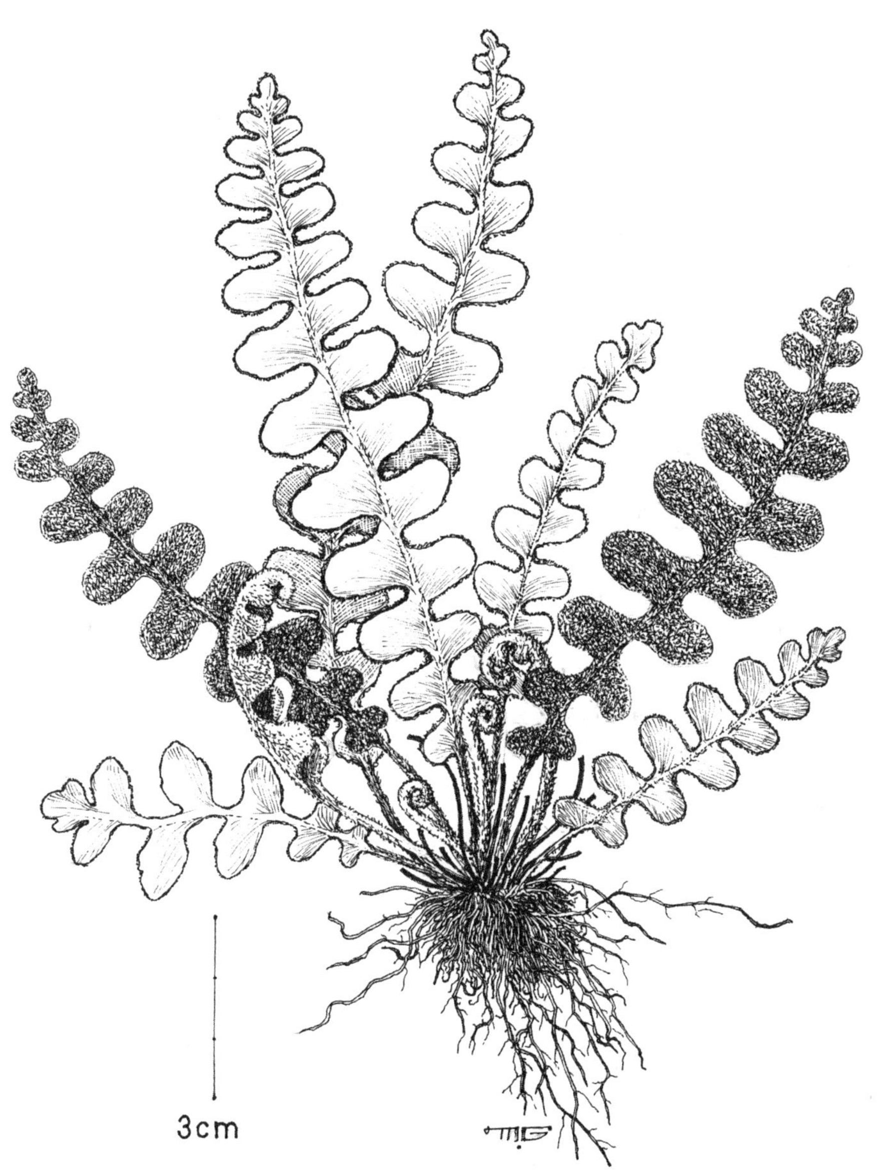

Ceterach officinarum

expel uroliths (Bedouins, Egypt). *Ref:* 5

***Pergularia tomentosa** L. *Area:*Egypt to Morocco.
Names: Arabic: Ghalqa (5, 40, 58, 62); Laban el-hamir (40, 62); Demia, Rouk, Louas, Umm el-laban (62). Berber: Tachkal, Dellakal, Tellakh, Sellaha (62).
Uses: Plant used as depilatory, poultice, laxative, anthelmintic, abortive, for skin diseases. *Ref:* 5, 40

Periploca laevigata Ait. *Area:* Libya to Morocco.
Names: Arabic: Hallaba (5, 62). Berber: Asslift, Sellouf (62).
Uses: Decoction of seeds rubbed on skin as local analgesic, especially for rheumatism. *Ref:* 5

* **Solenostemma arghel** (Del.) Hayne *Area:* Egypt, Libya, Algeria.
Names: Arabic: Argel (58, 62); Hargel (44, 58). Berber: Khallachem, Zellechem, Arellachem (62).
Uses: Effective remedy for cough. Infusion of leaves for gastro-intestinal cramps, stomachic, anticolic, for colds, urinary tracts, antisyphilitic if used for prolonged periods of 40 to 80 days (Bedouins, Egypt). *Ref:* 44, 62

Aspidiaceae

Dryopteris filix-mas (L.) Schott *Area:* Tunisia to Morocco.
Names: Arabic: Sarkhas (4, 42); Shurud (4). Berber: Ifilkou, Aoutem, Afersiou (42). English: Male fern, Male polypody (4). French: Fougère mâle (4, 24, 42); Polystic fougère mâle (4).
Uses: Rhizome anthelmintic, used for taenia and in veterinary medicine for distomatosis of sheep. Young fronds calmative, their tincture used by rubbing for rheumatism, sciatica, cramps, lumbago, cough. *Ref:* 24, 42, 45

Aspleniaceae

Asplenium adiantum-nigrum L. *Area:* Egypt to Morocco.
Names: Arabic: Berchenoussane, Zeita (23, 62); Sarkhas el-ballut (4). English: Black maidenhair fern (4, 24); Black spleenwort, Black oak fern (4). French: Capillaire noire (4, 23, 24, 62); Doradille noire (4).
Uses: Fronds expectorant, emollient, astringent; syrup from fronds for cough. *Ref:* 23, 45

Asplenium trichomanes L. *Area:* Tunisia to Morocco.
Names: Arabic: Kezber es-sakhr, Sha'ar el-ghul (62); Lihha el-ghul (4). Berber: Tamart (62). English: Bristle fern, Common spleenwort (4). French: Capillaire de maraille (62); Rue des murailles (23); Faux capillaire (4, 23); Capillaire rouge des officines, Polytric des officines (23).
Uses: Fronds expectorant, emollient, astringent; syrup from fronds for cough. *Ref:* 23, 45

Ceterach officinarum DC. *Area:* Egypt to Morocco.
Names: Arabic: Hashishet ed-dahab (4); 'Aqerban, Qesbir el-bir (23, 62). English: Scaly spleenwort, Rusty-back, Scale fern (4). French: Doradille (23, 62); Cétérach

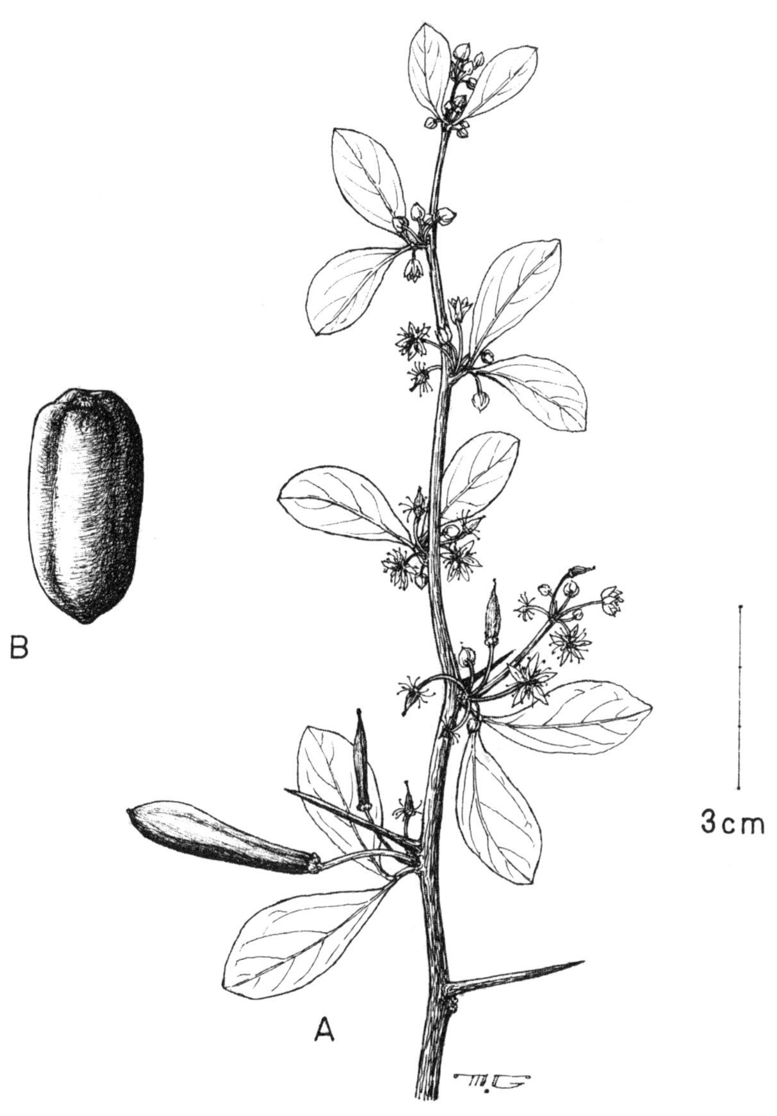

Balanites aegyptiaca
A. flowering branch with young fruits
B. ripe fruit

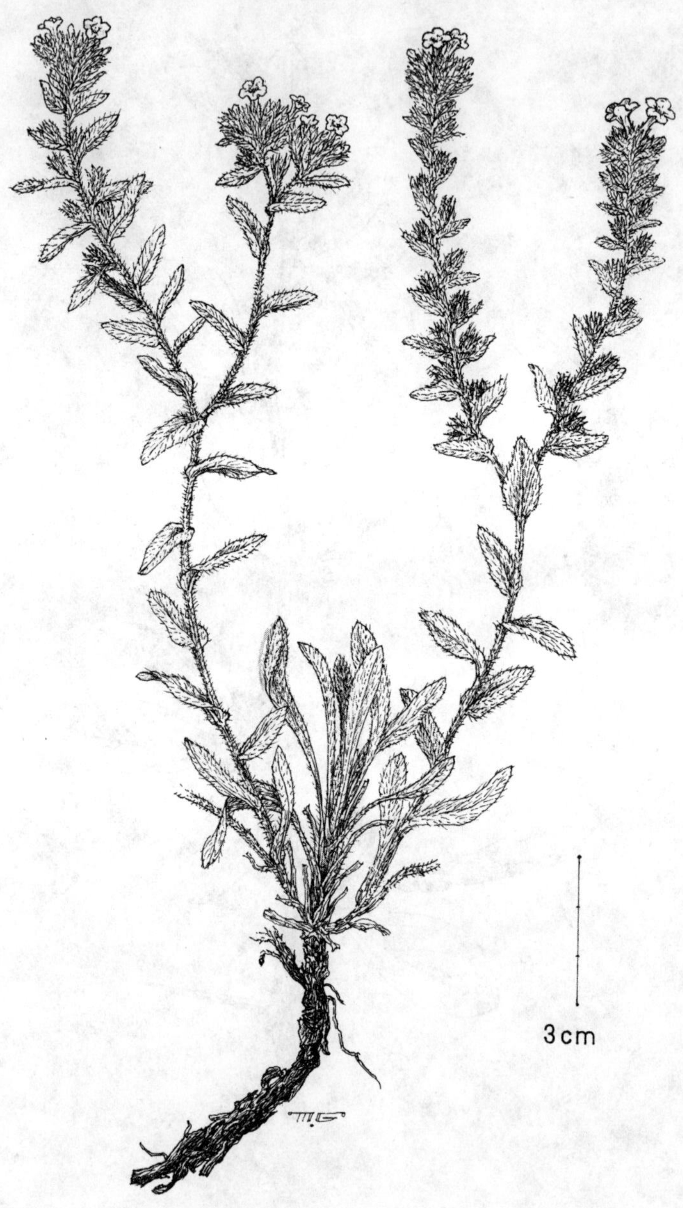

Alkanna tinctoria

officinal, Dorade (23); Herbe à dorer, Daurade (4).
Uses: Fronds astringent, diuretic, pectoral emollient, for spleen, kidney and bladder diseases, slightly bechic. *Ref:* 17, 23, 24

***Phyllitis scolopendrium** (L.) Newman *Area:* Tunisia to Morocco.
Names: Arabic: Lesan el-kheil, Lesan el-aiyel (23, 62); Kaff en-nesr, 'Uqruban (4).English: Hart's-tongue fern, Horse tongue (4). French: Scolopendre (4, 23, 24, 62); Langue de cerf (4, 23); Herbe à la rate (4).
Uses: Infusion of fronds diuretic, astringent, expectorant. *Ref:* 23, 24

Balanitaceae

Balanites aegyptiaca (L.) Del. *Area:* Egypt, Libya, Algeria, Morocco.
Names: Arabic: Heglig (4, 58, 62); Zaqqoum (5, 62); fruits: Balah harara (58). Berber: Taboraq, Teisset (5, 62); Addoua, Alo (62); fruits: Ebora, Ibororhen (62); Tugga (5). English: Thorn tree, Egyptian balsam, Zachum oil tree (4); Desert date, Soapberry bush (1). French: Dattier du désert, Hagueleg, Balanite d'Egypte (4).
Uses: Anthelmintic, purgative, boils, leucoderma, herpes, vermifuge, malaria, emetic, wounds, syphilis, colds, liver and spleen problems, aches, febrifuge. Kernel extracts have low activity against snail that harbors schistosomal worms; fruit kernels and fruits mild laxative; fruit antidote to arrow poison. Leaf cleans malignant wounds, bark fumigant to heal circumcision wound; root extract for malaria. *Ref:* 1, 2, 5

Berberidaceae

Berberis hispanica Boiss. & Reuter *Area:* Algeria, Morocco.
Names: Arabic: Barbaris (42, 62); Anbarbaris, 'Uqdah, 'Ud er-rihh (4); Ksila, Amirbaris (62); Bou seman (42). Berber: Tazgouart, Darrhis, Arrhis, Aizara, Ousmiche (62); root bark: Atrar, Argis (42). English: Barberry, Pipperidge, Berberry (4). French: Epine-vinette (4, 26, 42, 62); Vinettier (4).
Uses: Root and stem bark a bitter tonic, stomachic, antipyretic. Infusion of root bark used as eye bath for inflammations and pains of the eyes; same infusion used as a drink, depurative and antiscorbutic due to its febrifugal properties. *Ref:* 42, 45

Boraginaceae

Alkanna tinctoria (L.) Tausch *Area:* Egypt to Morocco.
Names: Arabic: Henna el-ghula, Kahla (4, 23, 58, 62); Sedira, Shendjar (23, 62); Rigl el-hamam, Shagaret ed-damm (4). English: Alkanet, Dyer's bugloss (4). French: Orcanette (4, 23, 62); Alkanna (2).
Uses: Bark astringent, used internally for ulcers. Root used as a coloring, water-insoluble tincture. *Ref:* 17, 23

***Anchusa azurea** Miller *Area:* Libya to Morocco.
Names: Arabic: Lisan el-thour (4, 23, 62); Sheikh el-boukoul, Shandjar (23, 62); Lisan el-hamal, Lisan el-qitt (4). Berber: Taharadjt (23, 62); Tirhounam, Sahtor

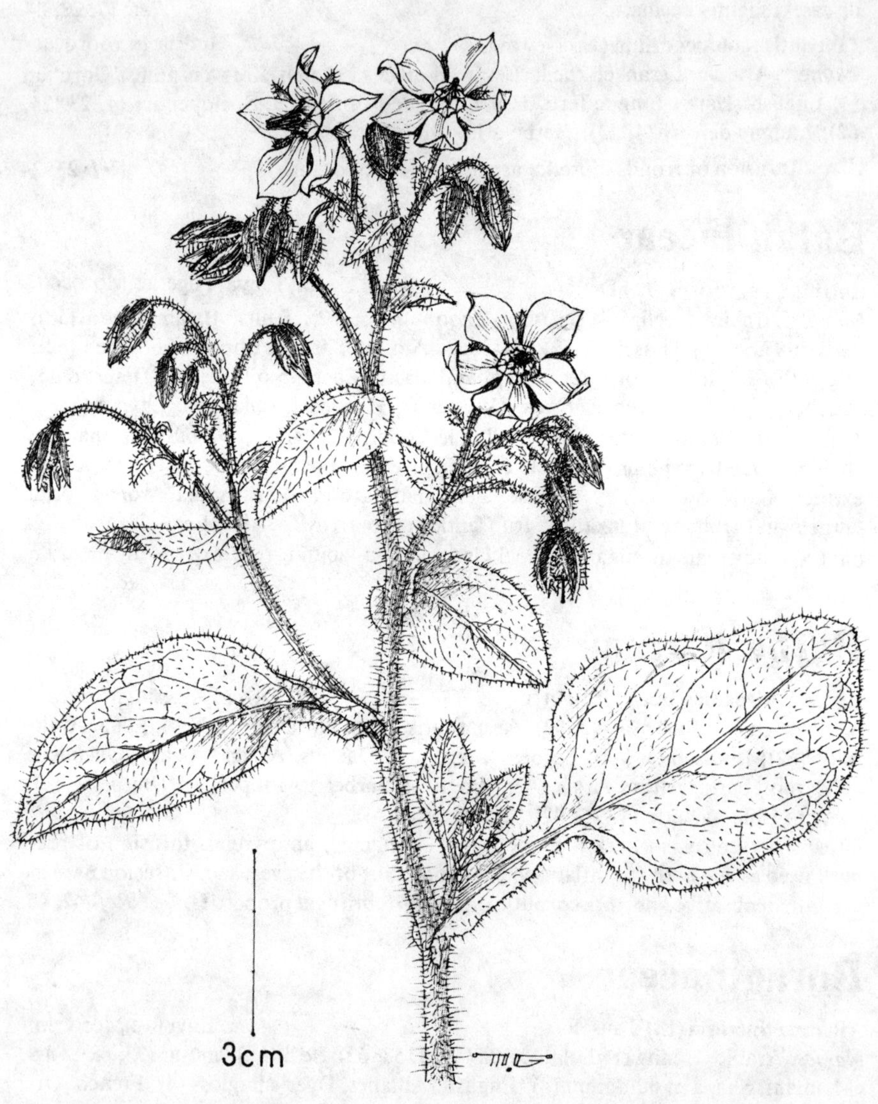

Borago officinalis

(62). English: Italian alkanet, Sea bugloss (4). French: Bourrache bâtarde (4, 23); Langue de boeuf (4); flowers: Buglosse (4, 23).
Uses: Flowers pectoral, sudorific, diuretic. *Ref:* 23

Borago officinalis L. *Area:* Libya to Morocco.
Names: Arabic: Lisan el-thour (4, 23, 62); Harsha, Bou shenaf, Bou krish, Bou sassal (23, 62). Berber: Tament, Tizizoua (23, 62). English: Common borago, Talewort (4). French: Bourrache (4, 23, 62), Bourrache officinale (4).
Uses: Leaves emollient. Flowers emollient, pectoral. Flowering branches sudorific and diuretic, useful for treating rheumatism, heart sedative. Used internally for scurvy, dropsy and jaundice, externally for inflammations of eyes; poultice for swellings and bruises in lotions and skin tonics; balsam vulnerary for ulcers and wounds, demulcent, refrigerant, diaphoretic. *Ref:* 22, 23, 56

Cynoglossum officinale L. *Area:* Tunisia to Morocco.
Names: Arabic: Ouden el-arnab (4, 23, 62); Ouden esh-shah (23, 62); Adhan el-ghazal (4); Lisan el-kalb (6, 23); Lisan ed-dib (23, 62); Saboun el-'arais (62). Berber: Asfarar, Asfarfar (23, 62). English: Hound's tongue, Gipsy flower (4). French: Cynoglosse (23, 45, 62); Langue de chien (23, 62).
Uses: Root calmative, mild narcotic, emollient, mild astringent. Cataplasm, juice or decoction of fresh leaves and roots calmative for pains of burns, inflammations, wounds and ulcers. *Ref:* 23, 24, 45

***Echium plantagineum** L. *Area:* Libya to Morocco.
Names: Arabic: Lisan el-thour, Bou shenaf (62); Kahila (23); Adhan el-thour, Kaff el-thour (4). Berber: Ilès ougendouz (23, 62). English: Purple viper's-bugloss (4). French: Vipérine (4, 23).
Uses: Flowers sudorific, diuretic, pectoral. *Ref:* 23

***Heliotropium bacciferum** Forssk. *Area:* Egypt to Morocco.
Names: Arabic: Sedjra tenshama, Sga'a, Medeb (62). Berber: Lebalig (62); Lehbaliya (5).
Uses: Plasters from dried, powdered leaves used for abscesses, boils, sprains, contusions, oedema, and swellings of all kinds. Plasters also used for anti-scabies preparations in veterinary medicine. *Ref:* 5

***Moltkiopsis ciliata** (Forssk.) Johnst. *Area:* Egypt to Morocco.
Names: Arabic: Halama, Ghabsha (58); El-Henna (5).
Uses: Plugs made from fresh plant are hemostatic. *Ref:5*

Buxaceae

Buxus sempervirens L. *Area:* Algeria, Morocco.
Names: Arabic: Baqs (4, 13); 'Athaq, Shamshad (4). Berber: Ibiqis (13, 62); Beuqs (62); Azazzer (13). English: Common box tree (4). French; Buis (4, 23, 45, 62); Buis toujours vert (4).
Uses: Root bark for syphilis. Stem bark purgative, emetic, febrifuge, sudorific, depurative, for rheumatism. Leaves purgative. *Ref:* 13, 23, 24, 45

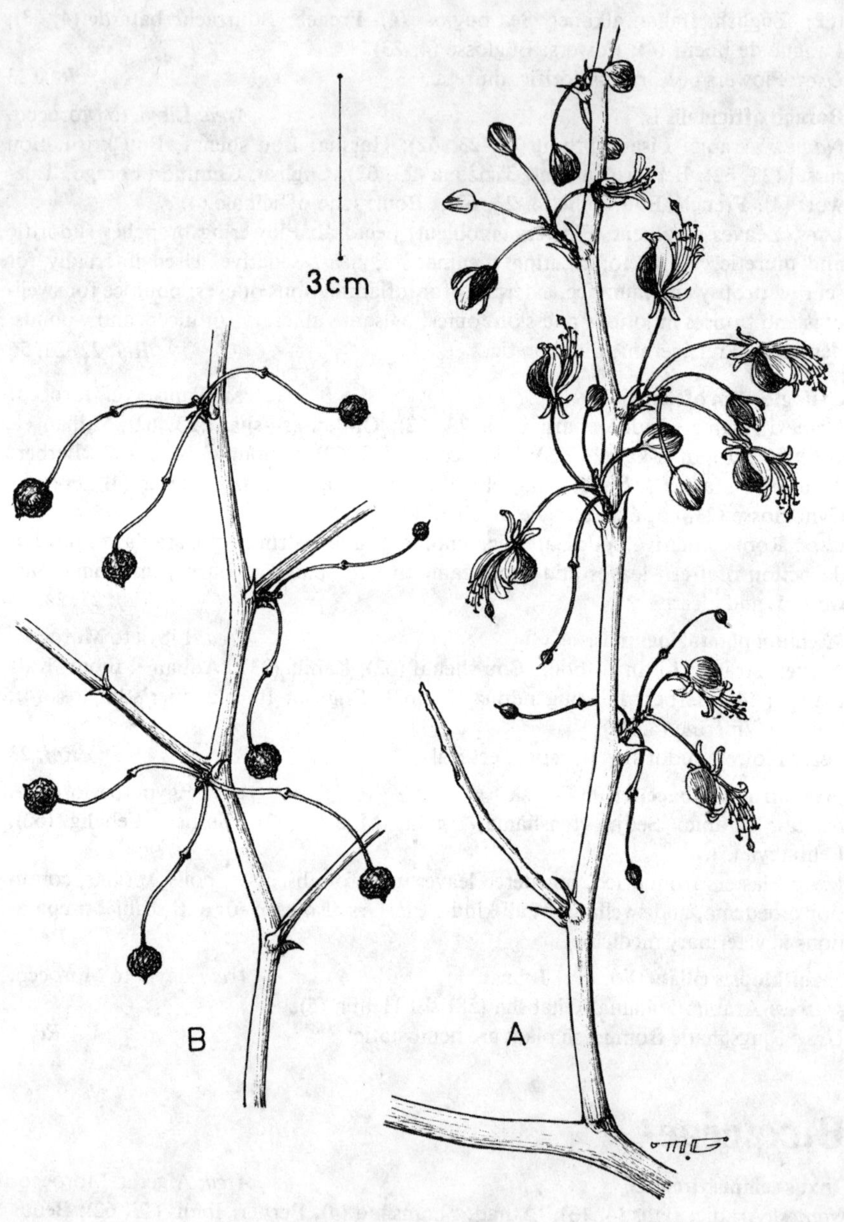

Capparis decidua
A. flowering branch
B. fruiting branch

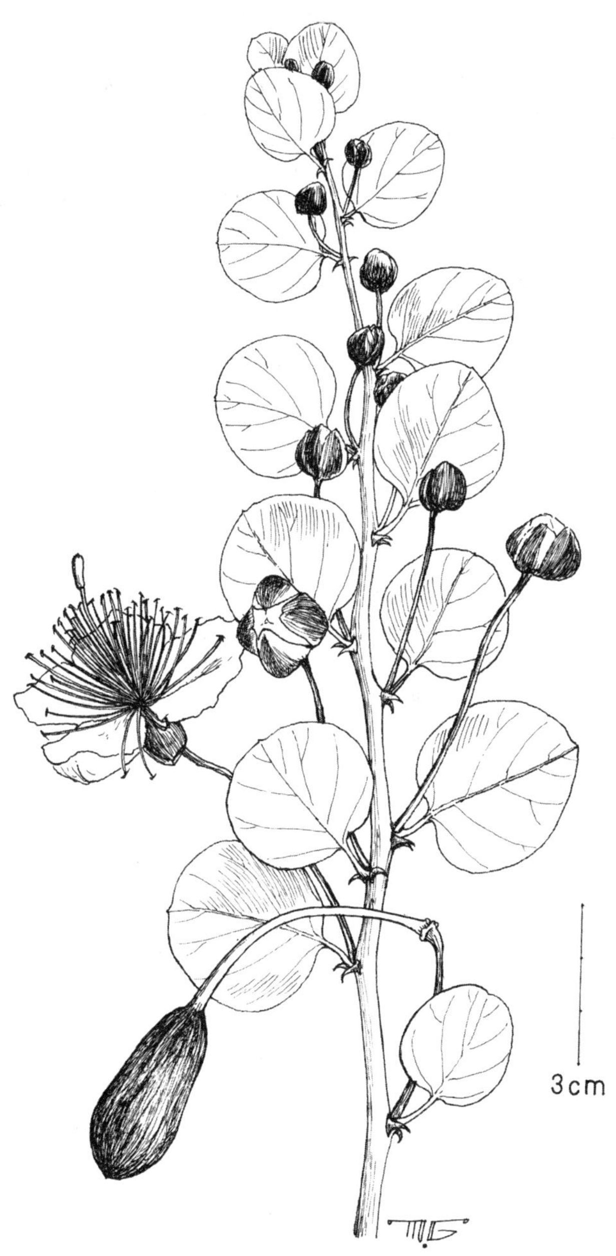

Capparis spinosa

Cactaceae

Opuntia ficus-indica (L.) Miller *Area:* Commonly cultivated in North Africa. Naturalized in Morocco.
Names: Arabic: Hendi (5, 23, 42, 62); Karmouz en-nsara (5, 23, 62); Tin shawki (4); spineless form: Seurti (23, 62); flowers: Nowara hindia, Nowaret el-karmouz (Rabat drug market). Berber: Sobbaira, Troumoucht, Amizzour (23, 62); Tihendit, Ihader, Aferoug (62). English: Prickly pear, Indian fig (4). French: Figuier de barbarie (5, 23, 42, 62); Figuier d'Inde (5, 62); Cactus raquette, Figuier nopal (4, 5).
Uses: Hot cataplasm of fleshy cladodes emollient. Infusion of flowers antidiarrhoeic; flowers used externally as antihemorrhagic; infusion of dried flower buds mixed with barley grains and maize silks used as remedy for gonorrhoea (Rabat drug market). Fruits astringent, anticolic, antidiarrhoeic. *Ref:* 5, 23, 42, 62

Cannabidaceae

Cannabis sativa L. *Area:* Cultivation prohibited by law in North Africa.
Names: Arabic: Qenneb (4, 5, 13, 42); Hashish, Kif, Chira (5, 13, 23, 62); Hashish el-fogara (13). Berber: Tifest (13, 42); Tifert (13). English: Indian hemp (4); Marijuana. French: Chanvre indien (4, 23, 42, 62); Chanvre (4).
Uses: Summits of female flowering plants analgesic, narcotic, sedative, anesthetic, hallucinogenic, aphrodisiac, antispasmodic. Resin has intoxicating, stimulating effects, in small quantities producing pleasant excitement, passing into delirium and catalepsy if the quantity is increased. *Ref:* 5, 23, 24, 42, 45, 64

Capparaceae

***Capparis decidua** (Forssk.) Edgew. *Area:*Egypt, Morocco.
Names: Arabic: Toundoub (58, 62); Habriga (62). Berber: Koussoms (62).
Uses: Ash of the bark hemostatic, astringent, disinfectant for wounds and sores. Green branches analgesic for rheumatism, also used for scabies in camels, astringent, cardiac problems, boils, swellings, toothache, laxative, diaphoretic, anthelmintic, cough, asthma, inflammation, fever, rheumatism. *Ref:*2, 5

***Capparis spinosa** L. *Area:* Egypt to Morocco.
Names: Arabic: Kabbar (4, 8, 16, 23, 62); Kabar (5, 8, 42, 58); Lassaf, Assaaf (4, 58); Asef, Shalem, Felfel el-djebel (62); Kronbeiza (23, 62). Berber: Tailoulout (5, 23, 62); Taybult (42); Amseilih (5); Tsailaloul, Ouailoulou, Belachem (62). English: Common caper-bush (4). French: Câprier (4, 5, 16, 42); Câprier commun (23); Câprier épineux (4, 24).
Uses: Root diuretic, astringent, tonic. Root bark appetizer, astringent; cataplasm externally applied for spleen troubles. Bark diuretic, astringent, tonic, for gout and rheumatism, laxative, expectorant, for chest diseases. Infusion of stem and root bark antidiarrhoeic, febrifuge. Flower buds and roots renal disinfectants, diuretic, tonic for arteriosclerosis as diuretic and for chills; used in compresses for the eyes.

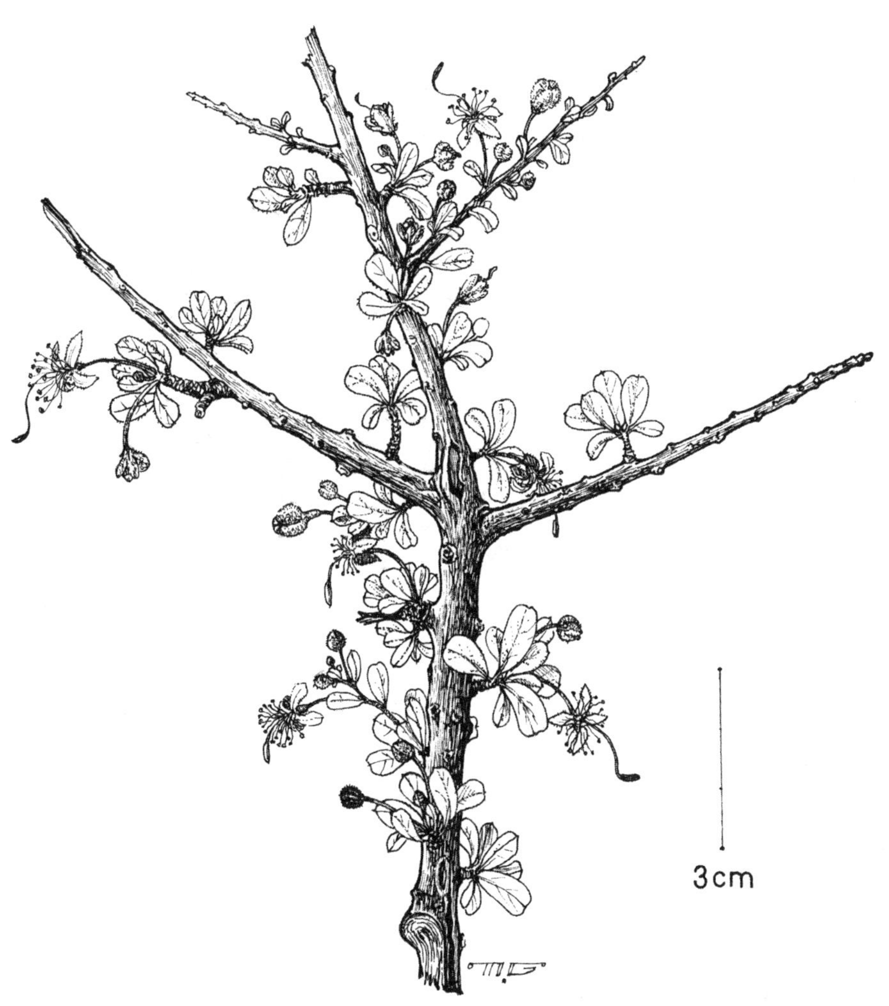

Maerua crassifolia

Fruits and leaves carminative, aphrodisiac. Fresh fruits consumed as antiscorbutic; infusion of fruits for sciatica and dropsy; powdered dry fruits mixed with honey, taken first thing in the morning for treating sciatica and colds of the back (Rabat drug market). Flower buds stimulant, slightly diuretic and refreshing agent, their decoction taken internally for sciatica. Seeds for feminine sterility and dysmenorrhoea; crushed seeds for ulcers, scrofula and ganglions.
Ref: 5, 8, 15, 16, 17, 23, 24, 42, 45, 56

Maerua crassifolia Forssk. *Area:* Egypt, Libya, Algeria, Morocco.
Names: Arabic: Sarkh (5, 11); Sarha, Sarah (58, 62); Mordjan (62). Berber: Adjar, Atil (5, 62); Arkerma, Adjem, Tereri, Tatil (62); Tagart (5); Arkenu (11).
Uses: Infusion of leaves for intestinal diseases. Decoction of leaves and bark febrifuge, for cephalalgia, toothache, infected hairy skins. Mixture of powdered leaves with henna leaves *(Lawsonia inermis)* and fat used for rapid healing of wounds and sores; cataplasm of this mixture reduces pain of bone fractures and aching parts of the body. *Ref:* 5

Caprifoliaceae

Sambucus ebulus L. *Area:* Tunisia to Morocco.
Names: Arabic: Khaman saghir (4, 13, 23, 62); Khelwan saghir, Rourawa (13, 23, 62); Khelwan (37). Berber: Agueridd, Ariouri (13, 23, 62); Mzertrioud (13, 62). English: Danewort, Dwarf elder, Ground elder (4). French: Hièble (4, 23, 24, 62); Petit sureau (4); Sureau hièble (37).
Uses: Bark purgative. Fruits antirheumatic, diuretic, purgative, sudorific, resolvent.
Ref: 23, 24, 37

Sambucus nigra L. *Area:* Tunisia to Morocco.
Names: Arabic: Bilasan, Khaman (4, 13, 23, 42, 62); Khelwan, Senbouqa (13, 23, 62); Khaman kabir, Damdamun (4). Berber: Akhilwan, Ageridd, Tourwagat, Bourrwabes, Timermenna, Arwari (13, 23, 62); Sahbakou, Hairuari, Wairurud (42). English: Elder tree, Arn tree, Boon tree (4). French: Sureau (4, 62); Sureau noir (4, 13, 23, 24, 37, 42); Sureau commun (23); Sulion, Haut bois (4).
Uses: Bark purgative, diuretic. Infusion of flowers sudorific, diuretic. Flowers and leaves diuretic, sudorific, emollient, vulnerary, resolvent. Fruits laxative, antirheumatic. *Ref:* 17, 23, 24, 37, 42, 45

Caryophyllaceae

Corrigiola telephiifolia Pourret *Area:* Morocco.
Names: Arabic: Serghina, Bokhour el-berber (5, 42, 62); Bokhour mourshka (62). Berber: Tassergint (5, 42, 62); Serient, Ouberka, Chellalah (26, 62). French: Sarghine (42, 45).
Uses: Root aromatic, only part of the plant used as a drug, enters into mixtures for cough, diuretic, aphrodisiac; fumes inhaled for influenza, colds and coryza; tonic, fortifier, reconstituent; used for skin diseases (Rabat drug market); used in local cosmetic powders. *Ref:* 5, 42

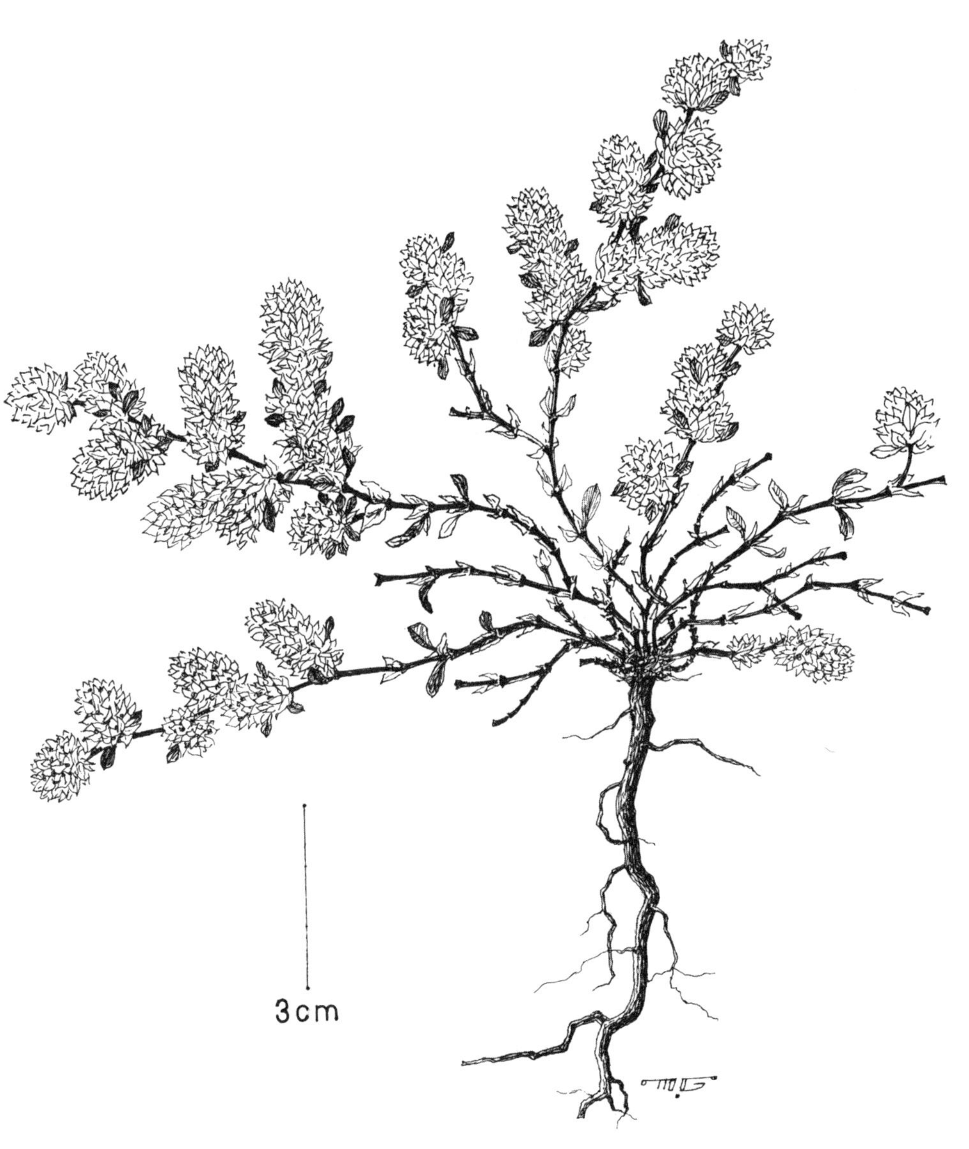

Paronychia argentea

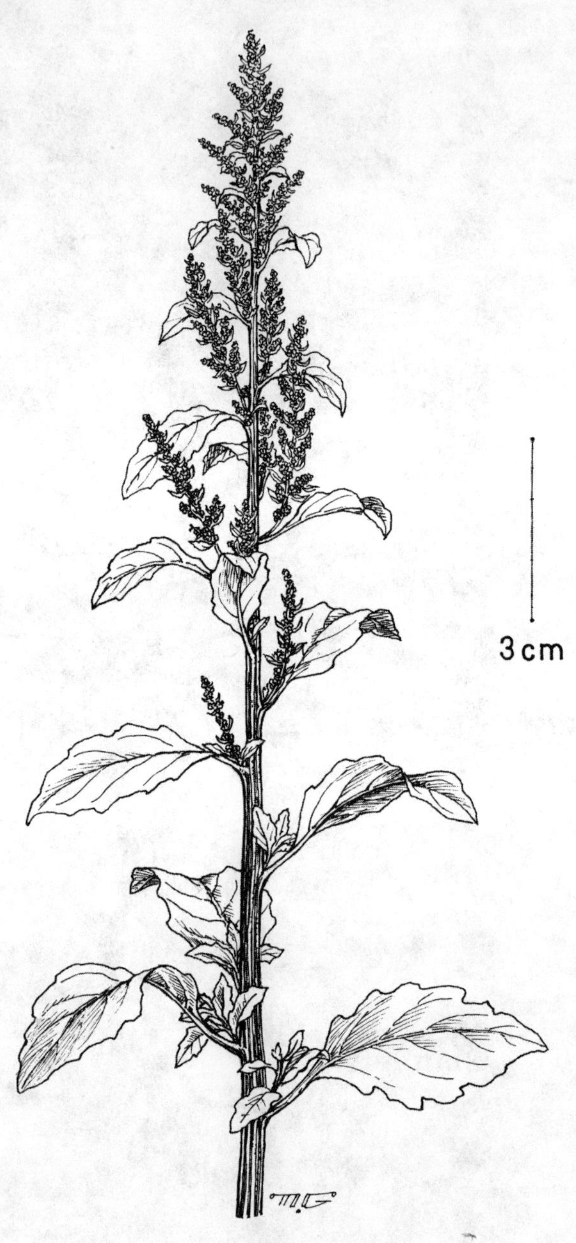

Chenopodium ambrosioides

Herniaria hirsuta L. *Area:* Egypt to Morocco.
Names: Arabic: Mouker, Makir (23, 62); Erq el-share'e (62). French: Herniare (23).
Uses: Entire plant used as diuretic, astringent, expectorant, depurative, antispasmodic. *Ref:* 23, 24, 65

Paronychia arabica (L.) DC. *Area:* Egypt to Morocco.
Names: Arabic: Ramram (5); Simreeb, Basees, Bassisa (58).
Uses: Entire plant used as stimulant, aphrodisiac. *Ref:* 5

Paronychia argentea Lam. *Area:* Egypt to Morocco.
Names: Arabic: Tai el-'areb (23, 62); Bessat el-ard (58, 62); Farsh el-ard, Kreisha, Rokheima (58); Ferash el-qa'a, Bessat el-qa'a, Hidouret er-ra'ai (62); Bessat el-melouk (Algiers drug market). Berber: Taoucatt (23, 62); Talsatt, Taoumiah, Tamiah, Tarmiga, Mzouchen (62). French: Thé arabe (23, 26, 62); Sanguinaire (23).
Uses: Infusion of entire plant, except the root, diuretic, febrifuge, appetizer, mild aphrodisiac, used to expel renal stones (Algiers drug market). *Ref:* 5, 23, 26, 42

***Spergularia media** (L.) C. Presl *Area:* Egypt to Morocco.
Names: Arabic: Bughlam, Dadaifa, Busweifa (5). Berber: Ourzima (62). French: Polygale de Syrie (5).
Uses: Root emetic-cathartic, expectorant. *Ref:* 5

***Spergularia rubra** (L.) J.& C. Presl *Area:* Egypt to Morocco.
Names: Arabic: Eshba hamra (4, 23, 62); Sherifa (23, 62). Berber: Ourzima (23, 62). English: Sand spurrey, Red sand-wort (4). French: Sabline rouge (23, 24, 62).
Uses: Whole plant used as diuretic, antiseptic, calmative, for catarrh. *Ref:* 23, 24, 45

Stellaria media (L.) Vill. *Area:* Egypt to Morocco.
Names: Arabic: Meshit, Habbeila (62); Qezaza (58, 62); Hashishet el-qizaz (4). English: Common chickweed (4). French: Mouron des oiseau (4, 62); Morgeline (4, 24); Mouron blanc, Stellaire (4).
Uses: Essence of fresh plant taken to relieve rheumatic pains and psoriasis; externally used as a rub to ease rheumatic pains, diuretic, emollient, mild astringent; decoction used externally for wounds and ulcers. *Ref:* 24, 56

***Vaccaria pyramidata** Medicus *Area:* Egypt to Morocco.
Names: Arabic: Foul el-'arab (4, 58, 62); Hamret er-ras, Tif es-sabounya (62). Berber: Tigigesht (5); Tiriresht (62). English: Cow-herb (4). French: Saponaire (5); Vaccaire, Buplèvre (4).
Uses: Root vulnerary for abscesses, furuncles, ulcers, scabies, mastitis, lymphangitis, emmenagogue and galactogogue, contraindicated in pregnancy. Decoction of root used to take care of wounds, sores, scabies and different dermal infections, taking into consideration its toxicity. Leaves and roots contain saponins which provoke, in strong doses, a general paralysis of muscles. *Ref:* 5, 34

Chenopodiaceae

Atriplex halimus L. *Area:* Egypt to Morocco.
Names: Arabic: Qataf (5, 23, 42, 62); Qtout (42); Qataf bahari, Maluh (4); Roghata

(58). Berber: Aramès (42, 62); Arams (5, 42, 62); Abougboug (42). English: Sea-orache, Sea purslane (4). French: Pourpier de mer (4, 23, 42, 50); Arroche, Halime (4).
Uses: Roots cut into long, narrow pieces used as toothbrush; remedy for hydropsy. Ash of plant is rich in alkaline salts, taken with water for gastric acidity. Seeds in small doses emetic, large doses poisonous. *Ref:* 5, 42, 50

Chenopodium ambrosioides L. *Area:* Egypt to Morocco. Naturalized from tropical America.
Names: Arabic: Natna (4, 58, 62); Sianama (23, 62); Bersiana (62); Zorbeih (58). Berber: Mkheinza (23, 42, 62, Rabat drug market). English: Mexican tea, Wormseed, Mexican goose-foot (4). French: Thé du Mexique (4, 23, 45, 62); Ambroisie (4); Ambroisie du Mexique (23).
Uses: Infusion of leaves digestive, carminative, stimulant, stomachic, antiasthmatic. Leaves and young shoots added to soups taken as febrifuge (Rabat drug market), galactogogue. Flowering and fruiting summits stomachic, diuretic, anthelmintic, antispasmodic, vermifuge, emmenagogue. *Ref:* 23, 24, 26, 42, 45

Chenopodium vulvaria L. *Area:* Egypt to Morocco.
Names: Arabic: Balia (23, 62); Muntinah (4); Melfouf el-kalb, Ghoumran (62); Qehaniya (58). Berber: Tahouet (23, 62). English: Stinking goose-foot, Dog's orache (4). French: Vulvaire (4, 23); Ansérine fétide (4).
Uses: Plant sedative, antihysteric, antispasmodic, antirheumatic, anthelmintic, emmenagogue. *Ref:* 23, 24

Cornulaca monacantha Del. *Area:* Egypt to Morocco.
Names: Arabic: Hadd (5, 58, 62); Djouri (62); Shawk ed-deeb (58). Berber: Tohar (62).
Uses: Decoction of leaves used for treatment of jaundice. *Ref:* 5

Haloxylon scoparium Pomel *Area:* Egypt to Morocco.
Names: Arabic: Remth (5). Berber: Assay (5).
Uses: Fruiting branches minced and mixed with camel's fat or butter used as cataplasm for treating snake bites. *Ref:* 5

Cistaceae

Cistus albidus L. *Area:* Algeria, Morocco.
Names: Arabic: Atai (23, 62); Salmiah (Rabat drug market). Berber: Touzzalt (23, 62); Touzzala (62). French: Ciste blanc (23).
Uses: Infusion of leaves and young shoots mixed with tea serve as digestive after heavy meals (Rabat drug market).

Cistus ladanifer L. *Area:* Algeria, Morocco.
Names: Arabic: Werd (23, 62); Umm aliya, Shedjeret el-aden, 'Ain if (62); Ladan, Shaqwas, Qistus (4). Berber: Touzzalt (62); Zouzzalt (23). English: Common cistus (4, 24); Ladanum-resin tree (4). French: Ciste à ladanum, Ladanier, Ladanum de Crête, Ambre végétal (23); Ciste ladanifère (4, 45); Ciste d'Espagne (4).
Uses: Plant stimulant, astringent, hemostatic, revulsive, yielding a resinous material

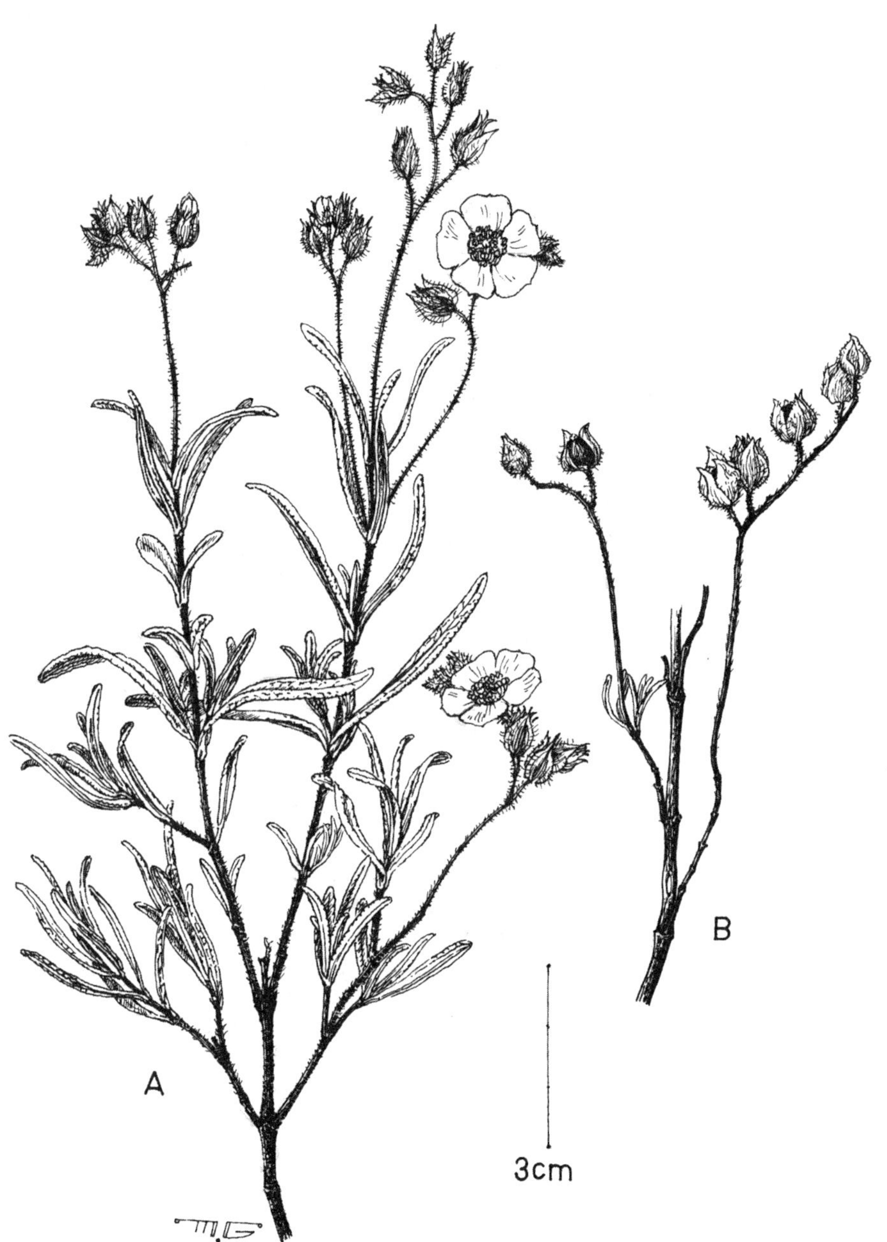

Cistus monspeliensis

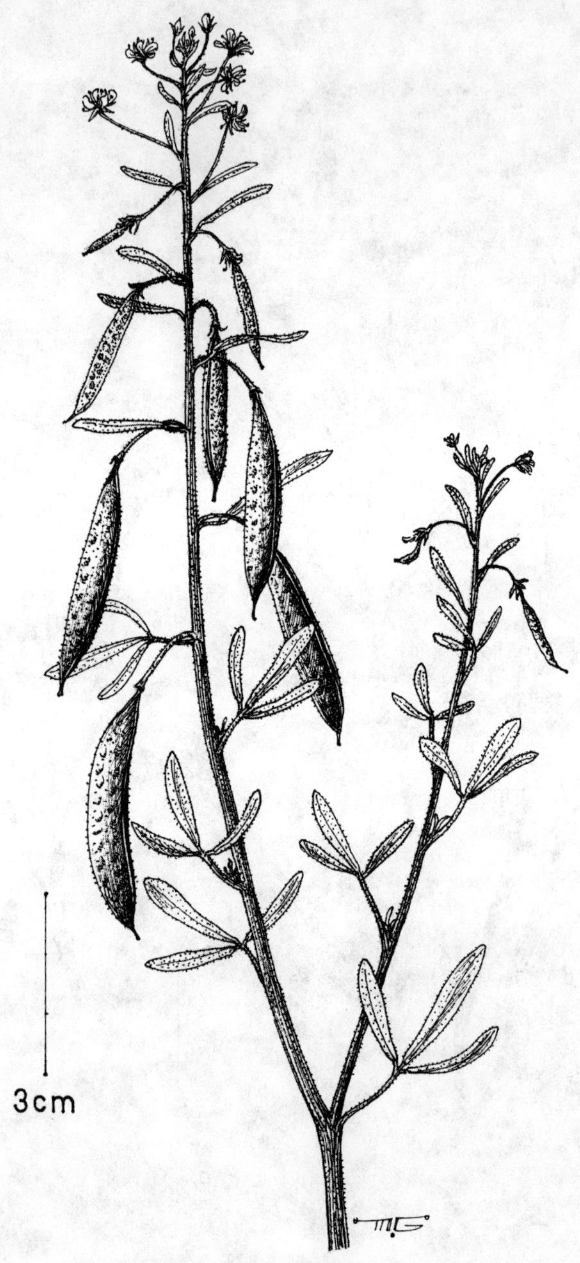

Cleome amblyocarpa

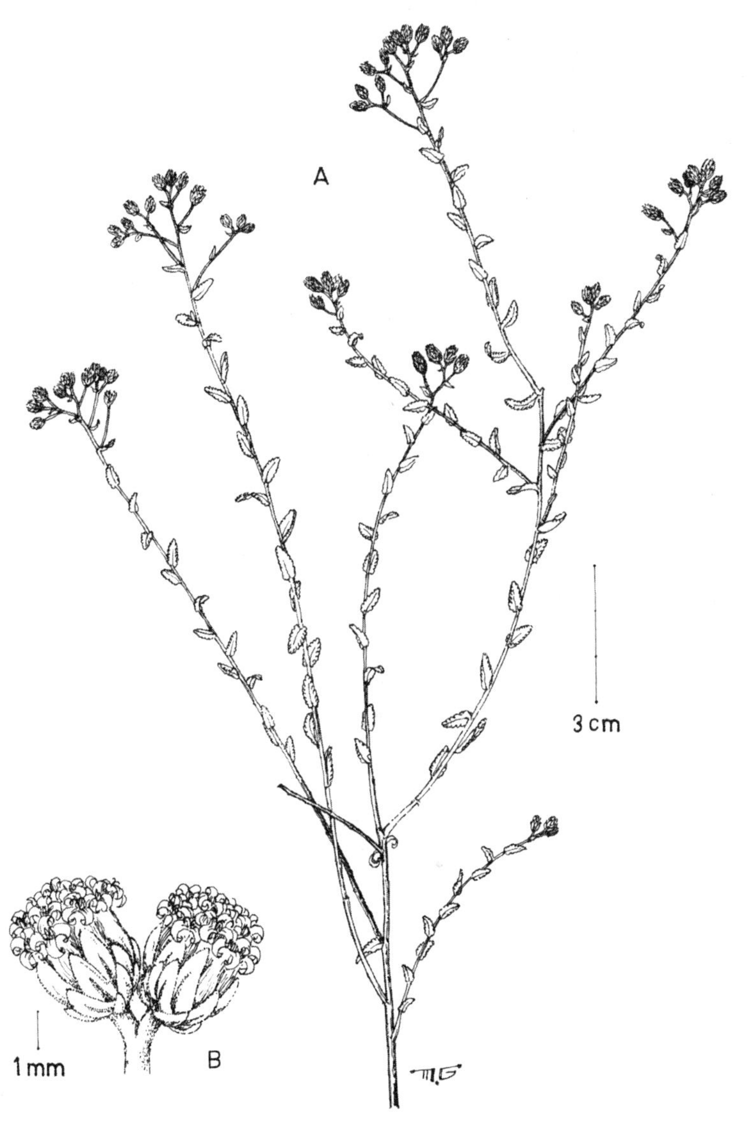

Achillea fragrantissima
A. flowering branch
B. two heads, enlarged

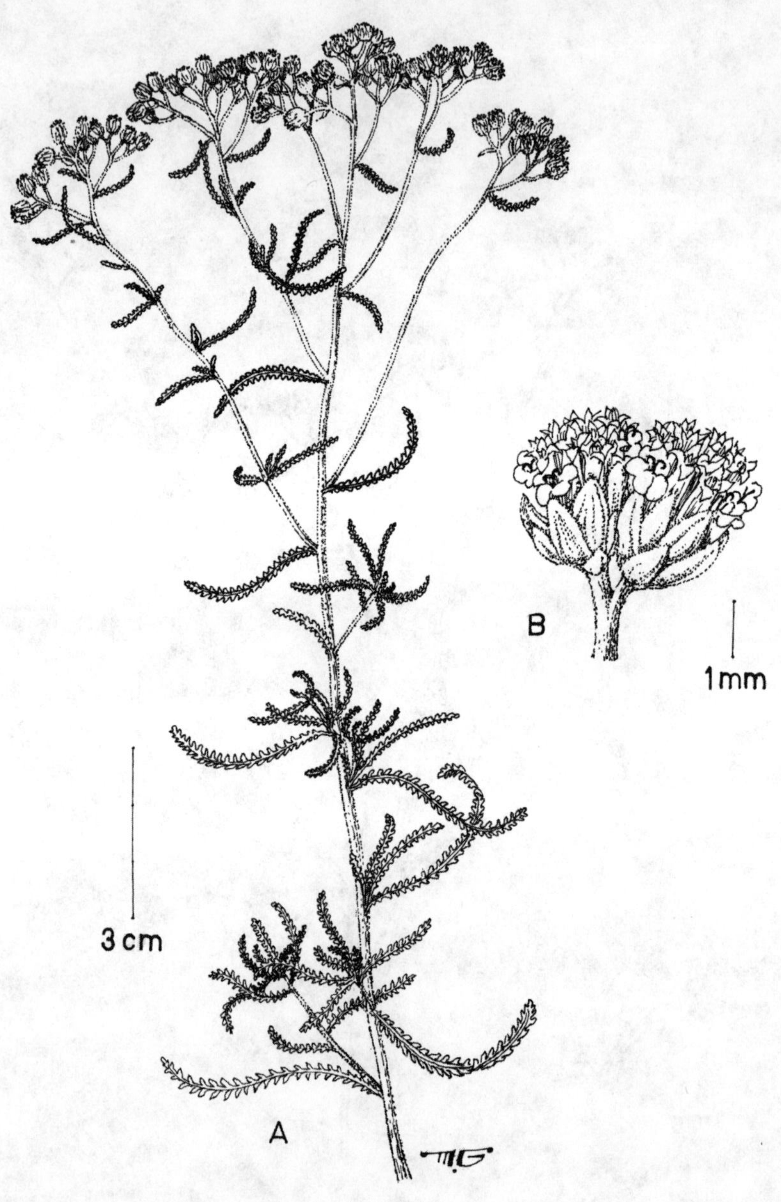

Achillea santolina
A. flowering branch
B. two heads, enlarged

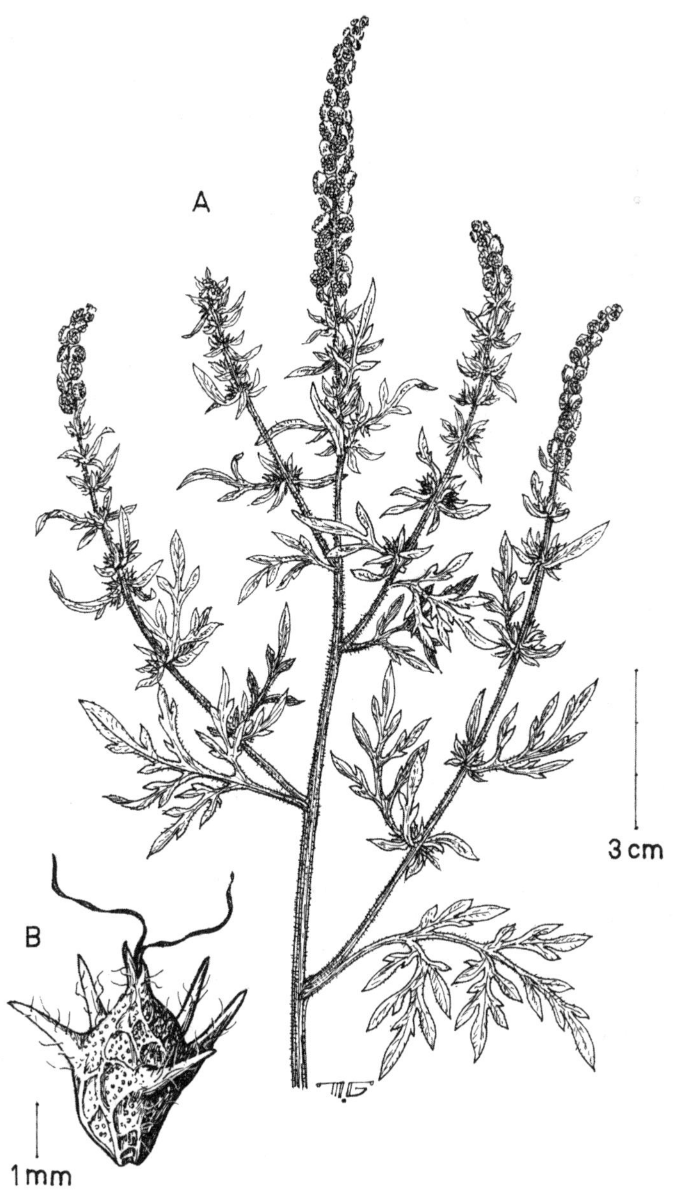

Ambrosia maritima
A. flowering branch
B. fruit, enlarged

"ladanum" used against dysentery, catarrh and asthma. Grains used as a condiment. *Ref:* 23, 24, 62

Cistus monspeliensis L. *Area:* Tunisia to Morocco.
Names: Arabic: Umm aliya (23, 62). Berber: Zamechttibt (23); Tamechttibt, Irgel (62); Tuzelt (Algiers drug market). French: Ciste de Montpellier (23).
Uses: Infusion of leaves replaces tea. Decoction of flowering branches for asthma (Algiers drug market). *Ref:* 23

Cleomaceae

***Cleome amblyocarpa** Barr. & Murb. *Area:* Egypt to Morocco.
Names: Arabic: Magnuna (4, 58, 62); 'Atana, Shagaret wahhsh (58); Wahhsh (4); Lemkheinza (5); Shareka, Gouffaz, Umm djeladjel (62). Berber: Tichmougin, Tamazout, Oyok, Ahajjar (62). English: Spider flower (4). French: Cléome (4).
Uses: Infusion of leaves has an almost immediate effect on abdominal and rheumatic pains. *Ref:* 5

Compositae

Achillea fragrantissima (Forssk.) Sch. Bip. *Area:* Egypt.
Names: Arabic: Qaysoum, Babounig, Be'eitheran (4, 58); Gesoum (58); Qaysun (4). English: Lavender cotton (4). French: Garde-robe, Aurone femelle, Santoline (4).
Uses: Flowering branches anthelmintic, stomachic (Bedouins, Egypt).

Achillea santolina L. *Area:* Egypt to Morocco.
Names: Arabic: Chaihata, Qort, Orairyia (62); Bishrin, Ghobbeisha, Qaysoum, Be'eitheran (4, 58); Fliet Ghadir (8). English: Santoline (8). French: Santoline (4).
Uses: Plant reduces pain of toothache by rubbing young flowering branches against teeth or by chewing them; anthelmintic, stomachic. *Ref:* 8, 28

Ageratum conyzoides L. *Area:* Naturalized in Egypt.
Names: Arabic: Korink, Berqam, Borgoman (58). English: Goat weed, Bastard agrimony, Floss flower (4). French: Agérate, Célestine (4).
Uses: Decoction of root for abdominal problems, digestion, colic. Plant sudorific, antipyretic, tonic, stimulant, for fever, ulcers, uterine problems, sleeping sickness, wounds, syphilis, burns, rheumatism. Crushed leaves mixed with water drunk by diarrhoea patients, and rubbed on forehead to treat headache. Leaves for pneumonia in children, eye lotion, emetic, purgative. *Ref:* 1, 31

Ambrosia maritima L. *Area:* Egypt to Algeria.
Names: Arabic: Demsisa (4, 7, 58, 62); Hashish el-awinet (62); Ghobbeira, Na'na, Tannoun (4). English: Sea ambrosia, Oak of Cappadocia (4). French: Ambroisie (62); Ambrosie, Absinthe bâtarde (4).
Uses: Decoction of plant for rheumatic pains, asthma, bilharziasis, diabetes and to expel kidney stones. Flowering branches stimulant, stomachic, slightly astringent, emollient, vulnerary, diuretic, renal troubles (Cairo drug market). *Ref:* 7, 24

Anacyclus pyrethrum (L.) Link *Area:* Algeria, Morocco.
Names: Arabic: 'Oud el-'attas (5, 23, 62); Agargarha (4, 42, 62). Berber: Tigenthast

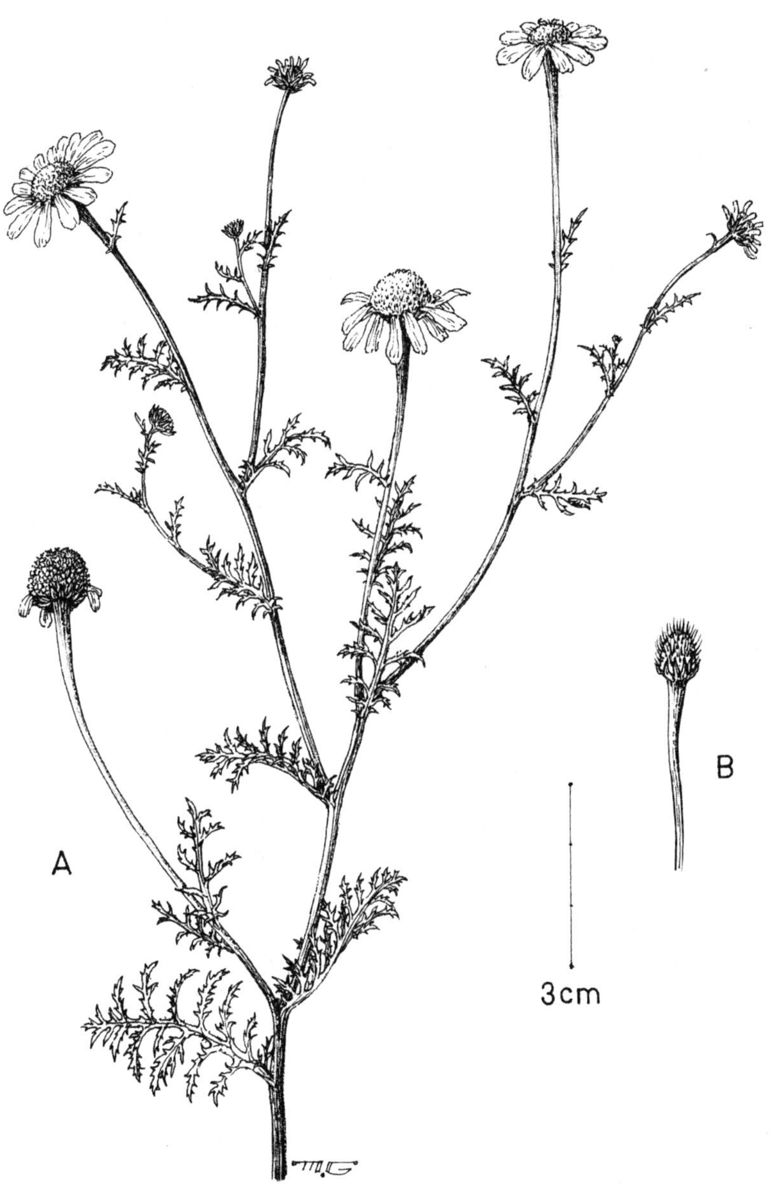

Anthemis pseudocotula
A. flowering branch
B. ripe fruiting head

(5, 42, 62); Genthus (5, 62); Ignens (62). English: Pellitory, Spanish pellitory, Roman pellitory, Spanish chamomile (32); Pellitory of Spain, Alexander's foot (4). French: Pyrèthre (4, 62); Pyrèthre d'Afrique (5, 23); Pyrèthre salivaire, Oeil de bouc, Pariètaire d'Espagne (43).
Uses: The root and lower part of the stem constitute the drug. Chewing of the root causes a remarkable flow of saliva (sialogogue), hence used as a masticatory, and in the form of lozenges for its reflex action on the salivary glands in dryness of the mouth and throat; relieves toothache due to its pungent efficacy. Tincture made from dried root relieves the aching of decayed teeth; a gargle of its infusion is prescribed for relaxed uvula and for partial paralysis of the tongue and lips, relief of neuralgia, rheumatism of the head and tongue, palsy. Root rubefacient and a local irritant when sliced and applied to the skin; it induces heat, tingling and redness; powdered root produces a good snuff to cure chronic catarrh of the head and nostrils and to clear the brain, by exiting a free flow of nasal mucous and tears; also used as a remedy for epilepsy, lethargy. Ointment made of the root with hog's lard helps to cure gout and sciatica; root stimulant, antineuralgic, sternutatory, for rheumatism; mixture of root with milk and honey has aphrodisiac properties and renders fertility to women; abuse of the drug may cause accidents as it contains a toxic principle which affects the brain causing loss of consciousness. Infusion of roots for asthma (Rabat drug market), diaphoretic. *Ref:* 5, 23, 32, 42

Anthemis pseudocotula Boiss. *Area:* Egypt, Libya.
Names: Arabic: Basoun (58); Ribyan (3).
Uses: Flower heads bacteriostatic, antifungal, antidiabetic, antitumor. *Ref:* 3

Artemisia absinthium L. *Area:* Algeria, Morocco.
Names: Arabic: Shadjret Mariam (13, 23, 62, Rabat drug market); Shaybet el-ajouz (5, 13, 23, 42, 62); Sheikh khorasani, Dagnat esh-sheikh (13, 23, 42, 62); Shih rumi, Afsantin, Dasisah, Kushuth rumi (4, 13); Eshbet Mariam (Algiers drug market). Berber: Siba, Shiba (23, 42, 62). English: Wormwood (4, 24); Absinthium, Old woman, Absinth (4). French: Absinthe (4, 5, 24, 42, 62); Grande absinthe, Alvine, Herbe aux vers (4, 23); Aluine, Absinthe menue (23).
Uses: Flowering summits anthelmintic, vulnerary; infusion vermifuge, diuretic, emmenagogue, digestive, stomachic, bitter tonic, febrifuge, antiseptic, appetizer, very effective against rheumatism, calefacient, chologogue; replaces mint to flavor tea; externally used in the form of fresh juice or decoction with salt or tincture for wounds and ulcers. *Ref:* 5, 13, 23, 24, 42, 45

Artemisia arborescens L. *Area:* Libya to Morocco. Often cultivated.
Names: Arabic: Shagaret (Shadjret) Mariam (8, 23); Shiba (4, 23, 42, 62); Dhaqn esh-sheikh (4). Berber: Tasetta Meriem (23, 62). English: Tree wormwood (4, 8). French: Armoise arborescente (42); Armoise en arbre (4); Absinthe arborescente (23).
Uses: Fresh leaves added to tea as a substitute for mint leaves, forming an infusion used as appetizer and diuretic; anthelmintic. Decoction of leaves for intestinal troubles; cataplasm of crushed leaves or snake and scorpion bites; powdered dry

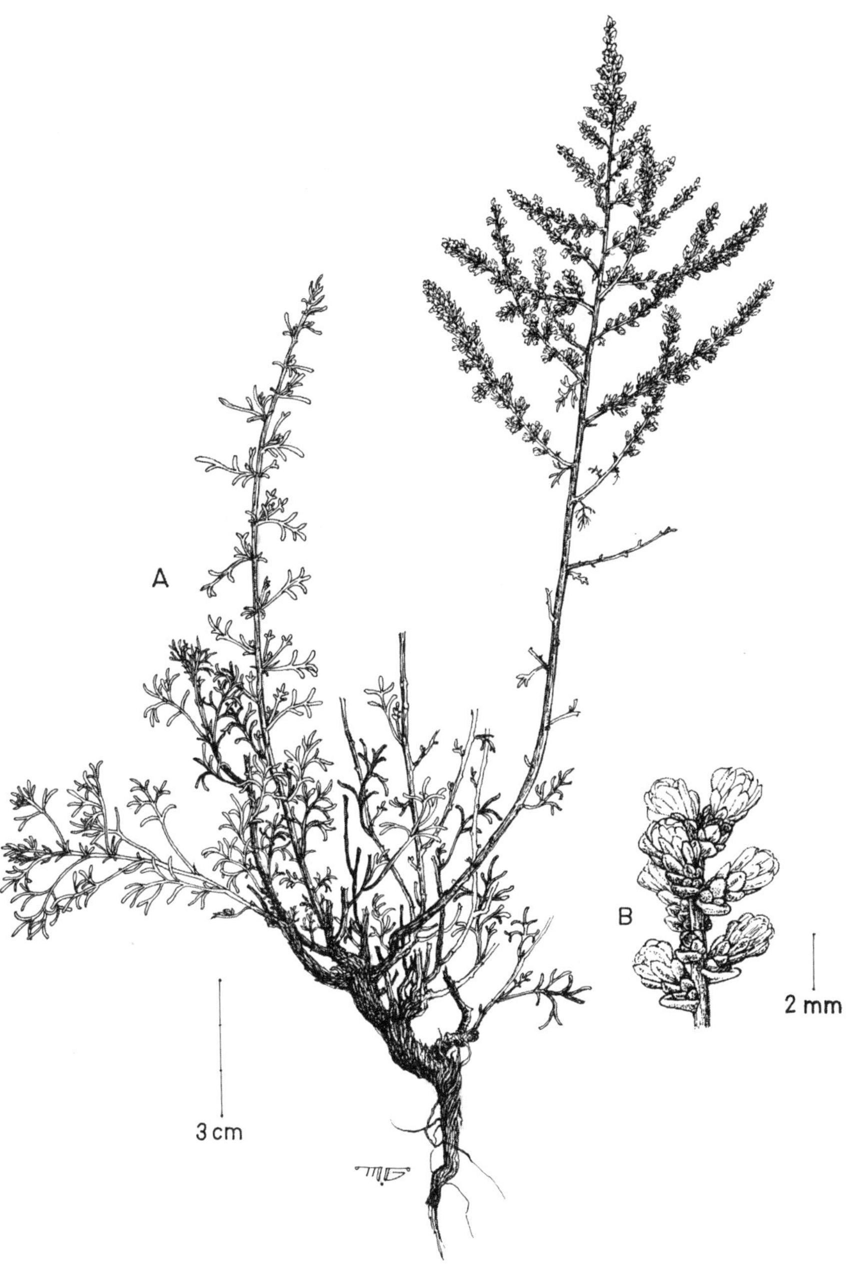

Artemisia herba-alba
A. flowering branch
B. branchlet, enlarged

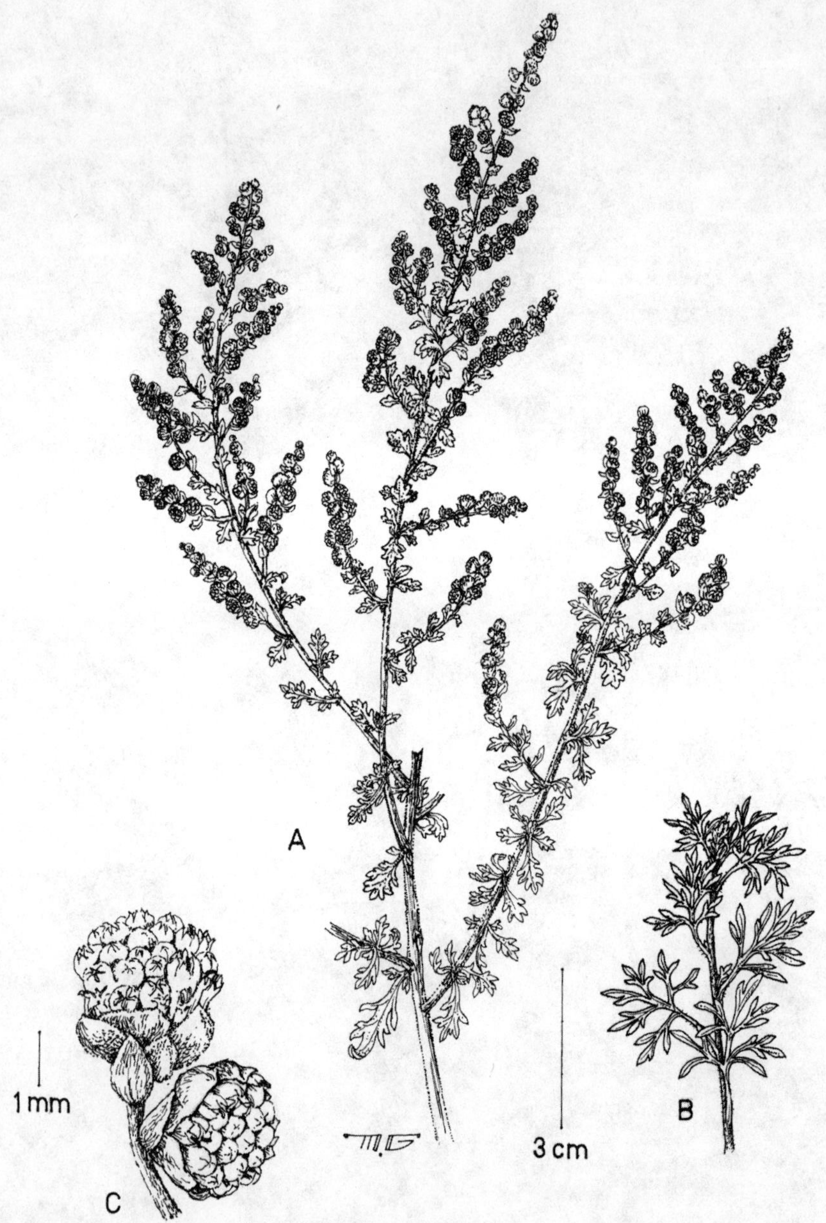

Artemisia judaica
A. flowering branch
B. basal leaf
C. two heads, enlarged

leaves applied to wounds and sores; infusion of leaves and young shoots antidiabetic (Rabat drug market). *Ref:* 8, 23, 42

Artemisia atlantica Coss. & Dur. *Area:* Endemic to Algeria and Morocco.
Names: Arabic: Chouaya (23, 47, 62).
Uses: Infusion of flowering branches vermifuge, emmenagogue. *Ref:* 23

Artemisia campestris L. *Area:* Libya to Morocco.
Names: Arabic: Degoufet, Alala, Sha'al, Khisoum (23, 62). Berber: Tagouft, Tagoug (23, 62); Tieredjeli (62). French: Aurone (62); Armoise rouge, Aurone des champs (23).
Uses: Used as a substitute for *Artemisia absinthium,* and has the same properties to a weaker degree. *Ref:* 23

***Artemisia herba-alba** Asso *Area:* Egypt to Morocco.
Names: Arabic: Shih (4, 5, 8, 16, 23, 42, 50, 58, 62); 'Alala (23, 62); Ghoreird (58). Berber: Ifsi, Zeri, Abelbel (23, 62); Izri (5, 62); Zezzeri, Odessir (62). English: Wormwood (4, 8). French: Armoise (4); Thym des steppes (23, 62); Armoise blanche (16, 23, 42).
Uses: Leaves and flowers febrifuge, calmative for stomach, cough and cephalalgia, cures nervous troubles and calms the emotions, used for ophthalmic diseases, enters in mixtures for treating hemorrhagic wounds. Infusion of flowering branches vermifuge, emmenagogue, tonic, stomachic. Dry powdered plant for healing wounds and burns, diuretic; infusion for rheumatism, bronchitis; cataplasm of boiled flowers used to ripen and cure abscesses, antidiarrhoeic (Rabat drug market); essential oil distilled from the plant good antiseptic and insecticide, also used as parasiticide in veterinary medicine. *Ref:* 5, 8, 16, 23, 42, 50, 62

Artemisia judaica L. *Area:* Egypt.
Names: Arabic: Shih (4, 44, 58); Shihan (4); Ba'athran (62). Berber: Techeredjili (47, 62). English: Judean wormwood (4); Wormwood (44). French: Absinthe de Judée, Armoise de Judée (4).
Uses: Leaves inhaled to relieve congestion of colds; smoke of burnt branches keeps snakes away; believed to prevent skin diseases if camels eat the plant. Infusion of flowering summits relieves gastro-intestinal cramps; infusion of flowering branches stomachic.

The subspecies *sahariensis* (Chev.) Maire, is known in North Africa from Libya to Morocco. *Ref:* 44, 57

Atractylis gummifera L. *Area:* Tunisia to Morocco.
Names: Arabic: Addad (5, 12, 13, 23, 42, 62); Heddad, Djerniz (23, 47, 62); Leddad (13, 23, 62); Shawk el-'elk (4, 13, 23, 62); Asad el-ard, Ashkhis (62). Berber: Tifroua (13, 23, 42, 62); Tifizza (5); Tabounekkart (23, 62); Tililsen (62); Ichkis (12). English: White chameleon, Spindle wort (4). French: Chardon à glu (5, 12, 13, 23, 42, 62); Chamoeleon blanc des anciens (23, 42, 62); Caméléon blanc, Carthame gummifère (4).
Uses: Decoction of dried root (highly toxic) stops hemorrhage in small doses, facilitates childbirth, purgative, emetic, for epilepsy and hysteria; in larger doses abortive. Cataplasm of powdered root for treating syphilitic cankers, abscesses,

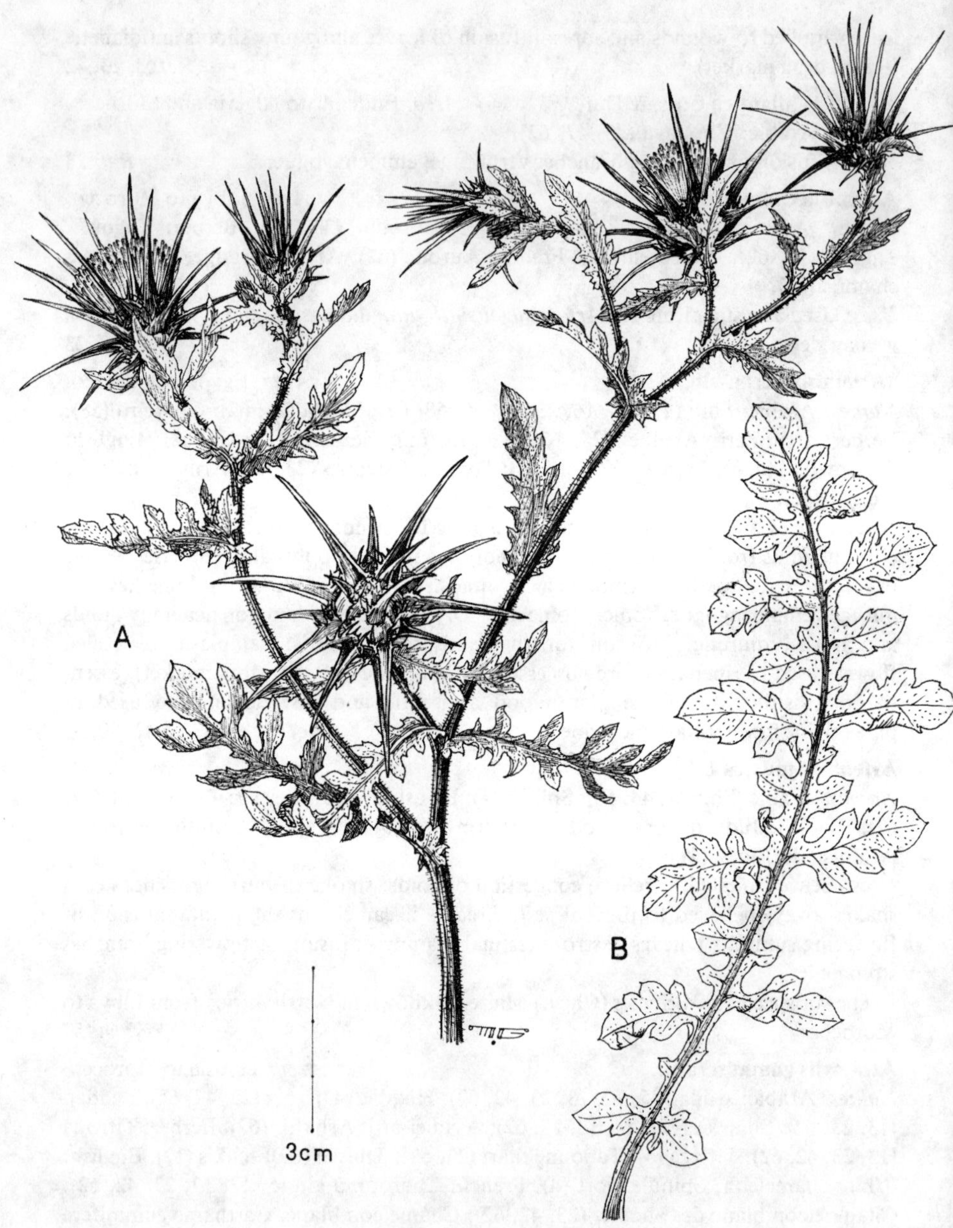

Centaurea alexandrina
A. flowering branch
B. Basal leaf

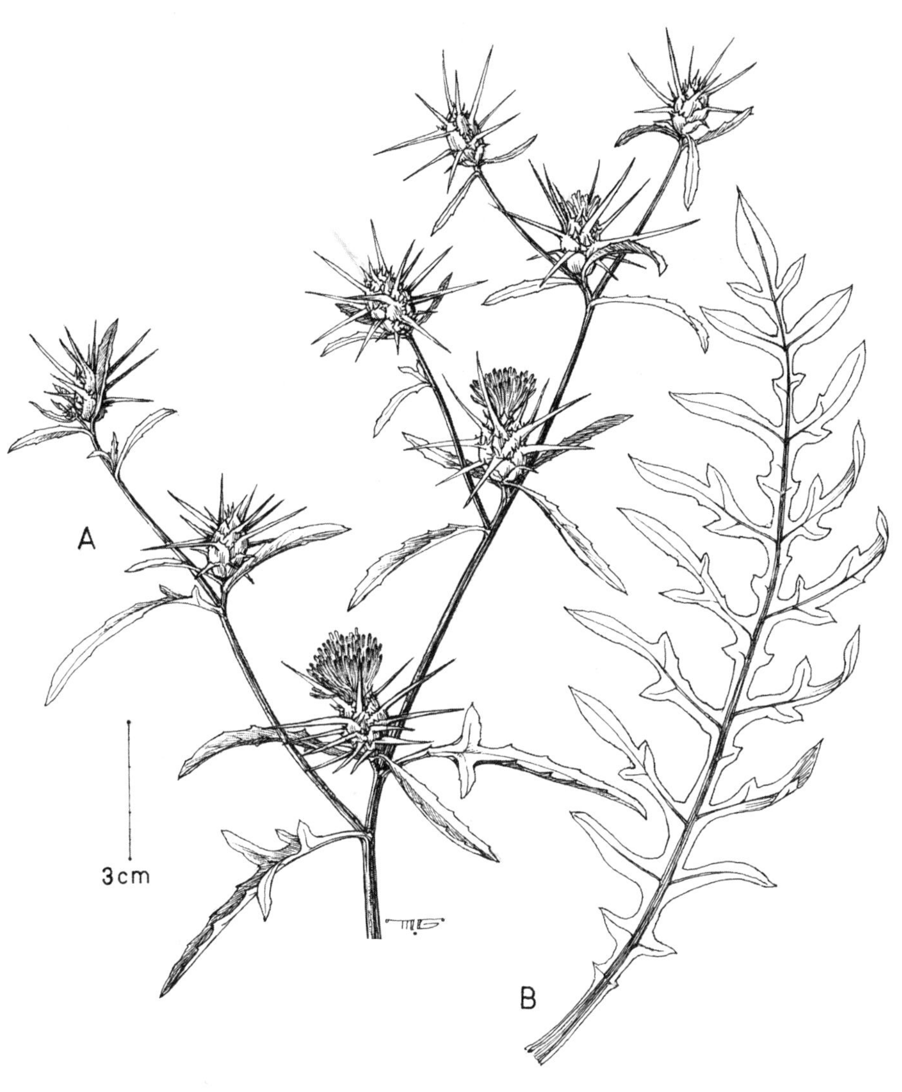

Centaurea calcitrapa
A. flowering branch
B. basal leaf

boils; root fumigant for paralysis, rheumatism, pulmonary troubles, insecticide. Root ashes boiled in water, then dried and mixed with semolina, mixed and heated with butter, eaten first thing in the morning for strengthening the body; eggs or beans boiled in the root infusion and consumed (without the liquid which is thrown away) to treat jaundice and chest diseases. Infusion of flowers for epilepsy and convulsions. *Ref:* 5, 12, 42

Calendula officinalis L. *Area:* North Africa. Mainly cultivated as ornamental plant and for cut flowers; often naturalized.
Names: Arabic: Djamir, Djoumaira, Gmredj, Zerzira, Lellousha (23, 62); Zobeida (4, 23, 62); Qawqhan, Qarqahan (4). Berber: Tousslat, Touzla guizgaren, Tahsoult (23, 62); Azouiout, Djemra, Djimri (62). English: Pot marigold, Hen and chickens (4). French: Souci (23, 62); Souci des jardins (4, 23); Souci officinal (23, 45).
Uses: Flower heads dried in the shade are used as emmenagogue, sudorific, chologogue, for curing wounds, homeopathic, stimulant, depurative, antispasmodic and antiemetic. *Ref:* 23, 24, 45

Centaurea acaulis L. *Area:* Tunisia to Morocco.
Names: Arabic: Ardjaqnou (6, 23, 62); Nagour, Tefrat el-kheil (23, 62); Argiqon (4). Berber: Ouzag, Ouerga (23, 62); Rejeguenu (6, 23, 62). English: Centaury (4). French: Centaurée acaule (23); Centaurée (4).
Uses: Root astringent, used as a yellow dye for wool. *Ref:* 6, 23, 62

Centaurea alexandrina Del. *Area:* Egypt, Libya.
Names: Arabic: Morrar (58).
Uses: Extract from flowering branches antibacterial, antidiabetic. *Ref:* 53

Centaurea calcitrapa L. *Area:* Egypt, Tunisia to Morocco.
Names: Arabic: Hassak, Bou neggar (23, 47, 62); Bou shweika, Nowar bellaremj (23, 62), Murrar (4, 58). Berber: Aceb (23, 62); Aboujoulj, Aourmela (62). English: Mouse-thorn, Star thistle, Caltrops (4). French: Chardon étoilé (4, 23); Chausse-trape (4, 23, 24).
Uses: Whole plant bitter-astringent, appetizer, vulnerary, antiophthalmic, antifebrile, stomachic, for intermittent fever, eye diseases. Leaves for cephalalgia. Flowering summits febrifuge; root and fruits diuretic. Seeds vulnerary, febrifuge, for renal stones and pains. *Ref:* 17, 23, 24, 33

***Chamaemelum nobile** (L.) All. *Area:* Drug imported from Europe. Often cultivated.
Names: Arabic: Babounag (4, 5, 62); Babounag rumi (5); Qurras, Mushraf (4). English: Camamel, Chamomile, Roman chamomile (4). French: Camomile (5, 62), Camomille romaine (4, 24, 45); Anthémis noble, Camomille odorante (4).
Uses: Flower heads yield bitter and aromatic tonic, stomachic, febrifuge, emmenagogue, vermifuge, vulnerary, stimulant, antispasmodic; infusion used against migraine, jaundice, digestive troubles. Oil of chamomile used as rub for rheumatism. *Ref:* 5, 24, 45

***Chamomilla recutita** (L.) Rauschert *Area:* Egypt to Morocco. Cultivated or naturalized.

Names: Arabic: Babounag (4, 42, 58); Babounig (58); Babnouj, Babnouz (Rabat drug market). Berber: Kourras (42). English: Wild chamomile, Dog's chamomile (4). French: Camomille commune, Matricaire camomille (4); Matricaire (45).

Uses: Infusion of flower heads carminative, stomachic, antispasmodic, vulnerary, soothing, antiallergic, tonic, febrifuge, stimulant, for bronchitis. *Ref:* 42, 45, 56

Chrysanthemum coronarium L. *Area:* Egypt to Morocco.
Names: Arabic: Rezaima (47, 62); Oqhowan (5, 58); Mandeliya (4, 58); Qurras (4); Asloudya, Gihwana, Djashwan, Kera'a ed-djaja (62); Mourara (47). Berber: Aouzed, Taoulzit (62). English: Crown daisy, Crown marigold, Garden chrysanthemum (4). French: Marguerite (5); Marguerite des champs, Chrysanthème à carène (4).
Uses: Flowers vermifuge, used against itch. *Ref:* 5

Cichorium intybus L. *Area:* Cultivated or naturalized in North Africa.
Names: Arabic: Seris, Shikouria (4, 23, 62); Tilfaf, Djouldjoulan (23, 62). Berber: Arhilon, Timerzouga, Mersag (23, 62); Timizagt, Tsalina (62). English: Wild chicory, Succory (4). French: Chicorée (4, 45, 62); Chicorée sauvage (4, 23); Barbede capucin, Chicorée amère, Cheveux de paysan (4).
Uses: Leaves and root tonic, stomachic, depurative, diuretic, laxative, chologogue, febrifuge; infusion an appetizer, for atony and digestive troubles, stimulates bile secretion. *Ref:* 5, 23, 24, 45, 56

***Conyza bonariensis** (L.) Cronq. *Area:* Egypt to Morocco. Naturalized from tropical America.
Names: Arabic: Gemliya (23, 62); Hashish el-gabal (4, 58); Zibl el-far, 'Ain elkatkout, Halouk baladi (58). English: Fleabane (4). French: Erigère, Erigéron (4); Conyze vulgaire, Herbe aux puces (23).
Uses: Flowering branches antirheumatic, diuretic. *Ref:* 23

***Cotula cinerea** Del. *Area:* Egypt to Morocco.
Names: Arabic: Ribyan (58, 62); Shiria, Robita (47, 62); Gertufa (5, 16), Rebruba (5), Shwikhia, Shwilia (62); Erbyan, Sekran (58). Berber: Takkilt (62). French: Camomille du Sahara (62).
Uses: Infusion of flower heads aromatic and very agreeable, stomachic and to flavor tea replacing peppermint, useful for broncho-pulmonary conditions, against scorpion bites, rheumatism, vomiting, nausea, stomach pains. *Ref:* 5, 16, 62

Cotula coronopifolia L. *Area:* Tunisia to Morocco. Naturalized from South Africa.
Names: Arabic: Babounig, Gertoufa (62).
Uses: Infusion anthelmintic (Rabat drug market).

Cynara cardunculus L. *Area:* Libya to Morocco.
Names: Arabic: Khorshef (12, 42, 47, 62); Genina (47, 62); Tinjara, Jenah en-nesr; stem: 'Asluj; midrib of leaf: Djimmar; florets: Haqq; head: Garnoun (62); Kharshaf barri, Hayshar, Shawk el-himir (2). Berber: Tagha (42, 62); Arhdon, Tardiut (62). English: Cardoon, Prickley artichoke (4). French: Cardon (4, 24, 42, 45); Artichaut carde (4); Artichaut sauvage (42).
Uses: Appreciated for its diuretic properties, aphrodisiac, mild purgative. Decoction of the plant made into lotion makes the offensive smell of the armpit and feet disap-

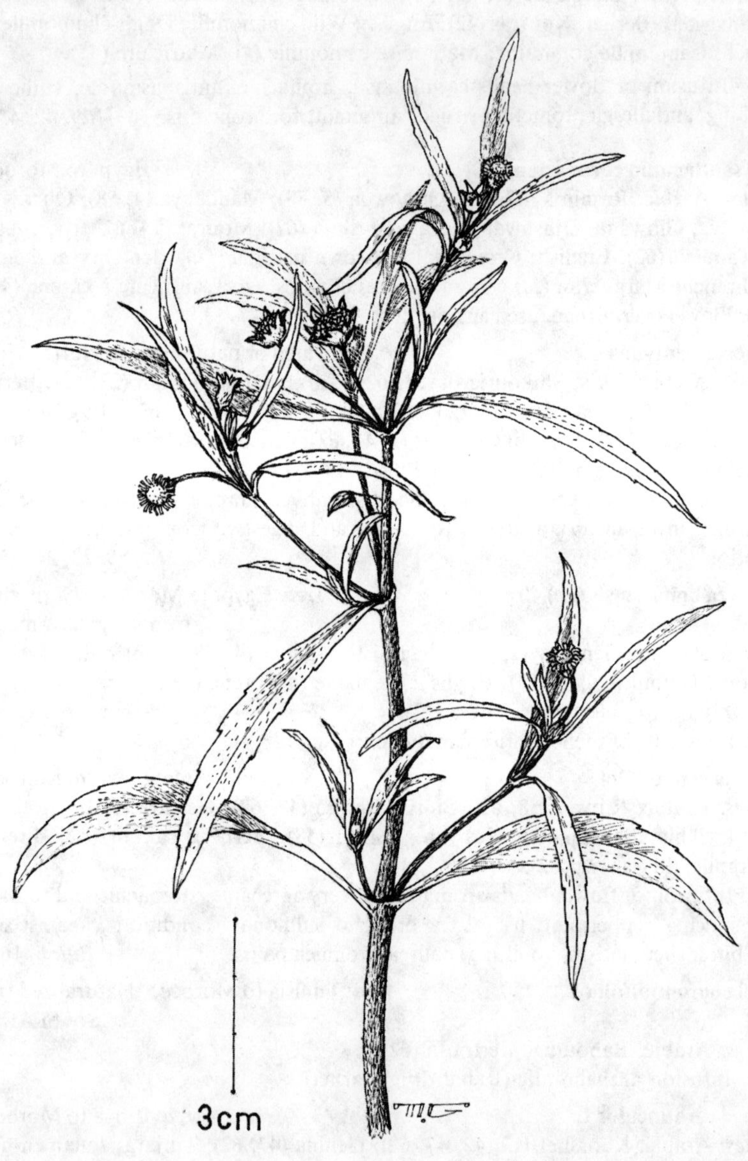

Eclipta prostrata

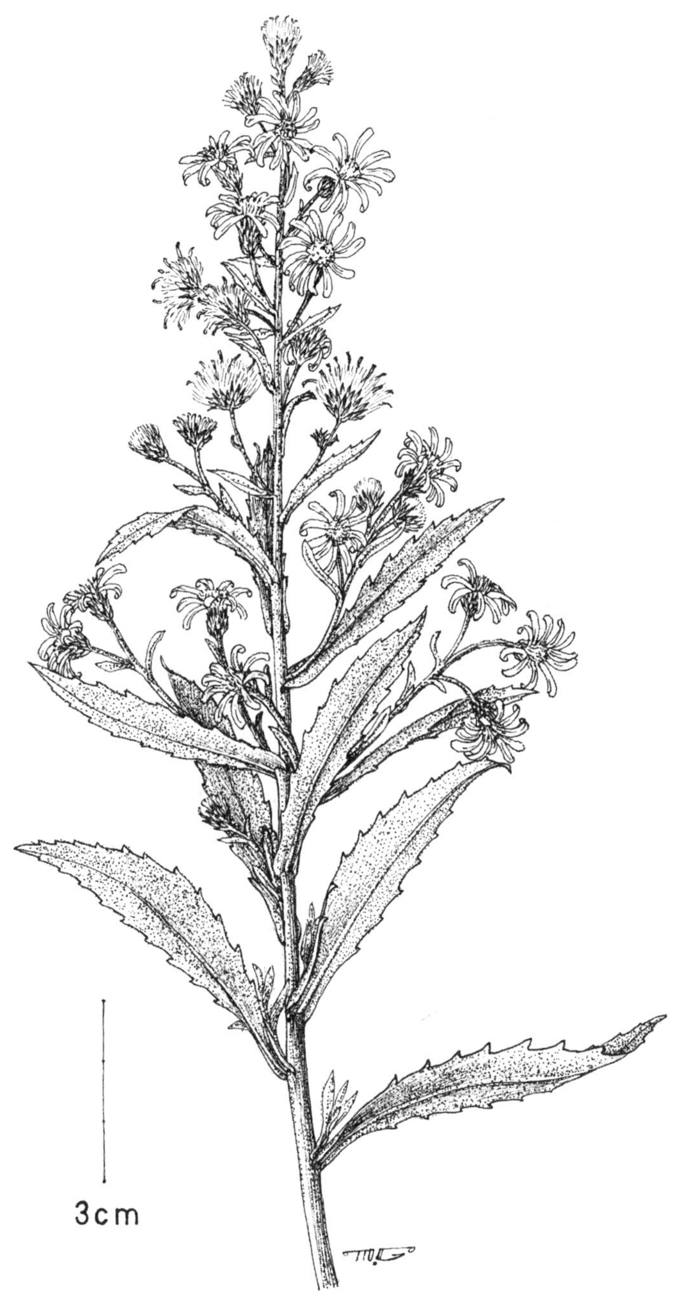

Inula viscosa

pear. Powdered leaves, roots and young flower heads cooked in small amount of oil applied in form of cataplasm on recent hernias four times a day for one month would bring patients to normal. *Ref:* 12, 42

Cynara humilis L. *Area:* Algeria, Morocco.
Names: Arabic: Feg'aa (47, 62); Khorshef (Rabat drug market).
Uses: Infusion of root used for liver inflation (Rabat drug market).

Cynara scolymus L. *Area:* Commonly cultivated in North Africa.
Names: Arabic: Kharshuf (4); Khorshef en-nasara, Qennarya (62). Berber: Tifrhout, Fegane, Taga (62). English: Artichoke (4, 24). French: Artichaut (4, 24, 62).
Uses: Leaves diuretic, tonic, stomachic, chologogue, stimulant, febrifuge, antirheumatic, for hepatic and renal affections, choleretic in cases of liver malfunction, jaundice, dyspepsia, chronic albuminurea, post-operative anemia, arteriosclerosis, skin disorders. *Ref:* 24, 45, 56

Echinops spinosus L. *Area:* Egypt to Morocco.
Names: Arabic: Shouk el-gamal (5, 13, 23, 42, 58, 62); Fougat el-gamal (13, 23, 62); Shouk el-hamir (5, 13, 23); Kashir, Ikshir, Shikaw, Sorr (13, 23, 62); Qatab, Asharab (58). Berber: Teskera (5, 13, 23, 26, 42, 62); Taskarat, Sarsor, Ameskelit (62). French: Echinops ritron (23); Teskra (5).
Uses: Decoction of root mixed with olive oil facilitates childbirth, hemostatic, diaphoretic. Stem, leaves and root abortive, diuretic, depurative, liver diseases, vasoconstrictor, for hypertension in large doses, dysmenorrhoea, metrorrhagia, prostatism, varices, varicocele. *Ref:* 5, 23, 42

***Eclipta prostrata** (L.) L. *Area:* Egypt. Naturalized from tropical and warm temperate America.
Names: Arabic: Suweid (4, 58); Hashish el-faras, Sa'aet el-naqa (58). English: False daisy (4). French: Eclipte droite (4).
Uses: Entire plant is astringent, hemostatic. Juice of fresh herb applied to scalp to promote hair growth; taken internally it blackens the hair and beard. *Ref:* 34

Eupatorium cannabinum L. *Area:* Algeria, Morocco.
Names: Arabic: Tebbaq (23, 47, 62); Ghafath, Khadd el-bint (4). English: Water hemp agrimony, Hemp weed (4). French: Chanvrine, Eupatoire d'Avicenne (4, 23), Eupatoire (62); Chanvre d'eau (4); Eupatoire chanvrine (23, 24).
Uses: Plant, including the root, appetizer, diuretic, sudorific, tonic, febrifuge, purgative; in large doses chologogue, emetic, vermifuge; externally used as resolvent, vulnerary. *Ref:* 23, 24

Helianthus annuus L. *Area:* Commonly cultivated in North Africa.
Names: Arabic: 'Abbad esh-shams (4); Daret esh-shams, 'Asheq esh-Shams, 'Ain esh-shams, Shemsia; seeds: Habb esh-shams (62). English: Sunflower, Golden flower of Peru (4). French: Hélianthe, Tournesol (4, 45); Grand soleil (4, 24).
Uses: Tincture of mature seeds very effective in treating constipation and urticaria; tincture used externally on bruises and wounds. *Ref:* 56

***Inula viscosa** (L.) Ait. *Area:* Egypt to Morocco.
Names: Arabic: Magraman (5, 42, Algiers drug market); Terhala (5, 42); Safsag, Mersit, Hafina, Amagraman (62); 'Erq et-tayyoun (58); Gafit, Tubbaq (42); Ter-

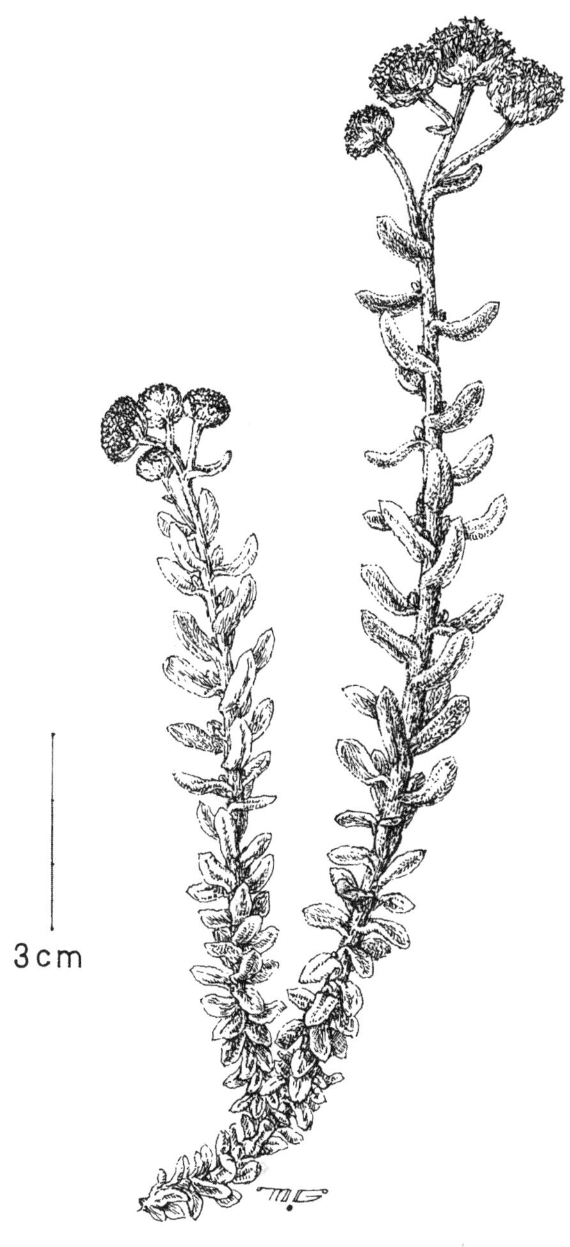

Otanthus maritimus

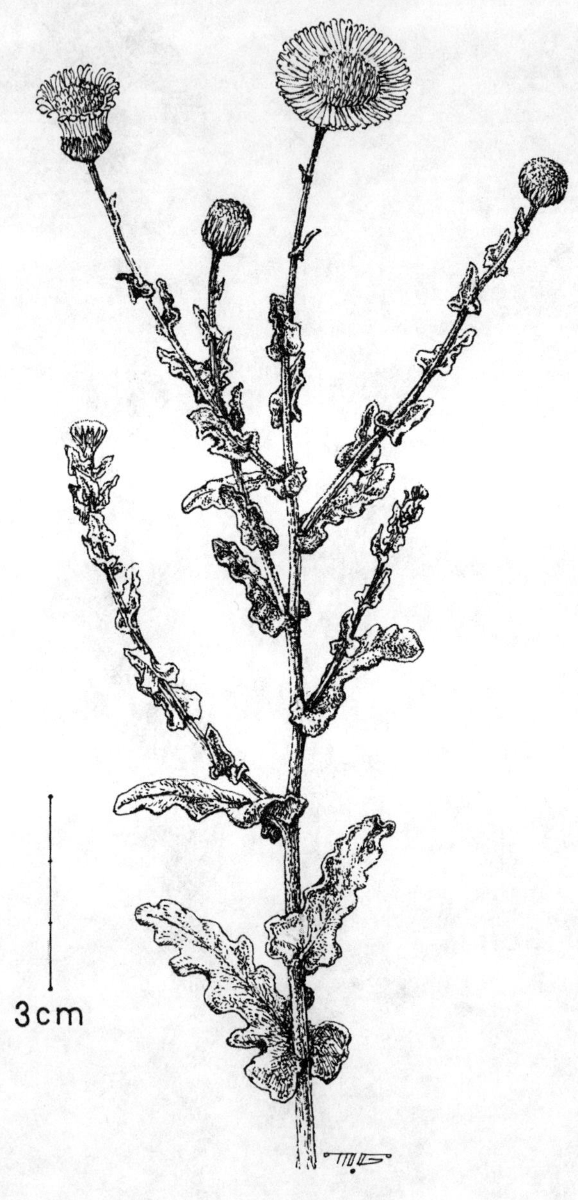

Pulicaria incisa

rehla (Rabat drug market). Berber: Afedjedad, Neiret, Tlirin (62). French: Aunée visqueuse (5, 42).
Uses: Flowering branches used for bronchitis, tuberculosis, anemia, astringent, fattening, for malaria and diseases of the urinary system; boiled in oil, the oil is rubbed on bruises and swellings; cataplasm for rheumatic pains; powdered and mixed with henna leaves, a cataplasm is made for sunstroke (Algiers drug market). *Ref:* 5, 24, 42

Lactuca sativa L. *Area:* Cultivated in many varieties in North Africa.
Names: Arabic: Khass (4, 62); Mesiouka, Harouka (62). English: Common lettuce (4). French: Laitue cultivée (4, 24, 62).
Uses: In homeopathy, a tincture extracted from the whole plant is used in treatment of impotence; symbol of fertility in Ancient Egypt. Leaves emollient, calmative, a valuable source of iron and vitamins. Seed oil aphrodisiac. *Ref:* 24, 43, 56

***Lactuca serriola** L. *Area:* Egypt to Morocco.
Names: Arabic: Mesalem (13, 42, 62); Seif el-ghorab (13, 62); Khass ez-zeit (4); Dafla sahrawia (13, 42). English: Oil lettuce, Prickly lettuce (4). French: Laitue scariole (4, 24); Laitue sauvage, Laitue d'huile (4).
Uses: Plant calmative; decoction antipoison for scorpion and snake bites, acting by hypotonic effect of the sap, emollient, antispasmodic, diuretic. *Ref:* 24, 42

Lactuca virosa L. *Area:* Algeria, Morocco.
Names: Arabic: Lebbein (4, 13, 42, 62). English: Acrid lettuce (4, 24); Wild lettuce (4). French: Laitue vireuse (4, 24, 45).
Uses: Same uses and effects as *Lactuca serriola;* calmative, diuretic, sudorific, slightly laxative, narcotic, mild hypotonic, calmative for babies cough. *Ref:* 13, 24, 42, 45

***Otanthus maritimus** (L.) Hoffmanns. & Link *Area:* Egypt to Morocco.
Names: Arabic: Shiba, Arhbita (23, 42, 50, 62). English: Cotton weed, Sea cud-weed (4). French: Herbe blanche (4); Herba buena des espagnols (42); Hierba buena (62).
Uses: Flowering branches febrifuge, emmenagogue, tonic, taenifuge.
Ref: 23, 42, 50, 62

***Pulicaria crispa** (Forssk.) Benth. ex Oliver *Area:* Egypt to Morocco.
Names: Arabic: 'Arfeg (47, 58, 62); Feliet el-hami (62); El-'attasa, El-'eteytesa (5); Sabad, Gettiat, Zibl el-far, Ghobbeira, Khanouf (58). Berber: Timetfest, Attasa, Tanater, Atoua (62); Shini (11). *Ref:* 5
Uses: Flowering branches for preparing sneezing powder, sternutatory. *Ref:* 5

***Pulicaria incisa** (Lam.) DC. *Area:* Egypt, Libya, Algeria.
Names: Arabic: Shay gebeli (44, 58); Rabal (11, 58); Raboul, Rabd, Ghobbeira (58). Berber: Taganasu (11), Ameo (62). English: Wild tea (44).
Uses: Infusion for heart diseases, replaces tea as used by Bedouins in Egypt.
Ref: 44, 57

Santolina chamaecyparissus L. *Area:* Tunisia to Morocco.
Names: Arabic: 'Araira (23, 62); Qaysun, Babuni (62). Berber: Tairart (23, 62). English: Lavender cotton, Ground cypress (4). French: Santoline (4); Aurone femelle (4, 23); Santoline blanche, Petit cyprès (23).
Uses: Flowering summits vermifuge, emmenagogue, antispasmodic, sedative, stomachic, stimulant, for hysteric affections, anthelmintic; its essential oil used with success for taenia. *Ref:* 23, 24

***Senecio anteuphorbium** L. *Area:* Endemic to Morocco.
Names: Berber: Shbarto, Ashbarto (5); Ashbardou (42).
Uses: Entire plant used against burns often occurring due to the caustic latex from the cactus-like Euphorbias common in SW Morocco, where the plant grows. Resinous sap prescribed as a calmative; internally for stomachache and enteritis; externally for rheumatic pains. Latex for sores and wounds, hemostatic, strong sedative for all pains including abdominal, dorsal, burns. Flower nectar acrid and rather bitter, good tonic. *Ref:* 5, 42

Senecio vulgaris L. *Area:* Egypt to Morocco.
Names: Arabic: Eshbet Salema (23, 62); Morrar (58); Muraya, Sheikh el-rabi, Babunig et-tuyur (4). Berber: Tidmamai (23, 62). English: Common groundsel, Flower of St. Macarius (4). French: Séneçon commun (4, 23, 24, 45).
Uses: Flowering branches emmenagogue, vaso-constrictor, vermifuge, emollient, hemostatic, mild laxative, resolvent. *Ref:* 23, 24, 45

Silybum marianum (L.) Gaertner *Area:* Egypt to Morocco.
Names: Arabic: Shouk en-nasara (4, 58); Shouk sinnari, Shouk el-gemal, Shouk el-ghazal, Lekhlakh (58); 'Akoub, Harshaf barri, Shouk el-diman (4); Shouk boulti; Shouket el-beida, Fouarek, Bou zerwal, Zaz, Baq, Lishlish, Hasoub (62). Berber: Tataoura, Doujnilourman (62). English: Milk thistle, St. Mary's thistle (4). French: Chardon Marie (4, 45); Chardon Notre Dame, Artichaut sauvage, Chardon argenté (4).
Uses: Plant bitter appetizer, tonic, febrifuge, resolvent. Tincture from seeds used for liver disorders, jaundice, gall stones, peritonitis, coughs, bronchitis, congestion of uterus and varicose veins. *Ref:* 24, 56

Convolvulaceae

Convolvulus althaeoides L. *Area:* Egypt to Morocco.
Names: Arabic: Luwwaya (5, 47, 62); 'Ulleiq (4, 62); Mesran lehwar (5); Maddad (58); Louzga, Tobbana (62). Berber: Tanesfalt, Anesfal (5). English: Mallow bindweed (4). French: Liseron de Provence (4); Liseron fausse-guimauve (24).
Uses: Flowering branches mild purgative, for cough, asthma, hydropsy. *Ref:* 5

Convolvulus arvensis L. *Area:* Egypt to Morocco.
Names: Arabic: Lebena, Ghorime, Douilat (47, 62); 'Ulleiq (4, 58, 62); Moddeid (4, 58); Tarbush el-ghorab (4, 62); Halib el-ghazal (62). Berber: Alouaich, Loueg, Anschfel (62). English: Lesser bindweed, Corn bind, Corn lily (4). French: Liseron des champs (4, 24, 37); Petit liseron, Vrillée (4).
Uses: Root extracts antihemorrhagic. Plant chologogue, febrifuge, one of the best purgatives. Leaves used externally as vulnerary. Flowering branches have same uses and effects as *Convolvulus althaeoides,* cathartic, purgative. *Ref:* 2, 5, 24

Convolvulus hystrix Vahl *Area:* Egypt.
Names: Arabic: Shibreq, Shobroq, Shibrim, Al-hilla (58).
Uses: Plant purgative. *Ref:* 2

Cressa cretica L. *Area:* Egypt to Morocco.

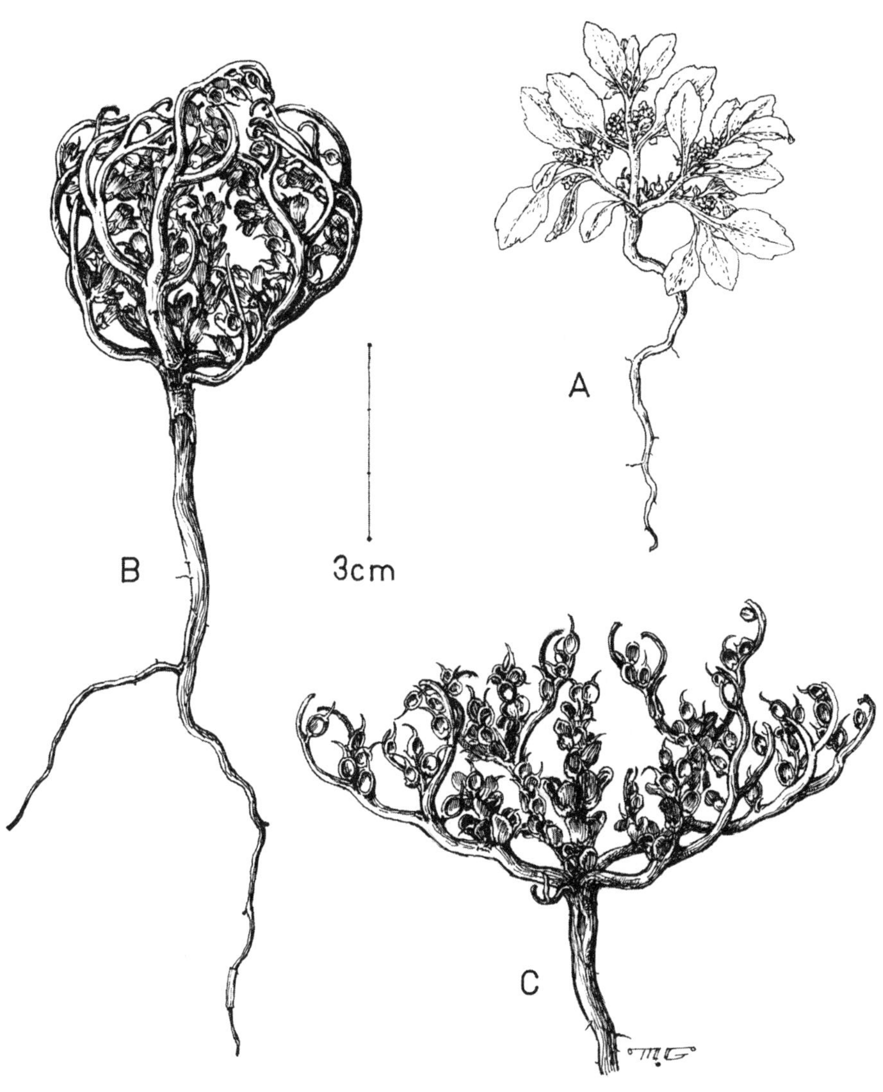

Anastatica hierochuntica
A. flowering plant, B. closed fruiting plant
C. opened fruiting plant

Names: Arabic: Melliha (5, 47, 58, 62); Nadwa (4, 47, 58, 62); Ghorara (4, 62); Melifa (62). English: Rosin weed (4). French: Cresse, Cresse à feuille d'herniaire (4).
Uses: Dried leaves crushed with sugar and taken as energetic purge for cases of jaundice, followed by a milk diet. *Ref:* 5

Cuscuta epithymum (L.) L. *Area:* Libya to Morocco.
Names: Arabic: Hummad el-arnab, Kashout (4, 37, 62); Shakuta (4). Berber: Akshout, Afistinoun (62). English: Lesser dodder, Clover dodder (4). French: Cuscute (37, 42); Petite cuscute, Epithym, Cuscute de thym (4).
Uses: Decoction of the entire parasitic plant depurative, stomachic, for intestinal troubles, chologogue, for jaundice, liver troubles, diuretic, mild laxative, purgative. *Ref:* 5, 37, 42, 45

Cuscuta planiflora Ten. *Area:* Egypt to Morocco.
Names: Arabic: Hariret el-za'atar (8); Kashout, Zouhmouk (62). Berber: Akshout, Aftimoun (62). English: Dodder of thyme (8).
Uses: Cold infusion of the entire plant an intestinal disinfectant, for jaundice, liver troubles, chologogue, diuretic, mild laxative. *Ref:* 5, 8

Coriariaceae

Coriaria myrtifolia L. *Area:* Algeria, Morocco.
Names: Arabic: Rouida, Redoul (13, 23, 62). Berber: Arouz, Rouiza (13, 23, 62). English: Myrtle-leaved sumach, Myrtle-leaved tanner's tree (4). French: Redoul commun, Corroyère à feuilles de myrthe (23); Corroyère, Redoul, Herbe aux tanneurs (4); Coriaire (13).
Uses: Plant toxic, intestinal astringent. Leaves rich in tannin. *Ref:* 13, 23, 62

Cruciferae

***Alliaria petiolata** (Bieb.) Cavara & Grande *Area:* Tunisia to Morocco.
Names: Arabic: Hashisha thawmiyah (4). English: Garlic mustard, Jack by the hedge (4). French: Alliare (4, 23); Alliare officinale (4, 24).
Uses: Plant antiasthmatic, rubefacient, stimulant, diuretic, sudorific, bechic, antiscorbutic, vermifuge. *Ref:* 23, 24

Anastatica hierochuntica L. *Area:* Egypt to Morocco.
Names: Arabic: Kaff Maryam (4, 6, 42, 58, 62); Shagret Mariam (4, 58); Kaff El-'Adra, Kufayfah (4); Kaff Lella Fatma, Yedd Fatma, Bint En-Nebi, Kemshet En-Nebi, Kemshe, Kershoud (62); Haddaq, Qebad, Kamaash (58); Kmisa (42); Shajaret et-talq, El-kemsha, El-kmisha (5). Berber: Akaraba (26, 62); Tamkelt (5). English: St. Mary's flower, Rose of Jericho (4). French: Rose de Jéricho (4, 5, 26, 42, 62); Main de Fathma (62); Jérose (4).
Uses: Infusion of dry plant reduces the pains and facilitates childbirth, emmenagogue, for epilepsy, colds (Rabat drug market). *Ref:* 5, 17, 26, 42

***Brassica nigra** (L.) Koch *Area:* Egypt to Morocco.
Names: Arabic: Khardal (13, 23, 47, 58, 62); Khardal aswad (4); Libsan, Libdan, Lifsan (58). English: Black mustard (4, 24). French: Moutarde noire (4, 23, 24, 45, 47, 62); Sénevé noir (4, 23); seeds: Chou noir (23).

Uses: Plant revulsive, stomachic, antiscorbutic, emetic, laxative, diuretic, stimulant, slightly febrifuge. *Ref:* 5, 23, 24, 45

Capsella bursa-pastoris (L.) Medicus *Area:* Egypt to Morocco.
Names: Arabic: Kis er-ra'i (4, 58, 62); Mikhlet er-ra'i (58); Harra el-berria, Shenaf (23, 62); Harra el-gharin, Lebsan el-khil, Khenfej, Kerkas (62); Barghoutha (37). English: Shepherd's purse, Mother's heart (4): Bourse à pasteur (4, 23, 24, 45, 62); Boursette, Bourse de capucin (4); Tabouret (23).
Uses: Plant astringent, hemostatic, vaso-constrictor. Infusion of dried plants effective remedy for menorrhagia, dysmenorrhoea, uterine haemorrhages. Homeopathic tincture is used for nasal and internal bleeding, in cases of cystitis and stones in the urinary tract. *Ref:* 23, 24, 37, 45, 56

Eruca sativa Miller *Area:* Cultivated and often naturalized in North Africa.
Names: Arabic: Gargir (Djerdjir) (4, 23, 58, 62); Kerkas (23, 62); 'Ai'afein (58, 62); Gery, Rawq, Shiltam (58); Bou kahli, Horf, Baglet 'Aisha, Rouka (62). Berber: Achnef (23, 62); Thorfel, Tanakfail (62). English: Rocket, Roquette (4). French: Roquette (4, 23, 62); Roquette vraie (24).
Uses: Leaves antiscorbutic, stimulant, rubefacient. Fresh plant eaten as a green salad considered aphrodisiac (Farmers, Egypt). *Ref:* 23, 24

Lepidium sativum L. *Area:* Cultivated and naturalized in North Africa.
Names: Arabic: Reshad (4, 23, 58, 62); seeds: Habb er-reshad (4, 5, 42, 58, 62); Horf (5, 23, 42, 62); Tseffa, Qerfa, Half (62). Berber: Belacheqine (23, 62). English: Garden cress, Tongue-grass (4). French: Cresson alénois (4, 5, 23, 42, 45, 62); Cressonnette (4, 23, 62); Passerage cultivé, Cresson des jardins (4).
Uses: Fresh plant eaten as antiscorbutic, nourishing, condiment. Seeds tonic, aphrodisiac, active expectorant, pulmonary stimulant. Crushed seeds mixed with honey or hot milk is taken for cough, tuberculosis, colds, pulmonary diseases, sterility, syphilis; also as a tonic, carminative, galactogogue. Flour from seeds enter in the composition of revulsive cataplasms against bronchitis and whitlow. Cataplasm of seeds used to heal scrofulous ulcers. Crushed seeds mixed with olive oil used as massage for rachitis. *Ref:* 5, 17, 23, 42

***Lobularia maritima** (L.) Desv. *Area:* Egypt to Morocco. Cultivated and often naturalized.
Names: Arabic: Aguerma (26, 42), Khurm el-ibrah (4); Agrima, Zerzira, Khenfdj el-hadjera (26). English: Sweet alison, Allison (4). French: Corbeille d'argent, Alysse argentée, Alysse maritime (4); Alysson maritime (26, 42).
Uses: Infusion of flowering plant is febrifuge. *Ref:* 26, 42

Nasturtium officinale R. Br. *Area:* Egypt to Morocco.
Names: Arabic: Qurrat el-'ayn (4, 62); Guernech (42, 47, 62), Karsun, Rashad, Horf, Harriqa, Djerdjir el-maa (62); Karsun mai, Horf el-maa, Abu khangar; seeds: Hab er-rashad (62). Berber: Grinouch, Timeskine, Icha, Iourzèz, Haldjamin, Taffa (62); Timegsin (42). English: Water cress (4, 24); Water grass (4). French: Cresson de fontaine (4, 24, 42, 47, 62); Santé du corps (4, 24).
Uses: Plant antiscorbutic, aphrodisiac. Young shoots stomachic, ease bronchitis and soothe some skin diseases, stimulant, diuretic, depurative, appetizer, anticatarrhal, febrifuge, antidiabetic. *Ref:* 24, 42, 45, 56

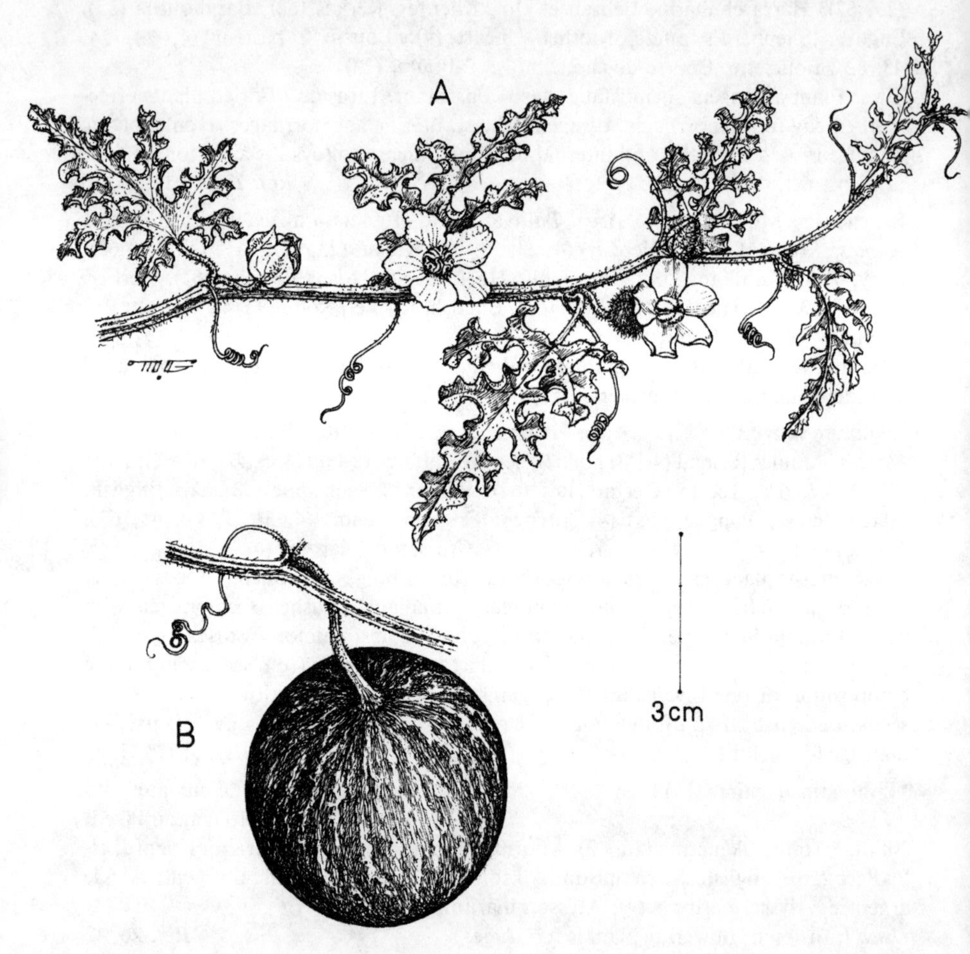

Citrullus colocynthis
A. flowering branch, B. fruit

Raphanus sativus L. *Area:* Frequently cultivated and often naturalized in North Africa.
Names: Arabic: Figl (4, 62); Mechtehiya (62). Berber: Left azouggar (62). English: Common cultivated radish (4). French: Radis cultivé (4, 24); Daikon (4).
Uses: Plant appetizer, stimulant. Fresh roots digestant, diuretic, antiscorbutic; dried root diuretic. Decoction of leaves antiphlogistic. Seeds stomachic, expectorant. *Ref:* 24, 34

Sinapis alba L. *Area:* Egypt to Morocco.
Names: Arabic: Khardal abiad (4, 13, 23, 62); Khardal, Kabar abiad (4); Horf el-babln (62); seeds: Toffa (13, 23, 62). English: White mustard (4, 24); Salad mustard (4). French: Moutarde blanche (4, 13, 23, 24, 45, 62); Sénevé blanc (4, 24); Plante au beurre (23).
Uses: Seeds used against chronic constipation, laxative; pulverized seeds purgative. *Ref:* 13, 23, 24

***Sisymbrium officinale** (L.) Scop. *Area:* Libya to Morocco.
Names: Arabic: Horf, Harif, Toudari (23, 62); Semmana (62); Sammarah, Tudharig, Figl el-gimal (4); El-harra (37). English: Hedge mustard, Common hedge mustard (4). French: Vélar (4, 23, 62); Herbe aux chantre (4, 23, 37); Tortelle (4); Vélar officinal (24).
Uses: Leaves and seeds expectorant, bechic, stimulant, antiscorbutic, diuretic. *Ref:* 23, 24, 37

***Zilla spinosa** (L.) Prantl *Area:* Egypt to Morocco.
Names: Arabic: Zilla (4, 62); Silla, Sirr (4); Shabrom, Shoubroq (62). Berber: Oftazzen, Ftozzer (62). French: Roquette épineuse (4).
Uses: Useful remedy in the treatment of ailments such as kidney stones. *Ref:* 20

Cucurbitaceae

Bryonia dioica Jacq. *Area:* Libya to Morocco.
Names: Arabic: Fashira (4, 5, 13, 23, 24, 62); Qeriou'aa (23, 42, 62); Lowwaya (5, 13, 42); Dalia beida (13, 42, 62); Karma beida (4, 13, 23, 62); 'Enab el-haiya, Bou tnia (4, 62); Terbuna (5); Bou Teriowa (62); Khiytah (4). Berber: Tailoula (13, 23, 42, 62); Tara bouchehen (13, 42, 62); Telmoumi (13, 62). English: Snake bryony, White wild vine, Common bryony (4). French: Bryone (13, 23, 42, 45); Navet du diable (4, 23); Bryone dioique, Bryone couleuvrée (4).
Uses: Whole plant is toxic, especially the berries and root. Root purgative, for itch, revulsive, antileprous; decoction of fresh roots purgative, diuretic. Red berries constitute a more violent purgative and possess doubtless vermifuge action, externally recommended for itch and leprosy, congestions, dropsy, rheumatism, cathartic, antitumor activity, depurative of blood, for epileptic crises. *Ref:* 5, 13, 18, 23, 42, 45

***Citrullus colocynthis** (L.) Schrader *Area:* Egypt to Morocco.
Names: Arabic: Handal (4, 8, 11, 13, 23, 42, 58, 62); Hadaj (4, 5, 13, 23, 42, 62); Hadja (13, 23, 47, 62); Hadaq, Qittat en-na'am (23, 62); dry fruits: Sise; seeds: Habid, Haguellet (23, 62); Merraret el-sekhour, Dingel, Marhoum (62); Hedej lehmar (5). Berber: Tadjellet, Alkat (13, 23, 62); Taferzizt (5, 13, 62); Tifersit (13,

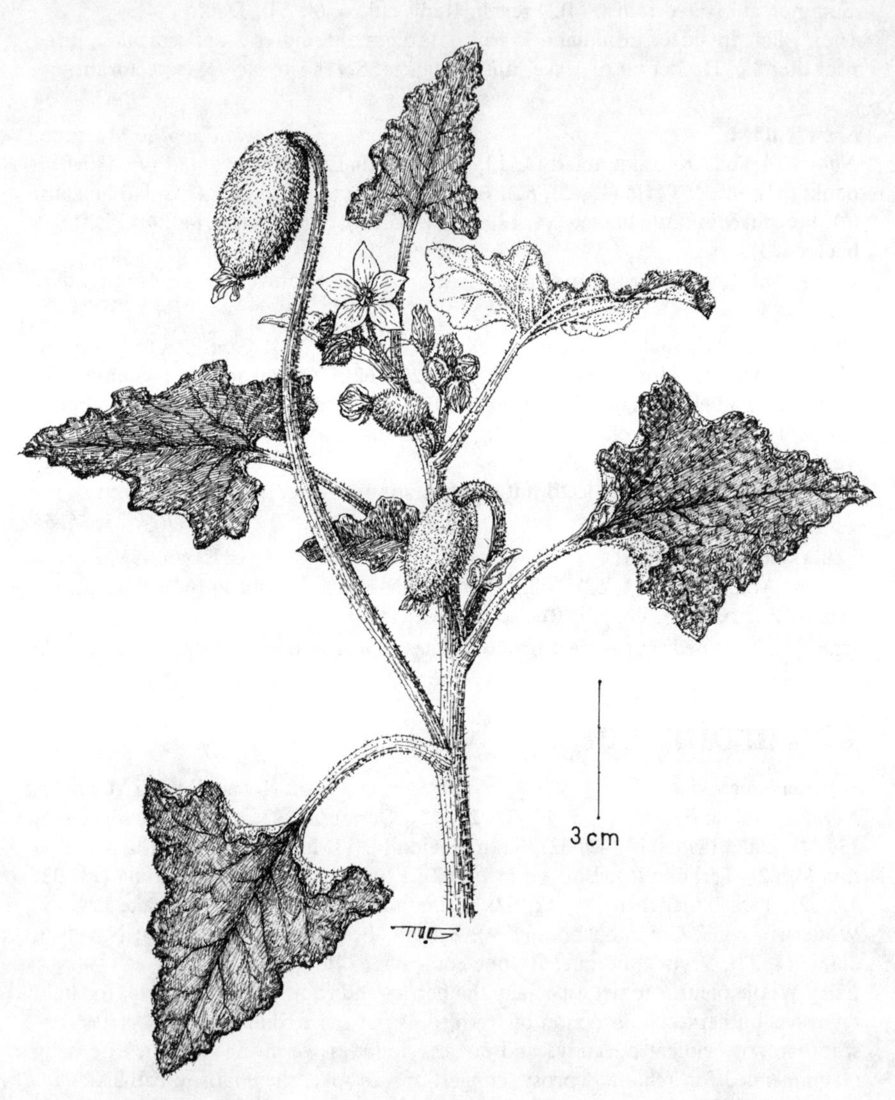

Ecballium elaterium

47, 62); Ubruzi (11); fruit: Abur (11). English: Colocynth (4, 8); Bitter apple, Bitter gourd (4). French: Coloquinte (4, 5, 13, 23, 42, 62); Chicotin (4).
Uses: Veterinary preparations used for itch very often contain colocynth; cataplasm of green or dried plant used as a remedy for leukoderma; cataplasm resolvent, astringent. Hot sap of plant used to cure certain skin diseases of camels. Decoction of roots mixed with garlic externally used against snake bites. Sap of unripe green fruits used against scorpion stings. Dry fruits effective insecticide especially for mites and weevils. Fruit pulp violent purgative, diuretic, antiepileptic, against gonorrhoea. Garlic added to extract of boiled seeds used against bites of poisonous snakes. Seeds anthelmintic, abortive, for gonorrhoea. One seed daily, swallowed without chewing, for 21 days, is a useful remedy for diabetes (Rabat drug market).
Ref: 5, 8, 13, 23, 42, 57

Cucumis melo L. *Area:* Commonly cultivated in North Africa. Several varieties are known, some usually restricted to certain regions.
Names: Arabic: 'Aggour (4, 62); Feggous, Bettikha (62); Qawoun, Shammam (4); Yaqtin, Bittikh (42). Berber: Tarrhsimte, Afqous, Bambous (62). English: Melon, Musk melon (4). French: Melon (42, 62); Musk melon (4).
Uses: Footstalk of fruit expectorant, emetic. Seeds vermifuge, digestive, refrigerant, antitussive. *Ref:* 34, 42

Cucurbita pepo L. *Area:* Commonly cultivated in North Africa.
Names: Arabic: Qar'a (5, 42); Qrei'a (62); Qar'a maghrabi, Qar'a rumi (4); Qar'a hamra, Lehshash, Lekshash (5); Kabouia, Kouaba, Djirouad (62). Berber: Kabéoualen, Sagadon (62). English: Pumpkin, Gourd (4). French: Citrouille (5, 42); Potiron (5); Giraumon (4); Courgette (62).
Uses: Embryo of the seed contains an isoprenoid compound which has remarkable antihelminthoid properties, capable of arresting cell division at metaphase and can be used to combat cancer in cases of hypertrophy of the prostate gland. Seeds anthelmintic; fresh peeled seeds vermifuge in association with a purgative.
Ref: 5, 34, 42, 56

Ecballium elaterium (L.) A. Rich. *Area:* Libya to Morocco.
Names: Arabic: Faggous el-hemar (4, 13, 23, 42, 62); Quittaa el-hemar (4, 13, 23, 62); Beid el-ghul (13, 23, 42, 62); Oumana (23, 62); Oufadia, Safirous (62); 'Awar-war, Qittaa barri (4). Berber: Afgous bourhioul (13, 23, 42, 62). English: Squirting cucumber (4). French: Concombre d'âne, (23, 42, 62); Momordique (24); Cornichon d'âne, Concombre sauvage, Concombre d'attrape (4, 24).
Uses: Plant toxic at low doses. Root used externally by rubbing for painful articular conditions. Root and fruit juice violent purgative, diuretic, emetic. Fruit dipped in oil used as a suppository against piles. Fruit juice used as nose drops (Algiers drug market), and for jaundice by nasal instillation, once a day for one week, during which period the patient eats one raw egg with an equal volume of oil.
Ref: 5, 13, 17, 23, 24, 42

***Lagenaria siceraria** (Molina) Standley *Area:* Frequently cultivated in North Africa.
Names: Arabic: Qar'a tawil (4, 42, 62); Dubb'a (42); Qar'a dubba, Qar'a duruf (4); Qar'a aslawiya (42, 62, Rabat drug market); Qer'aa, Qer'aa beida, Qer'aa gardousi, Qer'aa medwen, Qer'aa el-leben (62). Berber: Takhsaît, Ouowi, Laqttine, Tafe-

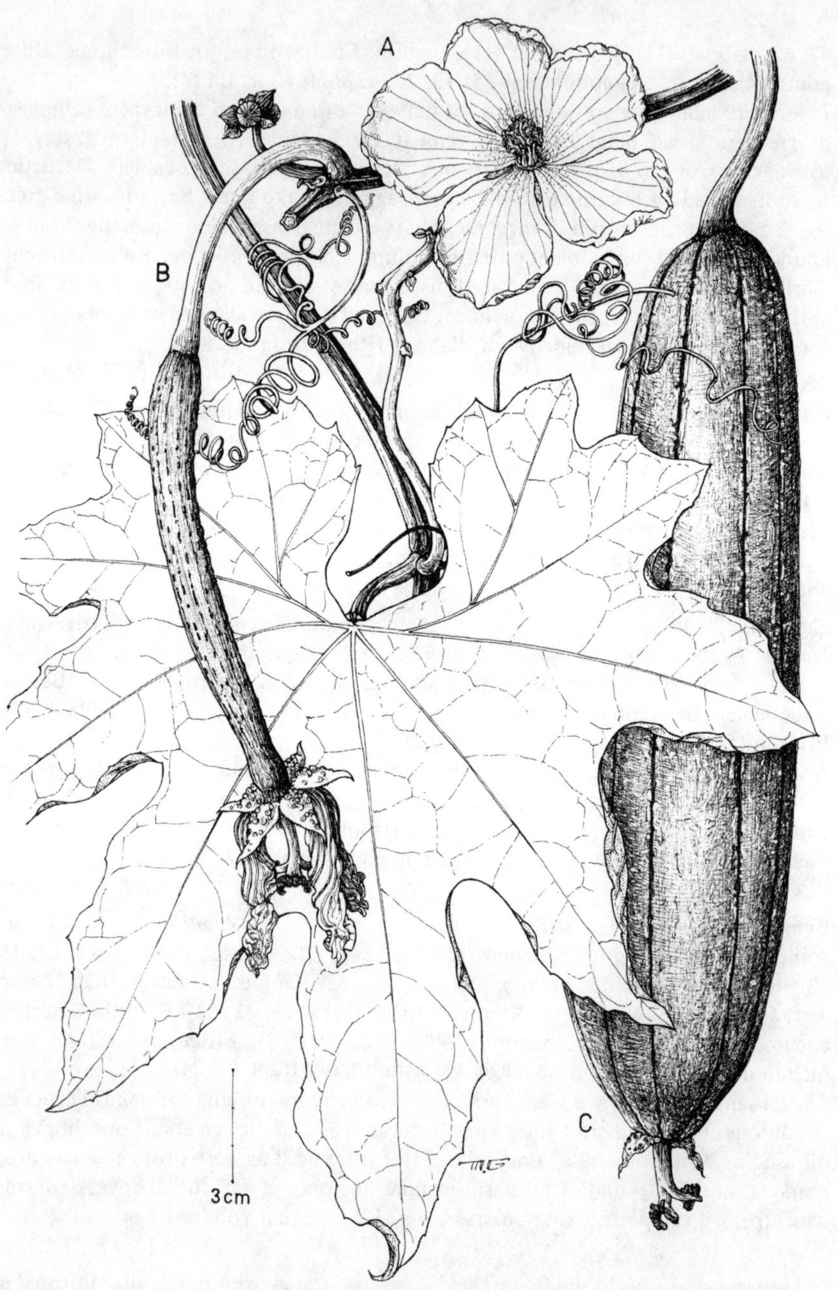

Luffa cylindrica
A. flowering branch with male flower
B. young fruit with remnants of female flower
C. immature fruit

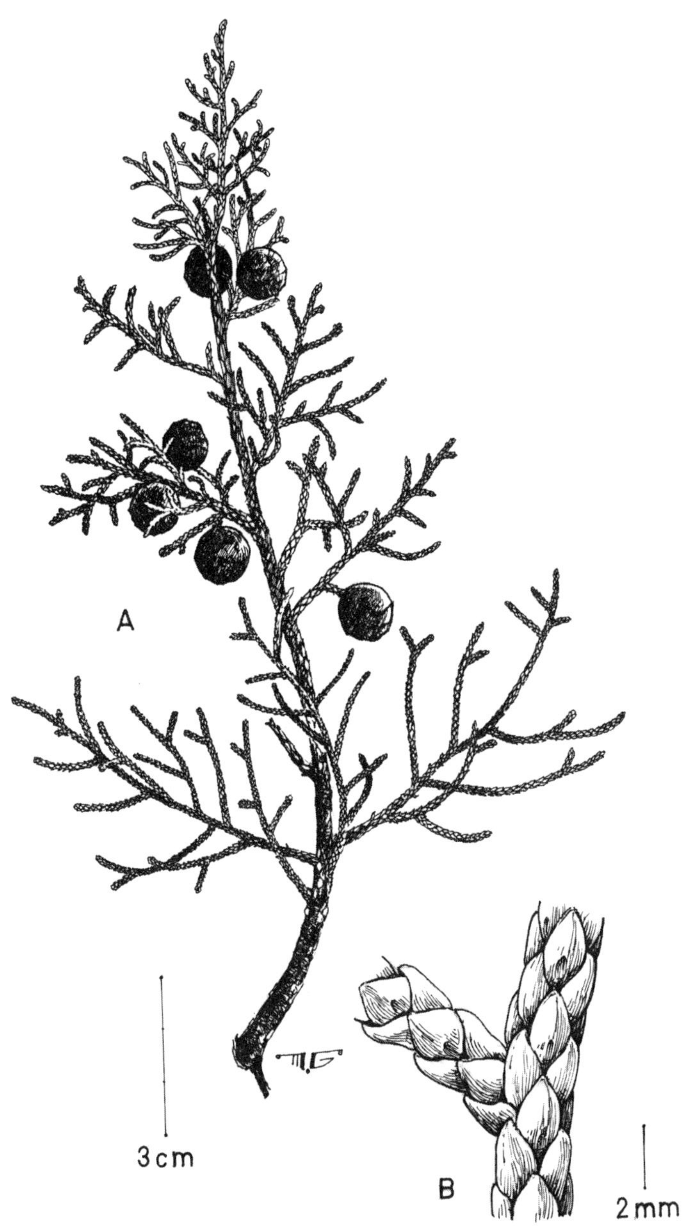

Juniperus phoenicea
A. fruiting branch, B. branchlet, enlarged

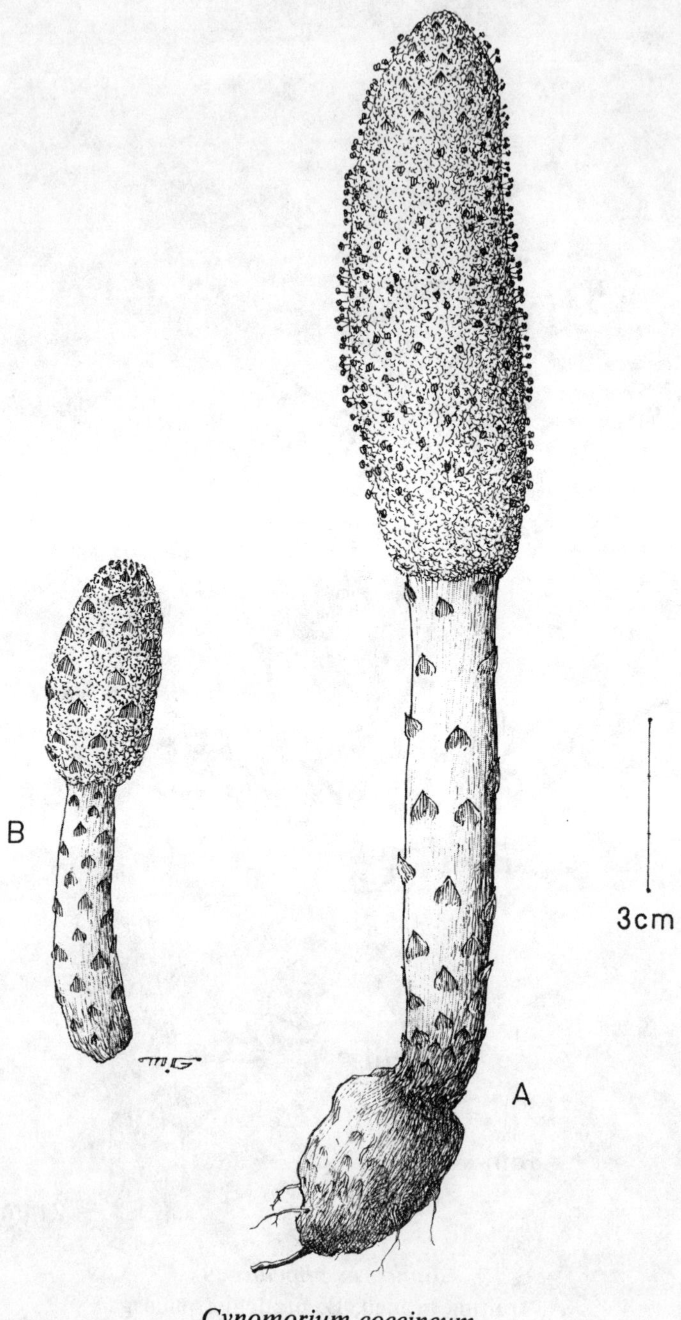

Cynomorium coccineum

qeloujla (62). English: Bottle gourd, Calabash cucumber (4). French: Calebasse (4, 42); Calebasse d'Europe, Bouteille, Congourde (4); Gourde (62).
Uses: Rind of mature fruit diuretic. Juice of the whitish-green fruit is much appreciated for its thirst-quenching qualities. Fresh peeled seeds mixed with honey is anthelmintic. *Ref:* 34, 42

***Luffa cylindrica** (L.) M. Roem. *Area:* Frequently cultivated in North Africa, especially in Egypt where it is mainly used as bath sponge.
Names: Arabic: Lufa (62); Luf (4). English: Egyptian towel gourd, Rag gourd, Vegetable sponge (4). French: Courge torchon (62); Torchon, Luffa d'Egypte, Eponge végétale (4).
Uses: Fruit fibres hemostatic and analgesic in enterorrhagia, dysentery, metrorrhagia, orchitis, hemorrhoids; also used to treat variola and boils. *Ref:* 34

Cupressaceae

Cupressus sempervirens L. *Area:* Libya, Tunisia, Morocco. Cultivated in Algeria and Egypt.
Names: Arabic: Sarw (4, 42, 62); Serwal (23, 42, 62); Shagaret el-hayat (4); Sa'ed, Bestana, Hayat (62). Berber: Tiddi (23, 42, 62); Arella (42). English: Cypress tree, Evergreen cypress (4). French: Cyprès (24, 37, 42, 62); Cyprès commun (4).
Uses: Cones astringent, sudorific, diuretic, slightly febrifuge, used against nocturnal incontinence of urine for children, sedative for cough, bronchital calmative, expectorant, bitter tonic, antidiarrhoeic, antihemorrhoid, antihemorrhagic.
Ref: 23, 24, 37, 42, 45

Juniperus communis L. *Area:* Algeria, Morocco.
Names: Arabic: Taga (13, 42); 'Ar'ar, Sarw gabali, Shizi (4). Berber: Tamerbout (13, 37, 42, 62); Tarka, Ir'en (62). English: Juniper tree (4). French: Genévrier (42, 45, 62); Genévrier commun (4, 37); Genièvre, Pétron (4).
Uses: Tar produced by distillation of dry wood used as antiseptic for skin diseases, for curing wounds and sores. Tincture of branches used as a rub for some skin conditions and to combat alopecia. Leaves abortive, used for hemorrhoids. Berries (small cones) used as condiment, diuretic, stomachic, tonic, carminative, rubefacient; infusion of berries disinfectant of urinary tracts. Use of the plant should be avoided by people with kidney inflammations. *Ref:* 13, 37, 42, 45, 56

Juniperus oxycedrus L. *Area:* Libya to Morocco.
Names: Arabic: Taga (37, 42, 47, 62); 'Ar'ar (4). Berber: Tamerbout (42, 62); Taka, Tagga, Teka, Tiqqi, Tirki (62). English: Prickly cedar, Sharp cedar (4). French: Cade (4, 62); Genévrier oxycèdre (4, 42); Oxycèdre (4, 24, 47); Cadier (37).
Uses: Tar produced by distillation of dry wood used as antiseptic for skin diseases, for curing wounds and sores, antiparasitic. Fruits diuretic, stimulant, vermifuge.
Ref: 24, 37, 42, 45

Juniperus phoenicea L. *Area:* Egypt to Morocco.
Names: Arabic: 'Ar'ar (6, 8, 16, 37, 62); Djineda (62). Berber: Zimeba, Aifz (62). English: Phoenician juniper (8); see note under French names. French: Genévrier rouge (62); Fausse sabine (16, 39). Mistakenly called Phoenician juniper or

Genévrier de Phénicie, as Linnaeus meant by "phoenicea" red, and not Phoenicia (62).
Uses: Hot infusion of leaves for children's diarrhoea and sedative for abdominal pains. Dry powdered leaves used to cure mild dermal inflammations, especially for babies, dialator for urinary tract, laxative, intestinal disinfectant (Algiers drug market). Leaves emmenagogue; help during childbirth by increasing the contractions of uterus, antidiarrhoeic. *Ref:* 8, 16, 37

Juniperus thurifera L. *Area:* Algeria, Morocco.
Names: Arabic: Sanina (42, 62). Berber: Aioual (42, 47, 62); Taoualt (42, 62); Adrouman (42); Adroumam, Takka, Tazenzena, Abaoual (62). French: Sabine à gros fruit (621); Sabine thurifère (42); Genévrier thurifère (47).
Uses: Decoction of leaves abortive, a dangerous product, used against hemorrhoids, emmenagogue, helps during childbirth by increasing contractions of the uterus. *Ref:* 37, 42

***Tetraclinis articulata** (Vahl) Masters *Area:* Tunisia to Morocco.
Names: Arabic: 'Ar'ar (42, 47, 62); Sandarus (4, 62); 'Ar'ar berboush (47); 'Ar'ar berhoush, 'Ar'ar el-ibel, Shagaret el-hayat (62). Berber: Irz, Irhkri, Tazout, Tarout, Tirarar, Tiranrat, Tifizza, Amelzi, Amkouk (62). English: Arar tree, Sandarach tree, Juniper-gum tree (4). French: Thuya (42, 62); Callitris (62); Thuia articulé, Thuia à la sandaraque, Vernix (4).
Uses: Tar produced from old or dead wood for dermal diseases, especially in veterinary medicine. Decoction of leaves abortive, dangerous to use; cataplasm of crushed leaves is locally applied against migraine, neck pains and insolation. *Ref:* 42

Cynomoriaceae

Cynomorium coccineum L. *Area:* Egypt to Morocco.
Names: Arabic: Zobb el-ard (4, 5, 42, 58, 62); Tartout (4, 5, 8, 42); Masrur (4); Mousowrar, Hawkal, Tartout el-beni-edem, Abushal, Zobb el-tourki, Zobb el-ghaba, Zobb el-qa'a (62); Mazrour, Marshoush (6). Berber: Afdad (42, 62); Tartous, Terzous (26). English: Maltese mushroom (4, 8); Scarlet synomorium (4). French: Champignon de Malte (4, 42, 62); Cynomoir écarlate (4).
Uses: Entire plant aphrodisiac, spermatopoietic, tonic, astringent. Dried plant powdered and mixed with butter used for bilary obstruction; powder added to meat dishes as a condiment. *Ref:* 5, 8, 34, 42, 62

Cyperaceae

Cyperus esculentus L. *Area:* Egypt to Morocco. Also cultivated in restricted areas in Egypt.
Names: Arabic: Habb el-'aziz (4, 58, 59, 62); Habb el-zalam (4, 5, 59, 62); Felfel es-sudan (5, 59); Soqqait barari, Soqqait (59). English: Earth almond, Edible cyperus, Rush-nut (4). French: Souchet comestible (4, 62); Almande de terre (4).
Uses: Tubers spermatogenic, aphrodisiac, galactogogue, pectoral, emollient, highly nutritious; fixed oil from tubers effective emollient for inflamed breasts of suckling

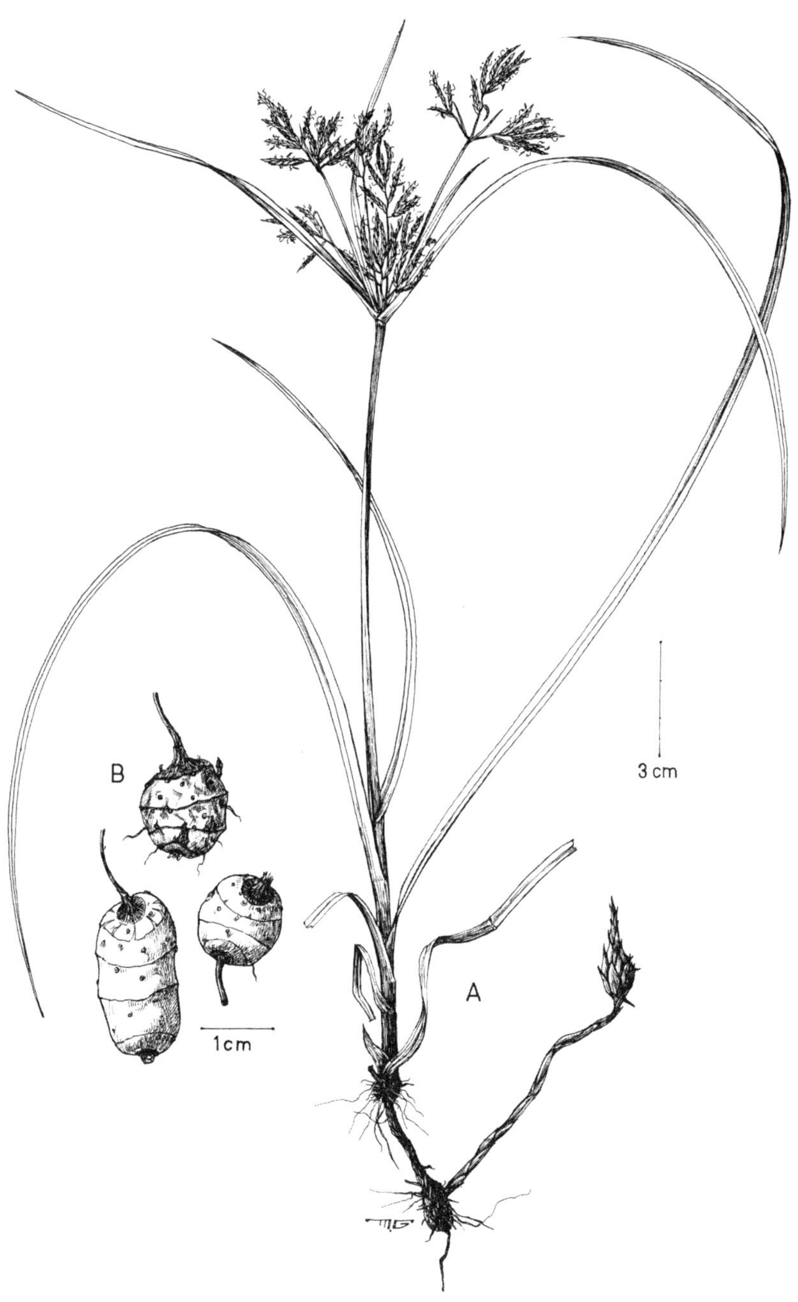

A. *Cyperus rotundus,* B. *Cyperus esculentus,* tubers

mothers; refreshing beverage prepared from crushed tubers soaked in water.

Ref: 5, 59

Cyperus papyrus L. *Area:* Cultivated in Egypt.
Names: Arabic: Bardi (4, 59); Qasab el-bardi (59). English: Papyrus, Nile papyrus, Paper reed (4). French: Papyrus, Jonc du Nil, Papier du Nil, Souchet à papier (4).
Uses: Ash of plant checks malignant ulcers from spreading in the mouth or elsewhere; if plant is macerated in vinegar and burnt, the ash heals wounds.

Ref: 59

Cyperus rotundus L. *Area:* Egypt to Morocco.
Names: Arabic: Sa'ad el-homar (4, 58, 59, 62); Saal (23, 42, 62); Sa'ad (42, 58, 59); Se'd (7); Zibl el-ma'iz (58, 59); Burbeit, Dis (59); Tara (42). Berber: Azdjmir (23, 62); Taselbou (62). English: Nut-grass (4). French: Souchet rond (4, 23, 42, 62).
Uses: Tubercles contain 0.5% of an essential oil used as aromatic stomachic in nervous gastralgia, dyspepsia, diarrhoea, emmenagogue, sedative, analgesic in dysmenorrhea, amenorrhea, chronic metritis, diuretic, carminative, stimulant, a colic remedy and to remove renal calculi, tonic, aphrodisiac, to increase the body weight, anthelmintic, analeptic, condiment, stomachic; in fresh state diaphoretic, astringent, for scorpion stings. Decoction of tubercles diaphoretic; infusion of tubers used for intestinal pains. *Ref:* 7, 17, 21, 23, 42, 59

Dioscoreaceae

Tamus communis L. *Area:* Libya to Morocco.
Names: Arabic: Ben memoun (13, 23, 62); Karma souda (4, 13, 62); Karm barri (4); Bou tania (13, 62). Berber: Fachirchin (23, 62); Tsminoun (13, 62). English: Black bryony, Ladies' seal, Mandrake (4). French: Taminier (23, 62); Bryone douce à fruit et racine noirs, Vigne noire, Racine vierge, Sceau de Notre Dame, Tamier (4).
Uses: All parts of plant purgative, diuretic, resolvent, emetic, rubefacient. Cataplasm of powdered root for contusions, rheumatism by rubbing. Red berries poisonous. *Ref:* 13, 23, 24, 45, 62

Ephedraceae

Ephedra alata Decne. *Area:* Egypt to Morocco.
Names: Arabic: 'Alenda (5, 8, 13, 23, 47, 62); 'Adam (61, 62); 'Alda, 'Alda el-gemal, 'Alda el-dabbaghin, Na'ad (61). Berber: Timaiart (13, 23, 62); Arzoum, Alelga (62). English: Ephedra (8). French: Alenda (62); Ephédra (23).
Uses: Plant depurative, for hypertension, antiasthmatic, sympathomimetic, astringent. Branches chewed for cephalalgia, cooked in butter and eaten by women for miscarriage, bronchodilator. *Ref:* 2, 5, 8, 23

Ericaceae

Arbutus pavari Pamp. *Area:* Endemic to Libya.
Names: Arabic: Shmary (9). English: Libyan strawberry tree (9).

Uses: Decoction of wood hypotensive (Shepherds, Gebel Akhdar, Libya). Fruit astringent.

Euphorbiaceae

Euphorbia balsamifera Ait. var. **sepium** N.E.Br. *Area:* Morocco.
Names: Arabic: 'Afernan, 'Agoua (62). Berber: Lfernan (5).
Uses: Latex of plant rather poisonous, enters into the composition of veterinary preparations for itch. *Ref:* 5

Euphorbia echinus Hook. fil. & Coss. *Area:* Endemic to Morocco.
Names: Arabic: Umm el-lbina (42); Daghmus, Zaqqum (5). Berber: Tikiut (5, 13, 42). French: Euphorbe cactoide (5).
Uses: Resinous latex of plant abortive, for gonorrhoea, purgative, cures warts and eczema, bites of poisonous animals. Diluted latex used as eye lotion, dangerous but much employed in ophthalmic treatments. Honey gathered by bees from the flowers has a very pungent taste, used as general tonic and calefacient. *Ref:* 5, 13, 42

Euphorbia falcata L. *Area:* Egypt to Morocco.
Names: Arabic: Hayat en-nefous (Rabat drug market).
Uses: Infusion mixed with milk recommended for colds and rheumatic pains (Rabat drug market).

Euphorbia granulata Forssk. *Area:* Egypt to Morocco.
Names: Arabic: Reda'a (62); Kbidet ed-dobb, Lembetha (5). Berber: Tellak (47, 62); Ttesses, Tehihans (62).
Uses: Latex locally applied against poisonous bites. *Ref:* 5

Euphorbia helioscopia L. *Area:* Egypt to Morocco.
Names: Arabic: Halib ed-diba (13, 23, 62); Sa'ada (4, 58); Rummadah (4). Berber: Ahon-n-igoura (13, 23, 62); Tafouri, Tanahout (13, 62); Kerbaboush (13). English: Water grass, Sun spurge, Wartwort, Cat's milk (4). French: Réveille-matin (4, 23, 62); Euphorbe hélioscope, Herbe aux verrues (4).
Uses: Latex laxative, purgative, vesicatory or causes formation of blisters on the skin. *Ref:* 23, 37

Euphorbia lathyrus L. *Area:* Morocco.
Names: Arabic: Habbet el-muluk (4, 13, 42); Tartaqah (4). English: Caper-spurge (4, 24); Myrtle spurge (4). French: Catapuce, Epurge, Catherinette (4); Euphorbe épurge (24, 42).
Uses: Seed oil purgative. *Ref:* 24, 42

Euphorbia peplis L. *Area:* Egypt to Morocco.
Names: Arabic: Kharrara, Halbita, Tsaboun ghett (62). French: Euphorbe peplis (24).
Uses: Latex diuretic, depurative, for asthma attacks, liver disorders, purgative, emetic, expectorant, for hydropsy, gout, chest diseases. *Ref:* 24, 56

Euphorbia resinifera Berg. *Area:* Endemic to Morocco.
Names: Arabic: Lubanah maghrabi (4, 42, 62); Ferbyoun, Zeggoum (26, 42, 62);

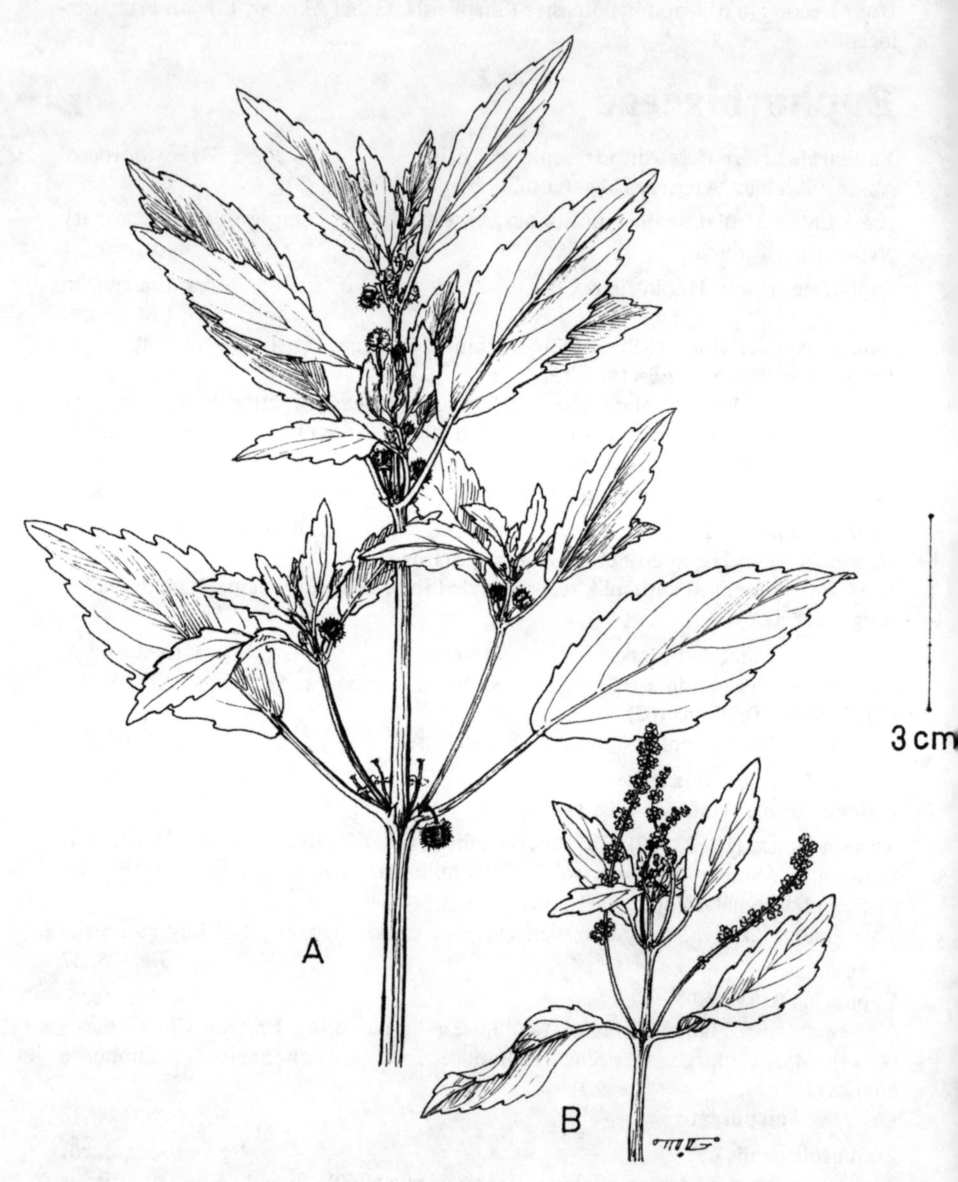

Mercurialis annua
A. branch of a female plant
B. branch of a male plant

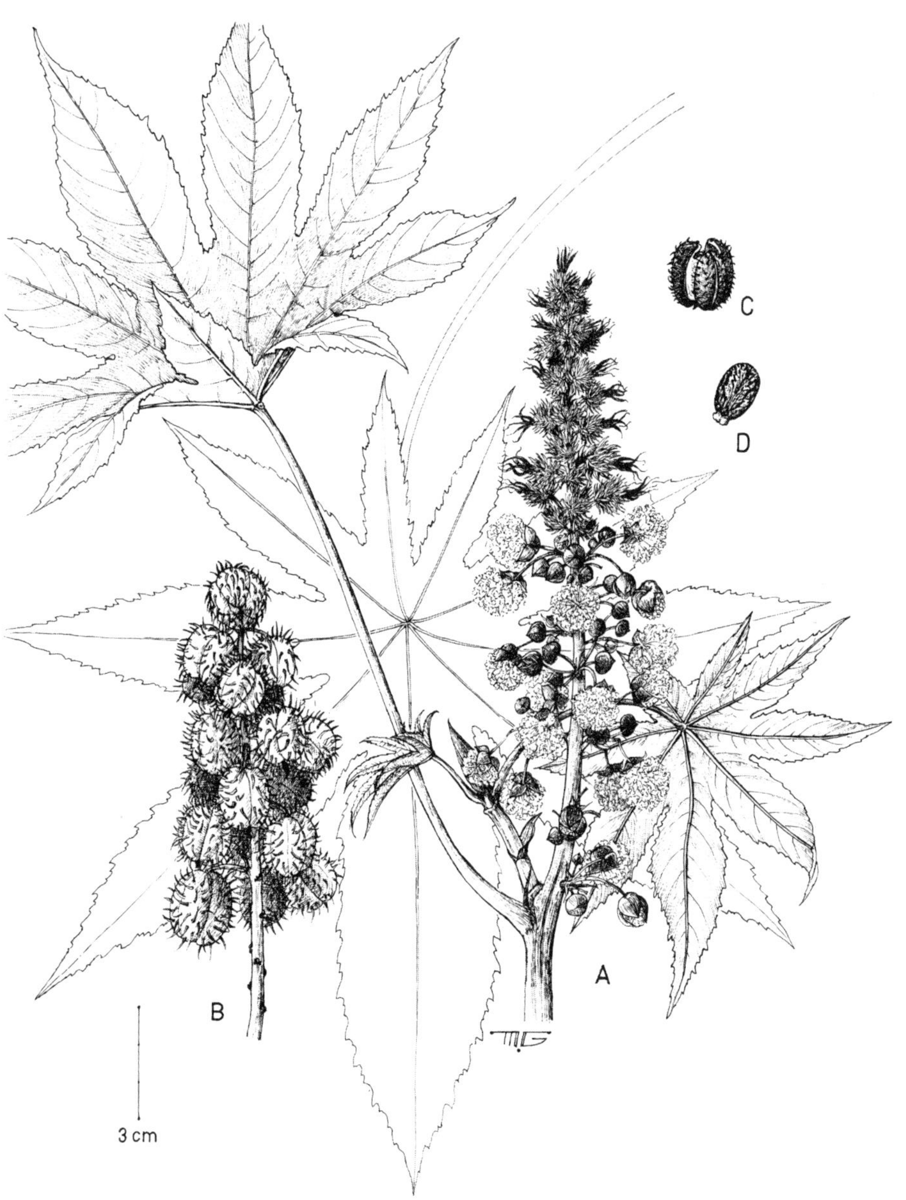

Ricinus communis
A. flowering branch with female flowers on top of male flowers
B. inflorescence with immature fruits
C. mature fruit, D. seed

Shawla beyda (4). Berber: Tikiout (26, 42, 62); Takout, Dermous (42, 62); Takert, Lagmez, Tanahot, Tanar'ant (62). English: Euphorbium gum-plant (4). French: Euphorbe résinifère (42); Euphorbe, Euphorbium (4).
Uses: Resinous latex revulsive, used against snake bites, dental pains, rheumatism, for alopecia, emetic, cathartic, mostly in veterinary medicine, violent purgative. Latex mixed with honey and titurated is used for the preparation of a decongestive eye lotion. *Ref:* 2, 42, 45, 62

Mercurialis annua L. *Area:* Egypt to Morocco.
Names: Arabic: Mourkeba (13, 23, 62); Halbub (4, 5, 13, 58); Khussa hermes (4, 62); Hashish el-line, Malfouf el-kelb, Bou zenzir, Zandjir, Habb geuzzoula, Laktounia, Hariq amless (13, 62). Berber: Touchanine (13, 23, 62). English: French mercury, Annual mercury (4). French: Mércuriale annuelle (5, 13, 23, 45, 62); Foirole (4, 23); Ortie bâtarde, Ramberge (4).
Uses: Tincture of plant recommended for rheumatism and gastric disorders. Fresh plant sometimes used as a laxative, purgative, diuretic. *Ref:* 13, 23, 45, 56

Ricinus communis L. *Area:* Egypt to Morocco. Cultivated and often naturalized. Spontaneous in southeastern Egypt and southern Hoggar.
Names: Arabic: Kherwa' (4, 5, 13, 23, 42, 62); Awrioun (5, 13, 42, 62); Shemouga (13, 62). Berber: Akhilwane (13, 23, 62); Krank (5, 13, 62); Ourioura (13, 42); Feni, Lirraiq (13). English: Castor oil plant (1, 4); Palma Christi (4). French: Ricin (4, 5, 23, 42, 62); Palma Christi (4, 23).
Uses: Root bark purgative. Root decoction for rheumatism, inflammatory affections, chronic enlargements, skin disease, abdominal pains, diarrhoea, nervous disorders, toothache, lumbago, sciatica, jaundice, kidney and bladder trouble. Leaves rubbed on joints relieve pain; emmenagogue; decoction purgative, has useful action on liver and kidneys, heated on head for feverish headache, on breast stop milk secretion, on abdomen promote menstrual flow, emetic in poisoning. Cataplasm of leaves for carbuncles, wounds, lacteral tumors, indurations of mammary gland, swellings, eye lotion, stomach ache, rheumatism, lumbago, sciatica; cataplasm of fresh leaves cures boils (Farmers, Egypt); infusion for itch. Powdered seeds toxic, applied externally to abscesses, carbuncles, prescribed in small doses for persistent constipation, used to treat buccal and pharyngeal inflammations, gastrointestinal hemorrhages, headaches, dizziness, stupor, hypothermy; the pollen is very allergic. Dried flowers mixed with honey antidiarrhoeic. Seed oil purgative, used against paralysis of arms and legs by rubbing. Seed oil for rheumatic pains by rubbing, emetic, colic, emollient, for tumor, boils, worms, headache, ophthalmia, wounds, rash, epilepsy, stomachache, itch, lumbago, jaundice, rheumatism, fever, diarrhoea, toothache, kidney and bladder trouble, asthma, cancer, leprosy, venereal and skin diseases. Seeds for scorpion sting, cathartic, emollient, fever, inflammatory affections, destroys mosquitos, parasitic skin diseases, leprosy, cancer.
Ref: 1, 2, 5, 7, 13, 34, 42, 45

Fagaceae

Quercus coccifera L. *Area:* Libya to Morocco.
Names: Arabic: Kerroush el-qermez (23, 62); Keshrt (37, 62); Ballout el-hallouf,

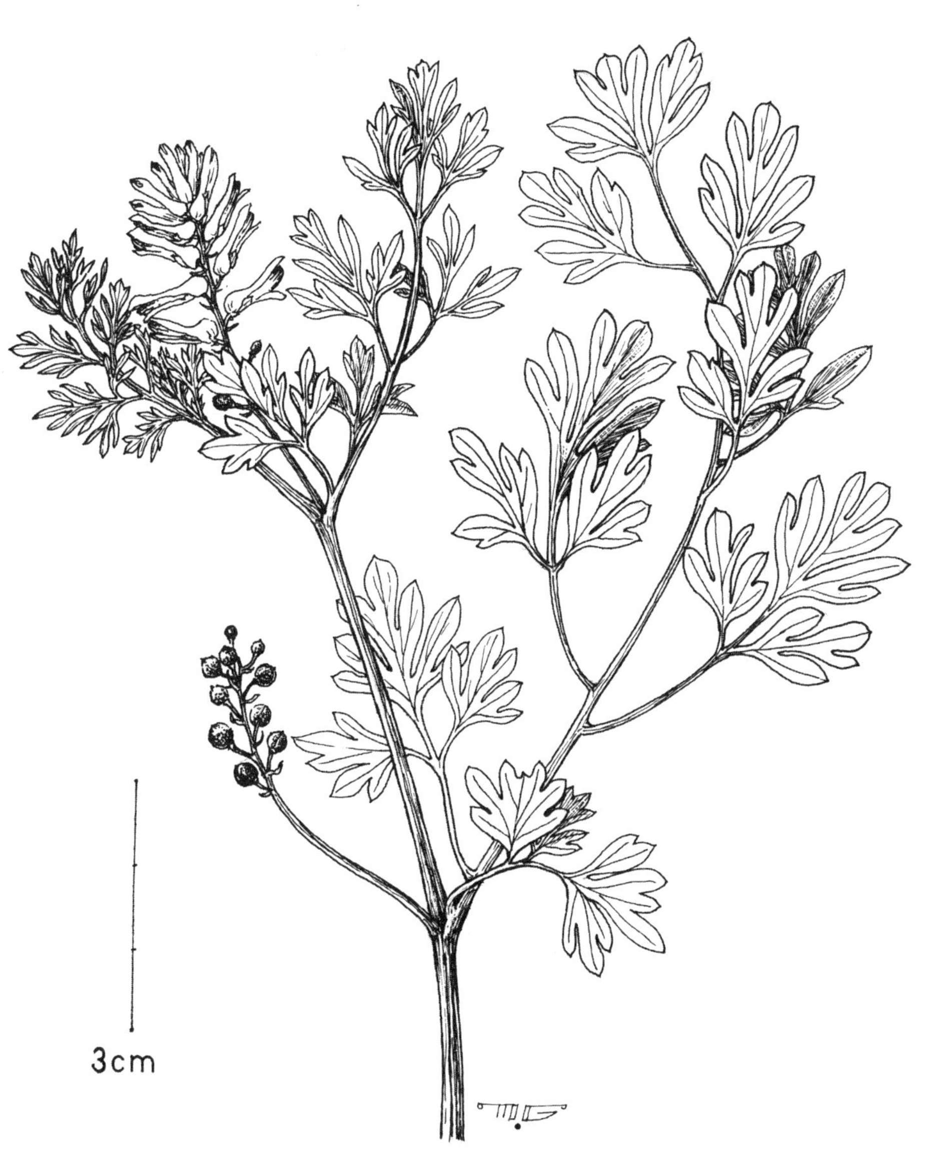

Fumaria judaica

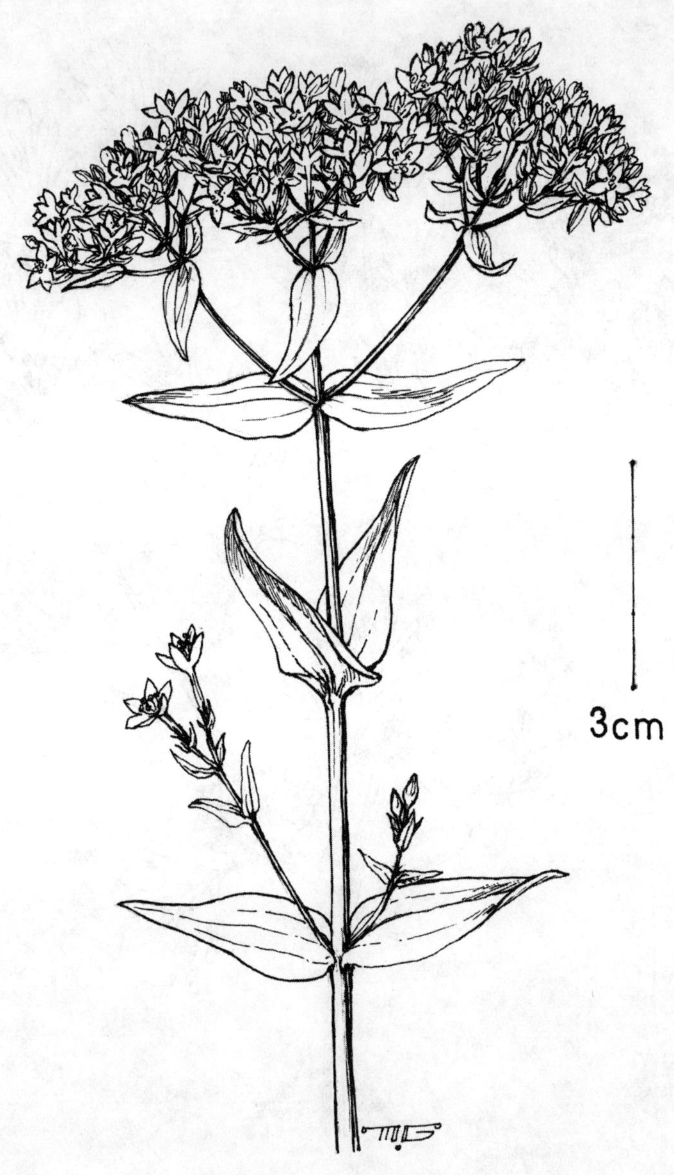

Centaurium erythraea

Kerkhash (62); Gidar (4). Berber: Tabellout igilef (23, 62). English: Kermes oak (4, 24); Scarlet oak (4). French: Chêne kermès (4, 13, 23, 37, 62); Chêne garouille (4, 62); Chêne cocciné (4).
Uses: Insect galls astringent; powdered galls mixed with honey used for treating wounds and sores. *Ref:* 23, 37, 42

Fumariaceae

Fumaria judaica Boiss. *Area:* Egypt, Libya.
Names: Arabic: Shahtarag (52).
Uses: The entire plant used for jaundice, hepatic fever, spleen obstructions; externally for scabies and dermatitis. *Ref:*52

Fumaria officinalis L. *Area:* Libya to Morocco.
Names: Arabic: Guessis (23, 62); Shahtredj (62); Satarag, Kusfarat el-himar (4). Berber: Tir'ad guisri (23, 62). English: Fumitory, Fumitere (4). French: Fumeterre (23, 45, 62); Fumeterre officinale (4, 23, 24).
Uses: Flowering branches used to cure eczema, dermatitis and exanthema, stomachic, laxative, diuretic, antiscrofulous, depurative, sedative, calmative, chologogue. *Ref:* 23, 24, 45, 56

Fumaria parviflora Lam. *Area:* Egypt to Morocco.
Names: Arabic: Hashishet as-sebyan (5, 62); Buqul as-sabiya (5, 42); Shatreg (58). Berber: Tijujar (62); Ijujer (5). French: Femeterre (5, 62).
Uses: Entire plant astringent, antipruriginous, sedative; infusion recommended to children to keep their vitality, depurative, laxative, diuretic. *Ref:* 5, 42

Gentianaceae

Centaurium erythraea Rafn *Area:* Libya to Morocco.
Names: Arabic: Qantarioun (23, 62); Murraret el-hanash (4, 23, 62, Algiers drug market); Goustt el-hayya (23, 42, 62, Rabat drug market); Hassak (42); Qantarioun saghir (4). Berber: Qelilou (23, 37, 62); Tikoukt, Tiouinet (23, 62). English: Centaury, Earth-gall, Feverwort (4). French: Petite centaurée (4, 23, 42, 62); Gentaine centaurée, Herbe au centaure (23); Erythrée centaurée (4, 37); Herbe à la fièvre (4).
Uses: Flowering and fruiting plants bitter tonic; infusion febrifuge, for anemia, gastralgia, depurative, for intermittent fevers, bilary stones, gastric troubles; decoction useful for diabetes (Rabat and Algiers drug markets); infusion for headache and fever (Algiers drug market). *Ref:*23, 37, 42

Centaurium spicatum (L.) Fritsch *Area:* Egypt to Morocco.
Names: Arabic: Hashishet el-'aqrab (4, 58); Qantarioun (35); Menash ed-dibban, Nashash ed-dibban, Qotaiba (58); Boubezzit, Ayate (62); Qushet el-hayya (5). French: Petite centaurée (5).
Uses: Flowering and fruiting plants used for hypertension, elimination of ureter and kidney stones, healing agent for wounds, enters in the ointments used for sciatica; infusion useful for diabetes (Cairo drug market). *Ref:* 5, 35

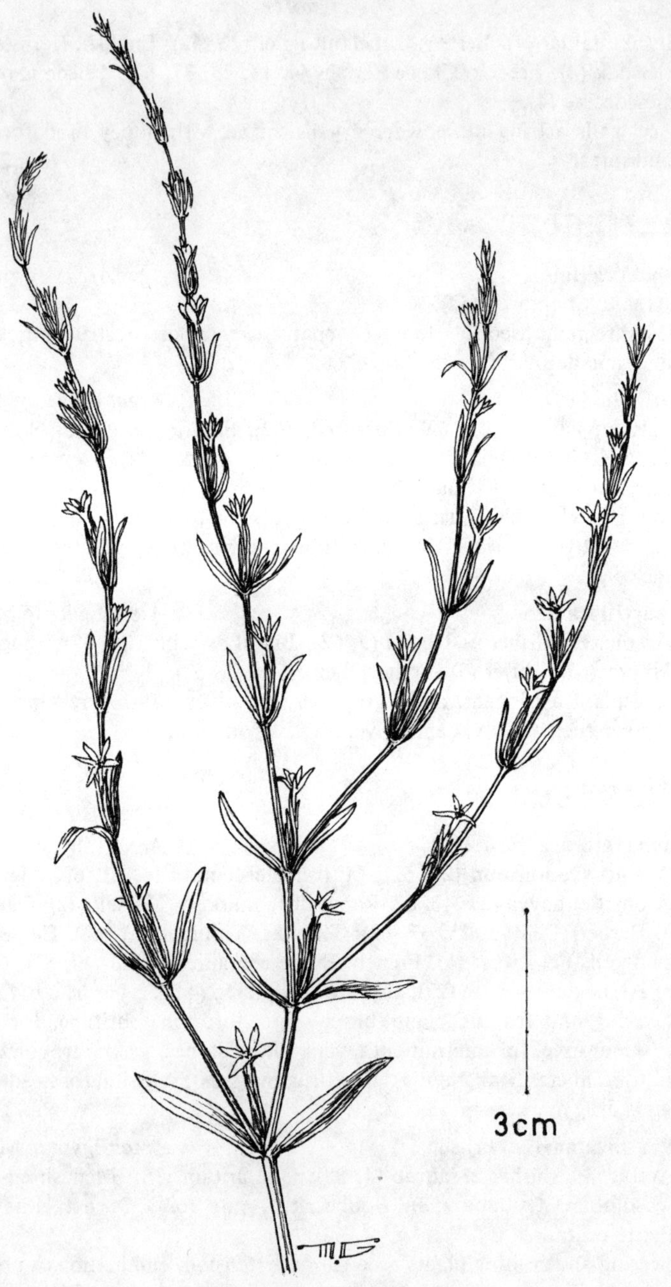

Centaurium spicatum

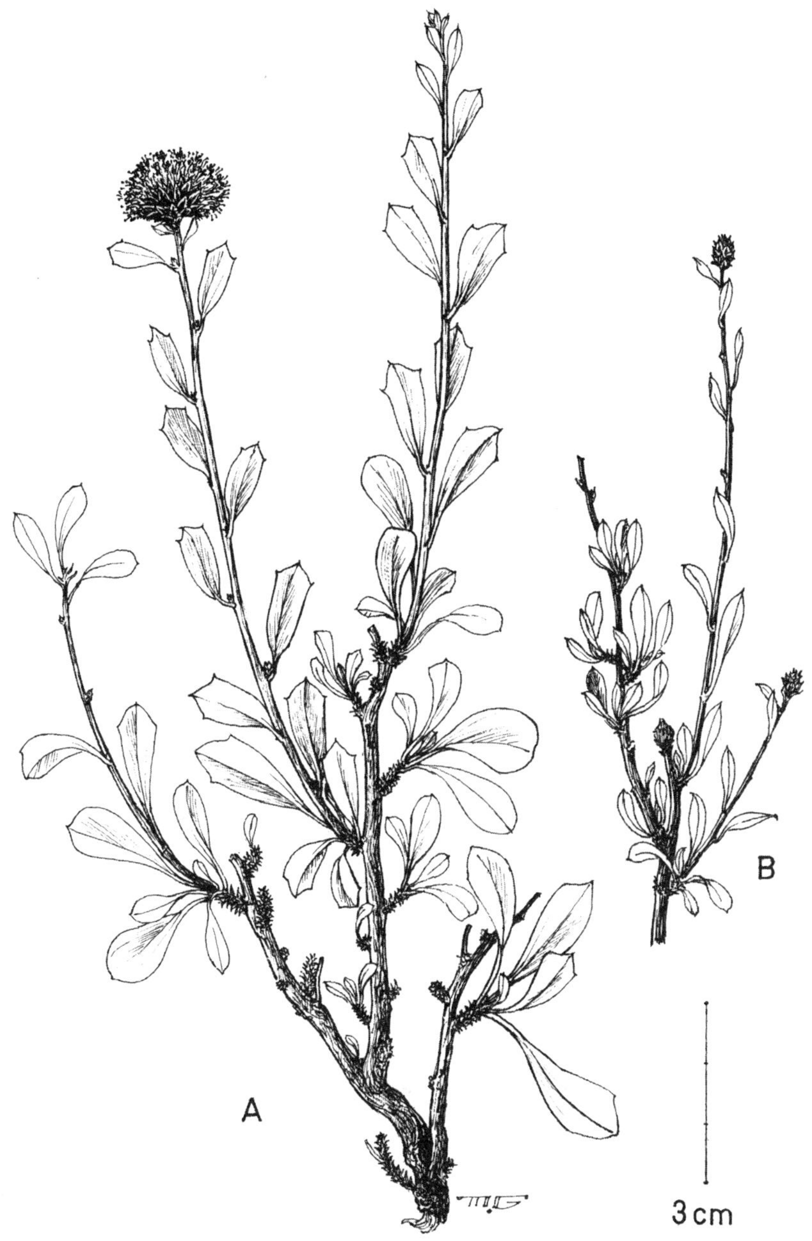

Globularia alypum
A. large-leaved form
B. small-leaved form

Geraniaceae

Erodium cicutarium (L.) L'Hérit. *Area:* Egypt to Morocco.
Names: Arabic: Regma (23, 62); Ghazil, Ibret el-'agouz (4); Mouchita (37). Berber: Tisermt ouakal (23, 62); Tisernas, Hammar tardjilel, Haroud tardjilel (62). English: Common stork's-bill, Hemlock geranium, Pick-needle, Pin-grass, Alfilaria (4). French: Erode, Erodion cicutin, Aiguille, Bec de cigogne, Bec de héron (4); Bec de grue (37).
Uses: Flowering branches hemostatic, healing agent for wounds, astringent, antidiarrhoeic, helps during childbirth by increasing contractions of the uterus.
*Ref:*23, 37, 45

Geranium robertianum L. *Area:* Libya to Morocco.
Names: Arabic: Requemaya, Talah, Djarna (23, 62); 'Etr, Ibret er-raheb (4). English: Adder's tongue, Herb Robert, Fox geranium (4). French: Herbe à Robert (4, 23, 62); Geranion (42); Aiguille (4).
Uses: Plant astringent, tonic, diuretic, antidiabetic, antihemorrhagic. Externally the plant provides a gargle effective against throat troubles, stomatitis, glossitis, tonsillitis, antidiarrhoeic, vulnerary. *Ref:* 23, 24, 45

Globulariaceae

Globularia alypum L. *Area:*Libya to Morocco.
Names: Arabic: Shelgha, Zerga, Zoweitna, 'Alk (13, 23, 62); Zerreiga (8, 62); 'Aynun (4, 5); Turbad (42); Senna beldi (5); Ghislah, Kahla (4); Zriga (38). Berber: Taselgha (5, 13, 23, 42, 62); Haselra (13, 23, 62); Oualbarda (13, 62). English: Alypo globe daisy, Globularia (4, 8). French: Globulaire (4, 23, 38); Globulaire turbith (5, 23, 42); Turbith blanc (5); Alype Séné sauvage, Herbe terrible, Turbith (4).
Uses: Decoction of branches boiled with dried figs or with jujube *(Ziziphus zizyphus)* fruits and sugar added, used as depurative, mild laxative, diuretic; weak decoction for urinary incontinence. Concentrated decoction of young branches and leaves used to cure boils and intermittent fever, decoction for ulcers. Decoction of leaves useful for rheumatism and arthritis, depurative, aphrodisiac. Leaves excellent purgative; infusion used as a substitute for senna. *Ref:* 5, 8, 12, 23, 38, 42, 50

Gramineae

Avena sativa L. *Area:* Egypt to Morocco. Cultivated or naturalized.
Names: Arabic: Hartaman, Shufan, Ziwan, Zummeir (4); Khortan (62). Berber: Taskrunt, Tamenzirt, Azekkoun (62). English: Oats (4). French: Avoine (4, 13, 45).
Uses: Tincture of fresh flowering plant used in treatment of arthritis, rheumatism, paralysis, liver infections, skin diseases. Plant tonic, diuretic, laxative, calmative, vulnerary. *Ref:*13, 56

***Cymbopogon proximus** (Hochst. ex A. Rich.) Stapf *Area:* Egypt, Libya, Algeria.
Names: Arabic: Half barr (58); Adkhar, Azkhar (8). English: Camel's hay (8).
Uses: Dried tufts of plant burnt and fumes inhaled against influenza and some

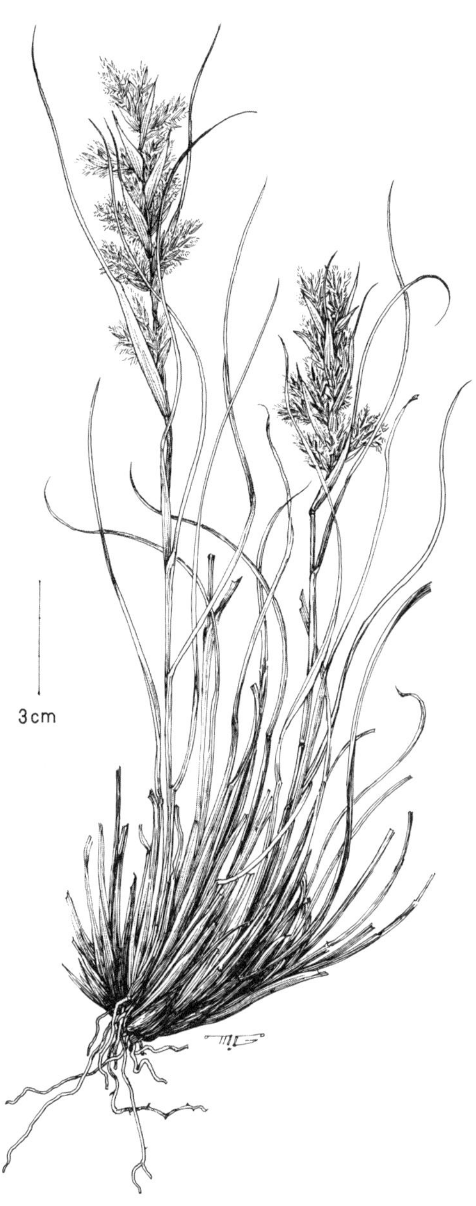

Cymbopogon proximus

neurotic diseases, or tufts soaked in water for one week and the cold infusion is drunk. Decoction of the lower part of the plant (without the flowers) for colic and fever; decoction of a mixture of the plant and *Ambrosia maritima* used for diabetes. Infusion of leaves diuretic, stomachic, lower the blood pressure (Cairo drug market).
Ref: 8, 61

***Cymbopogon schoenanthus** (L.) Spreng. *Area:* Egypt to Morocco.
Names: Arabic: Lemmad (23, 42, 47, 62); Hashma (58); Idkhir (4, 5, 61, 62); Mahareb (61, 62); Tibn Makkah (4, 5, 61); Halfet Makkah (5, 61); Sha'ret et-trab (5). Berber: Tiberrimt (16, 23, 62). English: Camel's hay, Scenanth, Geranium grass (4). French: Schoenanthe (4, 5); Scoenanthe officinal (23); Jonc aromatique (4, 23); Citronnelle, Jonc odorant, Paille de la Mecque (4).
Uses: Infusion of plant diuretic, emmenagogue, astringent, carminative, sudorific, antirheumatic; cataplasm for wounds of camels. Infusion of flowers febrifuge.
Ref: 5, 16, 42, 61

Cynodon dactylon (L.) Pers. *Area:* Egypt to Morocco.
Names: Arabic: Endjil (5, 23, 62); Nigil (4, 58, 61); Moddad (58); Nedjem (5, 61, 62); Rjel leghrab, Kar'a leghrab (5); Ndjil, Nadjir, Zabak, Kezmir, Tsil, Raifa, 'Akresh (62). Berber: Tizmit (23, 62); Affer, Agesmir (5); Tagamait, Imelzi, Haffar, Toungane, Agouzinir, Aoukeraz, Almès (62). English: Bermuda grass, Dog's-tooth-grass, Scutch-grass (4). French: Gros chiendent (4, 5, 23, 45, 62); Herbe du Bermudes (4); Chiendent pied de poule (4, 23); Chiendent d'Italie (23); Dactyle (5).
Uses: Decoction of rhizomes for renal and urinary troubles, depurative, emmenagogue, diuretic, refreshing agent, sudorific, emollient, for cough; used for supression of urine and vesical calculus, for purifying the blood, disinfectant, vulnerary. *Ref:* 5, 23, 24, 57, 61

Eleusine indica (L.) Gaertner *Area:* Egypt, Libya. Naturalized.
Names: Arabic: Negil (61). English: Wire-grass, Goose-grass (61).
Uses: Grass is used to strap broken limbs. Infusion eases vaginal bleeding. *Ref:* 31

***Elymus repens** (L.) Gould *Area:* Libya to Morocco.
Names: Arabic: Khafour (23, 62); Najem (4, 42, 62); Nedjil (4, 62); Thil (4); Seboulet el-far, Guzmir (62). Berber: Affar (23, 62). English: Couch grass, Quitch grass, Twitch grass (4). French: Chiendent (4, 42); Petit chiendent (23, 24); Racine de chiendent, Chiendent commun (23); Chiendent rampant (4).
Uses: Rhizome diuretic, refreshing agent, sudorific, depurative, emollient.
Ref: 23, 24, 42

Imperata cylindrica (L.) Beauv. *Area:*Egypt to Morocco.
Names: Arabic: Halfa (11, 58, 61); Deil el-qott, Silla (58, 61); Bodweya, Helein (58); Heish (61); Bou dweys (58, 61, 62); Deis, Silt, Sebet, Berdi, Halfa mt'a Kufra (62). Berber: Taicest (62); Uhri (11). English: Sharp grass (61).
Uses: Rhizome antipyretic, diuretic, hemostatic. Young shoots diuretic. Flowers used in hemoptysis and epistaxis of pulmonary diseases. *Ref:* 34

Lolium perenne L. *Area:* Egypt to Morocco.
Names: Arabic: Gazoun, Hashish el-faras (58, 61); Sammah (4, 61); Nusay (4); Zuwan, Qallab, Djelif (62). English: Ray-grass, Rye-grass, Red darnel, Lawn-grass (4). French: Ivraie vivace, Gazon anglais (4).

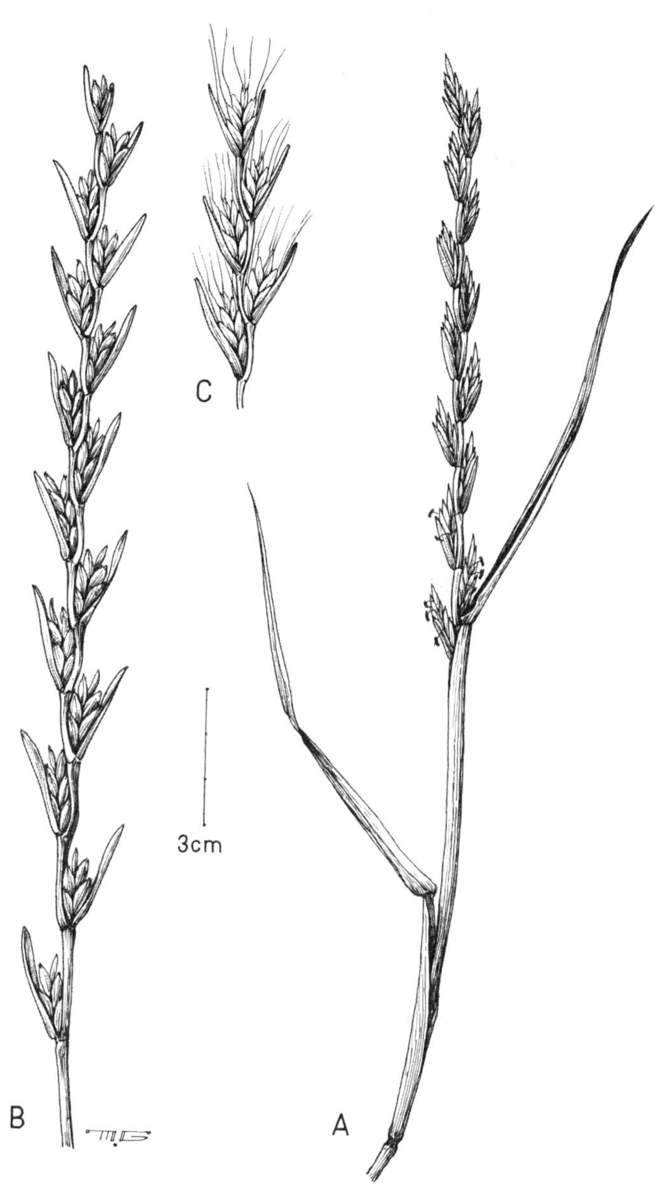

A. *Lolium perenne*
B. *Lolium temulentum* var. *leptochaeton*
C. *Lolium temulentum* var. *macrochaeton*

Uses: Plant contains several alkaloids, mainly perlolidine and perloline; perloline is sometimes suggested as a treatment for rheumatism. Infusion of plant drunk with an astringent wine for stopping diarrhoea and hemorrhage. *Ref:* 56, 61

Lolium temulentum L. *Area:* Egypt; Tunisia to Morocco.
Names: Arabic: Zuwan (4, 42, 61, 62); Shaylam (4, 62); Suwal, Sikra (42, 62); Danaqah (4); Samma (61). Berber: Laichour, Aqoullab (62). English: Darnel (4, 61); Ryegrass, Cheat, Ivary (4). French: Ivraie (4, 62); Zizanie, Lolium (4).
Uses: Decoction of entire plant prescribed for hemorrhage and incontinence of urine. Mature grains used to prepare a tincture in homeopathy to treat neuralgia, rheumatism and arthritis, nausea, nose bleeds, intestinal cramps and trembling limbs. *Ref:* 42, 56

Panicum turgidum Forssk. *Area:* Egypt to Morocco.
Names: Arabic: Bou rekba (5, 58, 61, 62); Tammam (5, 11, 58, 61); Umm Rekba (5, 62); Bokkar, Shush (58, 61, 62); Sabat, Dorran (58, 61); Hade, Safar (61). Berber: Goumshi (62); Goushi (11); grains: Afezou (62).
Uses: Plant used as a vulnerary agent and for removing white spots on the eye. *Ref:* 5, 61

***Phragmites australis** (Cav.) Trin. ex Steud. *Area:* Egypt to Morocco.
Names: Arabic: Qasba (4, 58, 61, 62); Bous, Ghab (4, 58, 61); Tra'a (62); Hagna, Heish moddeid (58, 61). Berber: Tiouli, Ilili, Tiranimine, Tagasiba, Djaboub, Tissendjelt, Aranim (62). English: Common reed (4, 61); Ditch reed (4). French: Roseau de maris (62); Roseau, Roseau commun, Roseau balais (4).
Uses: Rhizome stomachic, antiemetic, antipyretic, for acute arthritis, jaundice, pulmonary abscesses, food poisoning, diaphoretic, diuretic. *Ref:* 34, 61

***Stipagrostis pungens** (Desf.) de Winter *Area:* Egypt to Morocco.
Names: Arabic: Hasaknit (58, 62); Sbott, Drinn (5, 16, 62); Shouk el-ghazal (58); grains: Rechig, Loul (62). Berber: Sabat, Sebbit, Ibitt, Mioukou, Tarhi, Toulloult, Talout (62).
Uses: The strong, cylindrical, hollow culms are often used to probe wounds; used for rheumatic pains. *Ref:* 5, 16

Zea mays L. *Area:* Commonly cultivated in North Africa.
Names: Arabic: Dra (5, 23, 62); Dura shamiyah (4, 5, 61); Dra shami, Djabbar, Mstoura, Beshna, Qttania, Umm ghfara, Gafouli masri, Hdawa, Turkia, Hortania safra, Roum (62); the cob: Qwaleh, Qawleh (61); Draia, Qbala (62); the silky styles: Shurrabet el-dura (61); Hariret el-shami, Sha'ar el-dra (Rabat drug market); male panicles: Shawashi el-dura, Kaddab el-durra, Taratir el-dura (61). Berber: Assengar (5, 23, 62). English: Maize, Indian corn (4, 61); Turkey wheat (4). French: Maîs (4, 5, 23, 24, 62); Blé de Turquie (4, 24).
Uses: Infusion or decoction of styles very diuretic, calmative, frequently prescribed for urinary system diseases, particularly cystitis. Infusion of styles mixed with barley grains and dried flowers of *Opuntia ficus-indica* is taken for cases of retention of urine (Rabat drug market). *Ref:* 5, 23, 24, 45, 61

Guttiferae

Hypericum perforatum L. *Area:* Tunisia to Morocco.

Names: Arabic: Mesmoum (13, 23, 62); Hashishat el-jourh, Kheshkhash aswad (13, 42); Berslouna, Bersemoun (13, 62); Dadhi, Dadhi rumi, Hashishet el-qalb (4). English: Perfoliate St. John's wort (4). French: Millepertuis (4, 13, 23, 42, 62); Chasse diable, Herbe de Saint Jean, Herbe aux piqûres (4).
Uses: Flowering summits astringent, aromatic; infusion stimulant, digestive, chologogue, diuretic, anticatarrhal, emmenagogue, vermifuge, astringent, vulnerary, antiseptic. *Ref:* 13, 23, 24, 45

Iridaceae

Crocus sativus L. *Area:* Drug imported. Plant cultivated in a few restricted areas in North Africa.
Names: Arabic: Za'faran (4, 5, 23, 42, 60, 62); Kruku (4); Asfar (42). Berber: Kouzrkoum (23). English: Saffron, Crocus (4). French: Safran (4, 23, 42, 45, 62); Safran vrai (5); Safran cultivé (4).
Uses: Stigmas of the flower are the drug, used as condiment, stimulant, emmenagogue, tonic, aphrodisiac. Eight to ten filaments of the drug per one cup of tea used as a narcotic for cases of asthma, whooping-cough, hysteria. *Ref:* 5, 23, 42, 45

Iris foetidissima L. *Area:* Tunisia to Morocco.
Names: Arabic: Sif el-dib, Khenounat el-wsif (13, 23, 62); Qasuris (4). English: Gladdon, Roast-beef plant, Gladwin, Stinking iris (4). French: Iris fétide (4, 23, 24, 50); Xyris puant, Iris gigot (4, 24).
Uses: Rhizome and grains diuretic; rhizome appetizer, purgative, mild sedative, antispasmodic, for hydropsy. *Ref:* 13, 23, 24, 50

Iris germanica L. *Area:* Cultivated in North Africa. Subspontaneous in Morocco.
Names: Arabic: Sawsan azraq (5, 13, 23, 24, 62); Sisana (13, 23, 62); Zanbaq azraq, Kaff es-sabbagh (4); Sekkin ed-dib, Sif ed-dib (5); Benefsig (62); rhizome: 'Ambar ed-dor (62); 'Anbar (5, 13, 42, 60); 'Oud al-'anbar (5, 60); Irisa (4, 13, 62). Berber: Tafrut (5, 42). English: German iris (4, 60); Flowering flag (4). French: Flambe (23, 62); Iris commun, Grand iris (23); Lis bleu, Lis sauvage, Iris germanique (4).
Uses: Rhizome purgative, diuretic, used in perfumery. Decoction of rhizomes used by rubbing for rheumatism, dorsal pains and sciatica, orally taken as one of the most frequently used antidotes; women use it mixed with food to increase their girth. Aromatic rhizome used in composition of cosmetic powders and make-ups; rhizomes should be kept for several months before use as they acquire their smell by storage. Infusion of rhizome used for swelling of spleen and liver, colds and bronchitis, expectorant in weak doses, drastic purgative and emetocathartic in strong doses. *Ref:* 5, 13, 23, 42, 45, 50, 60

Iris pseudacorus L. *Area:* Algeria, Morocco.
Names: Arabic: Sawsan asfar (13, 23, 42, 62); Burbit, Siyaf (4). English: Yellow iris, Yellow water flag, Jacob's sword (4). French: Iris jaune, Iris des marais, Glaieul des marais (4, 23); Iris faux acore, Flambe d'eau, Flambe bâtarde (4); Flambe des marais (23).

Uses: Decoction of fragmented rhizomes boiled for several hours in water, used by rubbing for rheumatic pains, particularly sciatica. Pulverized rhizomes constitute one of the most general anti-poisons reputed in Morocco, also used as diuretic and purgative by mixing it with vinegar. Most currently used for its analeptic power. Minced rhizomes mixed with "couscous," a popular dish in North Africa, to serve as condiment and to increase the girth of women. Infusion of powdered rhizomes used against fall in the body temperature and hepatic ailments. *Ref:* 42

Juglandaceae

Juglans regia L. *Area:* Cultivated in some mountainous regions of North Africa. Fruits and bark exported from Morocco.
Names: Arabic: Djouz (4, 5, 23, 26, 62, Algiers drug market); Gerga' (5); root bark: Sowak (62). Berber: Tadjoudjte (23, 62); Tsouik (62). English: Walnut (4). French: Noyer (4, 5, 26, 45); Noyer commun (23).
Uses: Bark used for cleansing and whitening the teeth, to redden the lips and gums, to combat bad breath, gingivitis and pyorrhea. Infusion of leaves tonic, antidiabetic, astringent, antiscrofulous. Decoction of leaves used as hair shampoo against fall of hair (Algiers drug market). Fruits nourishing, provide high energy, aphrodisiac, antipoison. Fumes from burnt nut shells inhaled for influenza and coryza.
Ref: 5, 23, 42, 45

Juncaceae

Juncus acutus L. *Area:* Egypt to Morocco.
Names: Arabic: Samar (4, 59, 62); Asal (4, 58); Samar murr (58); Samar baladi, Kasba (59). Berber: Azeli, Sellbou (62). English: Sharp rush, Dutch rush (4). French: Jonc aigu, Jonc piquant (4).
Uses: Infusion of fruits mixed with barley grains useful for colds (Rabat drug market).

Juncus maritimus Lam. *Area:* Egypt to Morocco.
Names: Arabic: Samar (5, 62); Asal (5). Berber: Azemai (5,62); Taleggit, Tazmait, Arami (62). English: Sea rush (59). French: Jonc (5).
Uses: Rhizome recommended for insomnia. *Ref:* 5

Labiatae

Ajuga iva (L.) Schreber *Area:* Egypt to Morocco.
Names: Arabic: Shandgoura (5, 8, 37, 42, 62, Rabat drug market); Ga'ada (4, 58); Meskeh, Miseyka, Samseyk (58). Berber: Tuftolba (5, 42, 62). English: Herb ivy (4, 8); Musky bugle (4). French: Ivette musquée (4, 37, 42); Bugle (5).
Uses: Cold infusion of the herb antihelmintic, depurative, especially in spring time. Dried green plants powdered and taken aganist sinusitis and cephalalgia; this powder made into small balls is digested for its useful action against stomach and intestinal pains, the digestive tract and enteritis; considered a general preventive for all diseases and therefore added to the dough of "kesra," a local bread in Morocco. Powdered

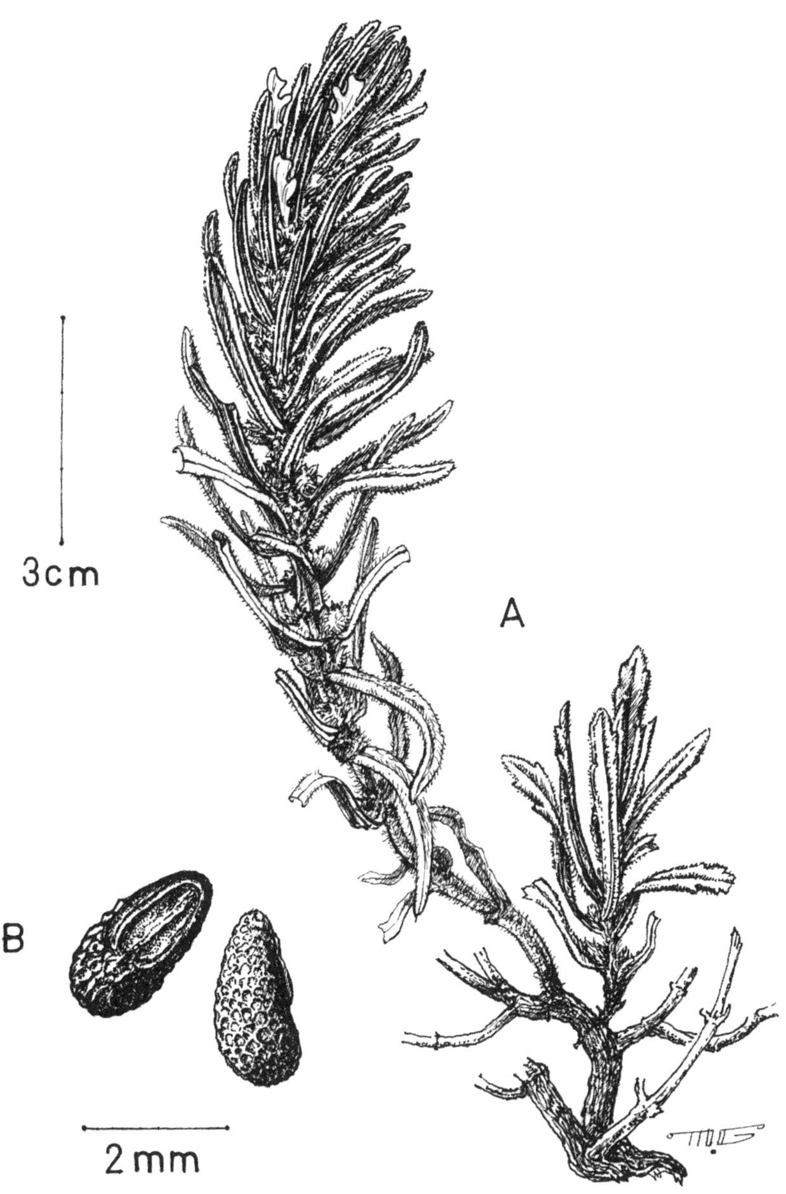

Ajuga iva
A. flowering branch, B. seeds

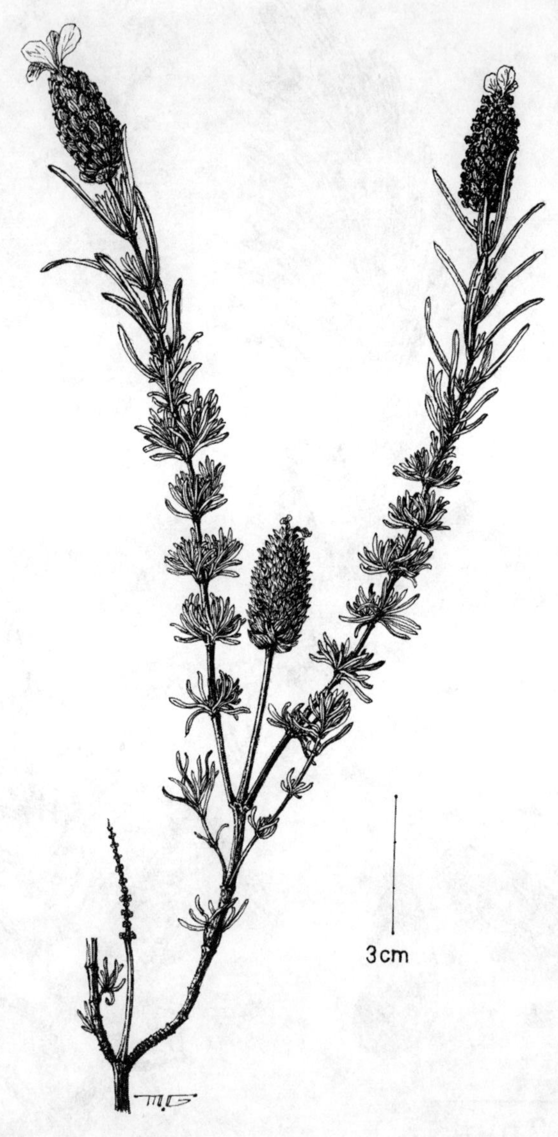

Lavandula stoechas

dried plant or its hot infusion taken after meals against diabetes (Rabat drug market). Infusion of flowering branches antidiarrhoeic, vulnerary, depurative, very effective vermifuge, for feminine sterility, colds, troubles of the digestive tract.

Ref: 5, 8, 37, 42

Ballota nigra L. *Area:* Libya to Morocco.
Names: Arabic: Ferasioun aswad (4, 23, 62); Sindiyan el-ard, Ballutah (4). English: Foetid horehound, Black horehound (4). French: Ballote fétide (4, 23, 37); Marrube noir (4, 23); Marrube puant (23).
Uses: Flowering branches antispasmodic, emmenagogue, tonic, vermifuge, for treatment of tinea, tranquilizer. *Ref:* 23, 37

***Lavandula angustifolia** Miller *Area:* Cultivated in restricted areas of North Africa. Also imported.
Names: Arabic: Khuzama (4, 5, 42, 62, Rabat drug market); Kuzama zarqa (42). English: Common lavender (4). French: Lavande (4, 5, 42, 62); Lavande officinale (24); Lavande vraie (4, 45).
Uses: Infusion of flowering summits stomachic, chologogue, stimulant, diuretic, sudorific, carminative, antispasmodic, vermifuge, emmenagogue (Rabat drug market); mixed with tea as a substitute for mint or other infusions for its agreeable smell. Lavender oil antispasmodic, stimulant, antiseptic. *Ref:* 5, 24, 42

Lavandula dentata L. *Area:* Algeria, Morocco.
Names: Arabic: Dj'eida (47, 62); Liazir, Helhal (62). Berber: Amezzour (62).
Uses: Infusion of flowering summits taken first thing in the morning and before going to bed, recommended for urine retention and to remove kidney or ureter stones (Rabat drug market).

Lavandula multifida L. *Area:* Egypt to Morocco.
Names: Arabic: Kammoun el-djmel (47, 62); Karawiet el-djmel, Khou helhal, Saraqtoun (62); Kohheila (Rabat drug market). Berber: Igigiz, Iggiz, Djei, Arssfa, Alanoudrag, Dehada (62).
Uses: Infusion of flowering branches for cough (Rabat drug market).

Lavandula stoechas L. *Area:* Tunisia to Morocco.
Names: Arabic: Halhal (5, 23, 42, 62, Rabat and Algiers drug markets); Halhal el-djebel, Meharga, Estakhoudes (23, 62). Berber: Amezzir (5, 23, 62); Imzir (23, 26); Timerzat (42); Iazir, Hamsdir (62). English: French lavender, Stoechas (4). French: Lavande stoechas, Quereillet (4).
Uses: Infusion of flowering summits tonic, resolvent, stomachic, for headache, vulnerary, for cases of irritability, epilepsy, blennorrhagia, diaphoretic, pectoral, diuretic, antispasmodic, antirheumatic (Rabat drug market). *Ref:* 5, 17, 23, 42

Lycopus europaeus L. *Area:* Tunisia to Morocco.
Names: Arabic: Zekza (23, 47, 62); Ferasioun (23, 62); Ferasioun mai (4). English: Gipsywort, Water horehound (4). French: Marrube d'eau (23, 62); Lycope des marais, Chanvre d'eau (23); Lycope, Marrube aquatique, Pied de loup, Lance du Christ (4).
Uses: Flowering branches antihemorrhagic, febrifuge, astringent. *Ref:* 23, 24

Marrubium vulgare L. *Area:* Egypt to Morocco.

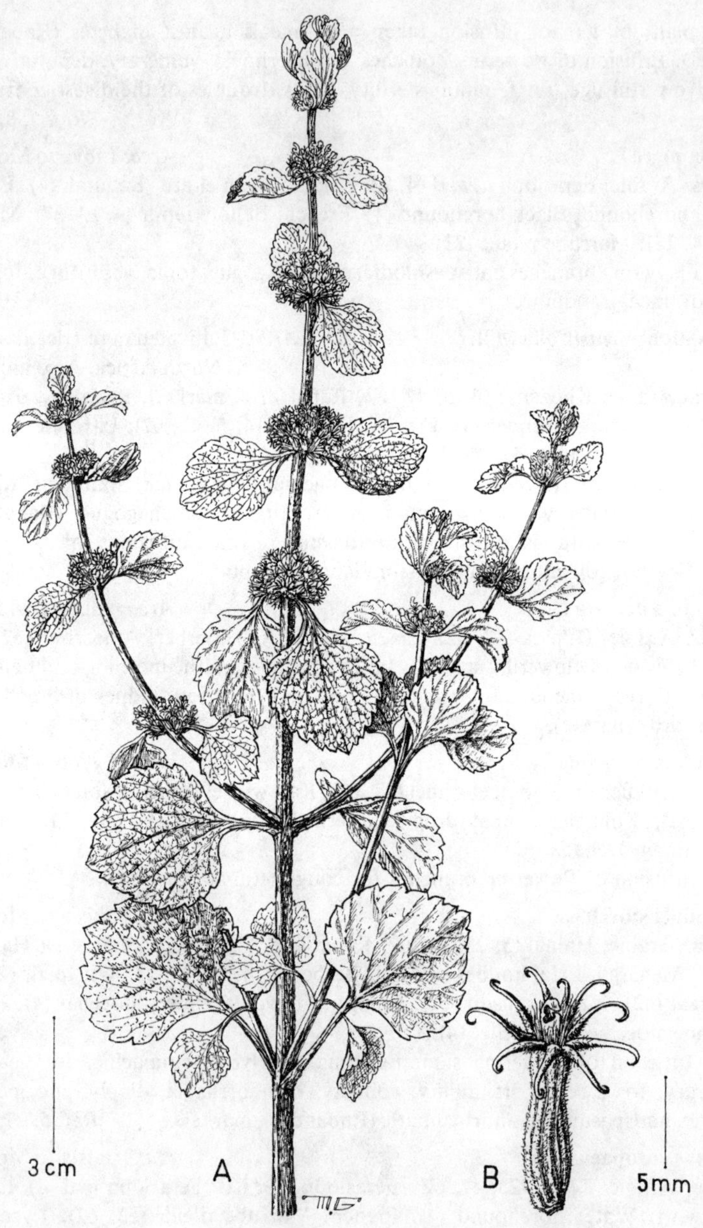

Marrubium vulgare
A. flowering branch
B. calyx enclosing fruit and withered corolla

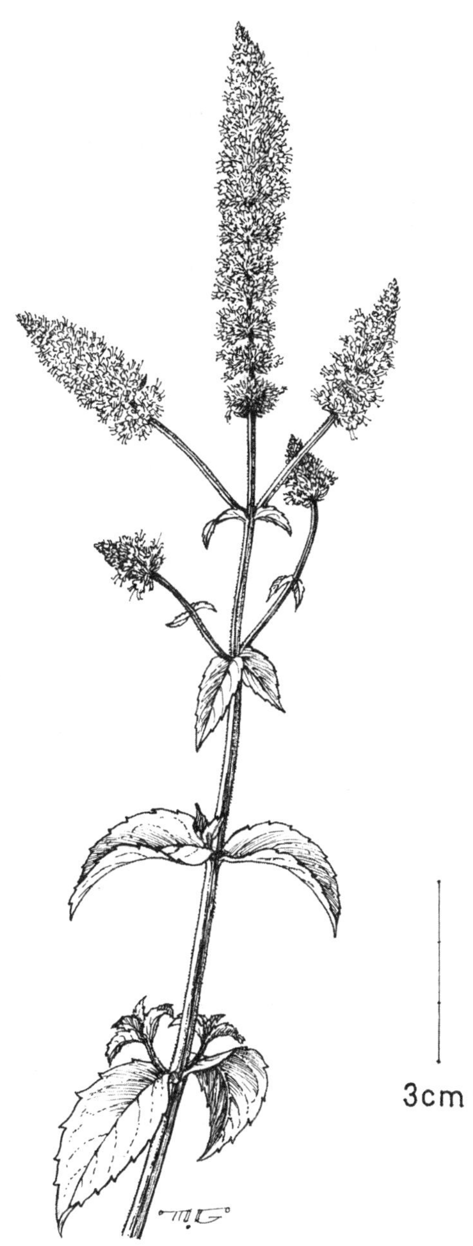

Mentha longifolia subsp. *typhoides*

Names: Arabic: Marriout (5, 23, 42, 50, 62, Rabat and Algiers drug markets); Marriout el-kelb (23, 42, 62); Umm re-roubia, Frasioun, Eshbet el-kelb (23, 62); Roubia (8, 58); Frasioun abiad, Sharir, Hashishet el-kelb (4); Merriwa (5). Berber: Timeriout, Timersat (23, 62); Ifzi (5, 62). English: Common white horehound (4, 8). French: Marrube blanc (4, 23, 45, 50); Marrube (42, 62); Herbe vierge, Marrochemin (23).
Uses: Infusion of leaves recommended for cases of jaundice, diabetes, fevers, typhoid, typhus, takes part in the treatment of otitis and eczema, reputed as diuretic and emmenagogue. Infusions or decoctions mainly of the fresh plant (easy to get throughout the year) mixed with dry raisins or honey, febrifuge used in the treatment of malaria, typhus and liver infections, particularly jaundice, pulmonary troubles, headaches, often by inhaling the fresh juice of the plant; tonic and stimulant in cases of anemia and convalescence, antidiabetic, of a regulatory action in cases of cardiac troubles; infusion after meals antidiabetic, antirheumatic and for colds (Rabat drug market), strong doses purgative and emetic. Infusion of the flowering summits expectorant for various respiratory disorders; tincture for gastrointestinal, hepatic and bilary disorders; hot infusion febrifuge, antidiabetic, stomach troubles, pectoral, tonic, chologogue. *Ref:* 5, 8, 23, 42, 45, 50, 56

Melissa officinalis L. *Area:* Tunisia to Morocco. Often cultivated.
Names: Arabic; Touroudjan (4, 23, 47, 62); Tzndjan (23, 62); Badarendjabouya (4, 23, 62); Na'na' et-teroundj (42, 62); Hashishet en-nahl (4); Louiza (26, 42); Merzizou (37). Berber: Tizizwit (23, 62); Merzizua (26, 42). English: Lemon-balm, Beebalm, Balm-leaf (4). French: Mélisse (4, 23, 26, 42, 45, 62); Citronelle (4, 23); Mélisse officinale (23, 37); Herbe du citron, Thé de France (23).
Uses: Infusion of leaves antispasmodic, stomachic, carminative, vulnerary, digestive, stimulant, antiviral. *Ref:* 23, 37, 45

***Mentha longifolia** (L.) Huds. subsp. **typhoides** (Briq.) R. Harley *Area:* Egypt, Algeria, Morocco.
Names: Arabic: Nemdar, Na'oudh (62); Habaq, Habaq el-bahr (4, 58); Habaq el-maya (58); Dabbab, Safira (4). Berber: Tahindest (62). English: Wild mint, Horse mint (4). French: Menthe sauvage, Menthe silvestre (4).
Uses: Plant added to water of hot bath useful for skin diseases. Infusion of leaves and flowering summits carminative (Farmers, Egypt).

Mentha pulegium L. *Area:* Egypt to Morocco.
Names: Arabic: Fliou (5, 13, 23, 37, 47, 62, Rabat and Algiers drug markets); Fulayya (4, 58); Fulayha, Habaq, Fudang (4). Berber: Afligou, Felgou, Moursal, Temarsa (13, 23, 62). English: Pennyroyal, Pudding grass (4). French: Menthe pouliot (4, 23, 24, 37); Pouliot (4, 13, 23, 62); Herbe aux puces, Herbe de Saint-Laurent (23); Chasse puce (13).
Uses: Infusion of leaves and flowering branches antispasmodic, antiseptic chologogue, bechic, insecticide. Infusion, cataplasm or inhaling the fresh plant for colds, catarrh, infections of the throat, bronchia and lungs. Flowering branches carminative (Rabat and Algiers drug markets), expectorant, anticatarrhal, disinfectant; infusion for abdominal ailments. *Ref:* 5, 13, 23, 24, 37

***Mentha spicata** L. *Area:* Cultivated in North Africa. Naturalized in some humid regions.

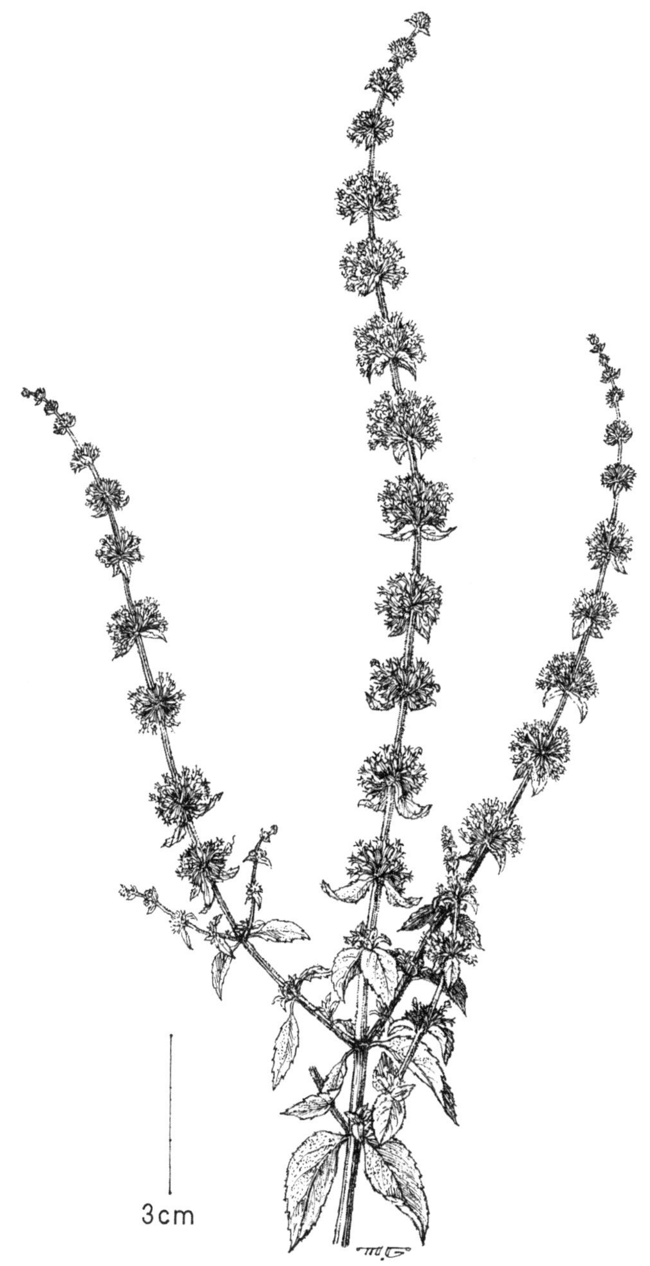

Mentha pulegium

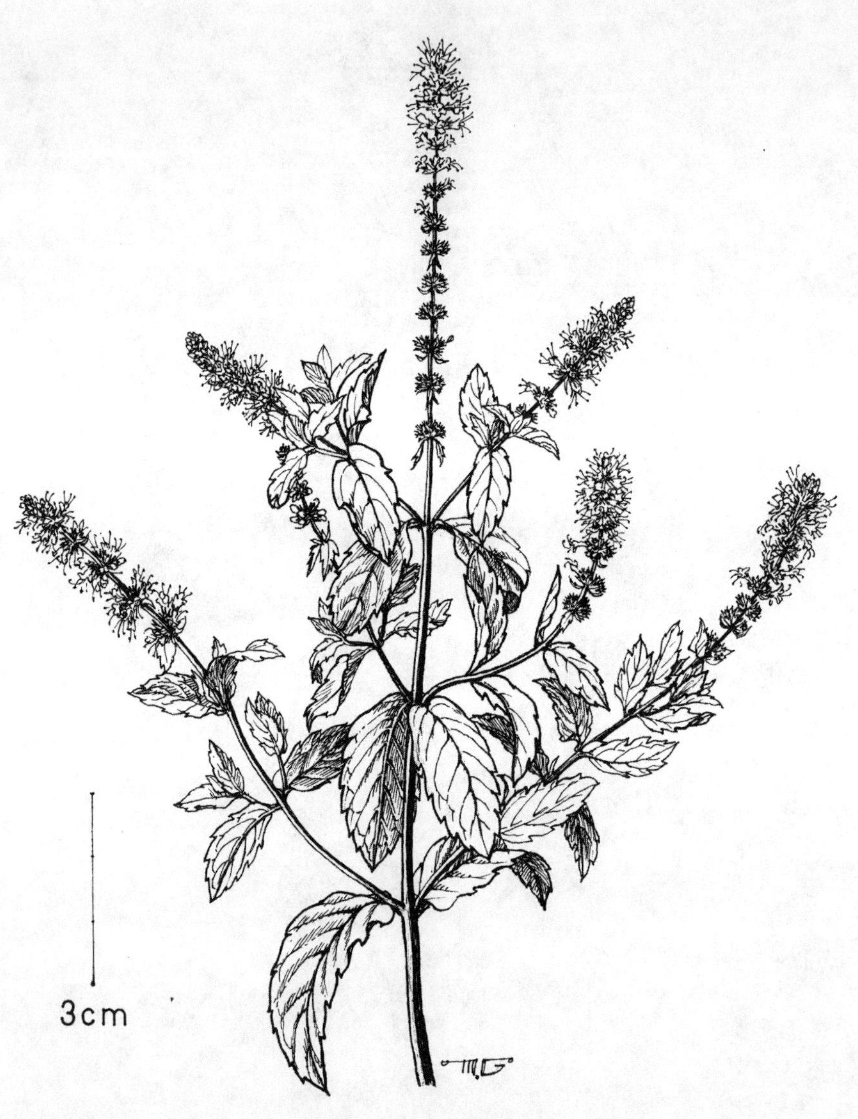

Mentha spicata

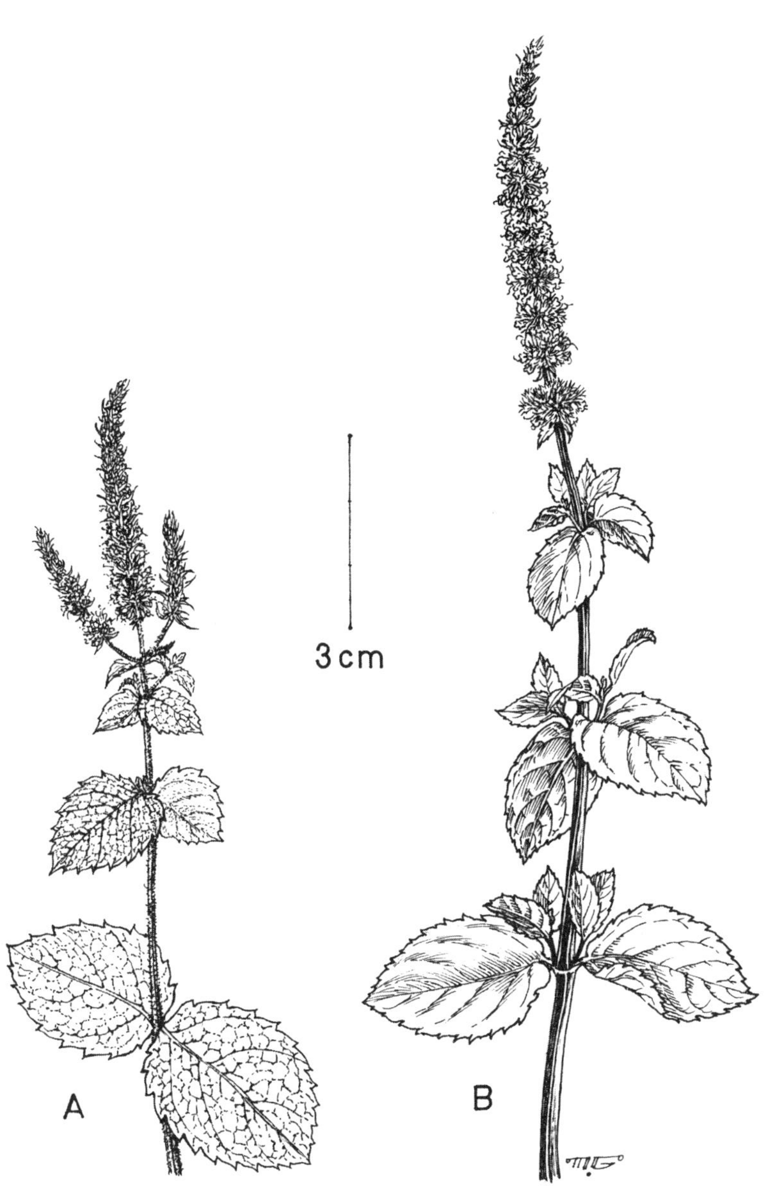

A. *Mentha suaveolens.* B. *Mentha* x *villosa*

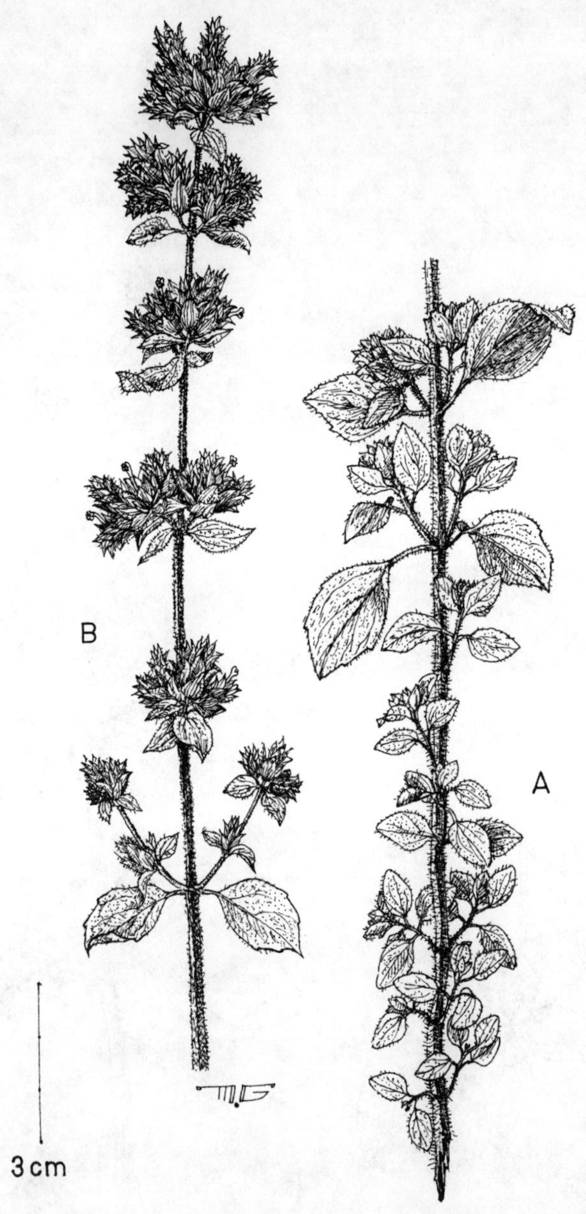

Origanum compactum
A. vegetative branch, B. flowering branch

Names: Arabic: Na'na' (4, 5, 37, 42, 47, 62); Na'na' akhdar, Nemdar (62); Lemmam (4); Hana (47). Berber: Liqamt (62). English: Common mint, Spearmint, Whorled mint (4). French: Menthe (42, 62); Menthe verte (4); Menthe douce (37).
Uses: Infusion of leaves refreshing, carminative, stomachic, aphrodisiac, odontalgic, appetizer, especially when mixed with tea; mixed with vinegar and indigo it forms an emetic. *Ref:* 5, 37, 42

***Mentha suaveolens** Ehrh. *Area:* Tunisia to Morocco.
Names: Arabic: Mersit (47, 62); Domran (62); Mersita, Mesistrou (Rabat drug market). Berber: Timijja (47, 62); Timersitine, Timersidi, Timersat, Nahari (62).
Uses: Leaves and young branches mixed with dough to give calefacient properties to bread; also used for preparing mint tea (Rabat drug market).

***Mentha** x **villosa** Huds. *Area:* Cultivated in North Africa.
Names: Arabic: Na'na' (Rabat drug market).
Uses: Infusion of leaves alone, or mixed with tea, digestive, carminative, for colds (Rabat drug market); makes the best mint tea in Morocco (Dr. R.M. Harley, personal communication).

Ocimum basilicum L. *Area:* Commonly cultivated in North Africa.
Names: Arabic: Habaq (23, 24, 62); Rayhan (4, 5); Za'ater hindi (4); Habaq el-ayalet, Hamahim (62). English: Basil, Sweet basil (4). French: Basilic (4, 5, 42, 62); Grand basilic (45).
Uses: Plant for fever, cough, worms, stomach complaints, gout, tumors of the eye, as ointment for sclerosis of spleen and liver. Twigs for stomach cancer as hot bath. Leaves or flowering summits gastric antispasmodic, stomachic tonic, carminative, galactogenic; infusions recommended for sinusitis, hemorrhoids, stomach troubles, stimulant, diuretic. Leaves for skin diseases, nasal douche, fungus infections, cataplasm for tumors. Flowers carminative, diuretic, stimulant, demulcent. Infusion of seeds for gonorrhoea, dysentery, chronic diarrhoea, constipation, piles.
Ref: 1, 5, 17, 42, 45, 56

Origanum compactum Benth. *Area:* Morocco.
Names: Arabic: Za'ater (5, 26, 42, 62). French: Origan du Maroc (42, 50).
Uses: Dry plant fumigant, antiseptic, disinfectant; fumigation used for colds, bronchitis, cephalalgia. Infusion or powdered plant excellent remedy for diarrhoea, stomach and intestinal troubles, digestive (Rabat drug market). Infusion of leaves and inflorescences tonic, antidiarrhoeic, slightly aphrodisiac. *Ref:* 5, 42

Origanum majorana L. *Area:* Cultivated in North Africa. Subspontaneous in Algeria and Morocco.
Names: Arabic: Mardaddoush (42, 62, Rabat drug market); Mardaqoush, Rayhan Dawoud (4); Za'ater (42); Bardaqoush (Cairo and Algiers drug markets). Berber: Arzema, Mloul (62). English: Sweet marjoram, Knotted marjoram (4). French: Marjolaine (4, 26, 42, 62); Amaracus, Marjolaine à coquille (4).
Uses: Plant soaked in hot olive oil and cooled, this oil used as ear drops for ear ailments, especially those in connection with colds (Algiers drug market). Leaves and flowering summits cephalic, pectoral, resolvent, vulnerary, sudorific, emmenagogue, aphrodisiac, condiment; infusion a tonic. *Ref:* 17, 26, 42, 45

***Origanum vulgare** L. subsp. **glandulosum** (Desf.) Ietswaart *Area:* Tunisia, Algeria.

Names: Arabic: Za'ater (23, 62). French: Origan (23).
Uses: Leaves and flowering summits stimulant. *Ref:* 23

Otostegia fruticosa (Forssk.) Schweinf. ex Penzig *Area:* Egypt.
Names: Arabic: Sharam, Ghassa (58).
Uses: Infusion or cataplasm of flowering branches a good remedy for sunstroke (Bedouins, Egypt).

Rosmarinus officinalis L. *Area:* Libya to Morocco. Cultivated in Egypt.
Names: Arabic: Iklil (8, 23, 62); Iklil el-gabal (4, 5, 42); Hassalban (4, 23, 62); Hatssa louban (23, 42). Berber: Azir, (5, 23, 42, 62); Iazir (23, 62); Ouzbir, Aklel, Touzala (62); Touzzal (42). English: Rosemary (8); Common rosemary (4). French: Romarin (4, 5, 23, 42, 45, 62).
Uses: Infusion of fresh plant diuretic; young shoots used for preparation of aromatic baths. Leaves emmenagogue, chologogue, carminative, stomachic, abortive, antispasmodic. Rosemary oil used in preparation of ointments for rheumatism, to soothe sprains, bruises, scrofulous ulcers, wounds and eczema. Infusion of leaves used externally to cure abscesses and wounds, as a gargle for mouth ulcers. Leaves added to bath water are thought to strengthen the weak and to help rheumatism sufferers, the volatile oil used with other drugs as antiseptic and insecticide. Dry powdered leaves mixed with olive oil used for healing wounds, antiseptic and vulnerary for recent wounds and at the moment of circumcision; decoction depurative; infusion remedy for cough. *Ref:* 5, 8, 23, 38, 42, 56

***Salvia fruticosa** Miller *Area:* Libya. Cultivated and subspontaneous in Algeria; probably cultivated in other regions of North Africa.
Names: Arabic: Khayat el-djurhat, Na'ama, Hobeiq es-sedr (62); Teffah (8); Khokh barri (4); Shay gabali (54). Berber: Agourim imeksawen (62). English: Three-lobed sage (8); Sage apple, Apple-bearing sage (4). French: Pomme de sauge (4).
Uses: Infusion of leaves and young shoots used for influenza, cough, rheumatic pains. *Ref:* 54

Salvia officinalis L. *Area:* Cultivated mainly in Algeria and Morocco.
Names: Arabic: Salima (5, 42); Salmiya (5, Rabat drug market); Salma (13, 42, 62); Selmia (62); Mofassa (42, 62); Mufassiha (42); Sowak En-Nebi (13, 47, 62); Kharnah, Maryamyah, Asfaqs (4); Kheyyat el-jrah (13). Berber: Tazzourt (13, 42, 62); Timijja, Mrennebo (13, 42). English: Common sage, Garden sage (4). French: Sauge officinale (4, 5, 24, 42, 45); Sauge, Thé de Grèce, Herbe sacrée (4).
Uses: Leaves and summits emmenagogue, diuretic, cholagogue, general antiseptic, infusion astringent, sudorific, stimulant, tonic, digestive, antispasmodic, febrifuge, resolvent, vulnerary, carminative; used for colds (Rabat drug market).
Ref: 2, 5, 17, 24, 42

Salvia sclarea L. *Area:* Tunisia, Algeria.
Names: Arabic: Kaff ed-dubb (4). Berber: Tsifsfa (23, 47, 62). English : Clary (4). French: Sclarée (62); Sauge sclarée, Toute bonne (4, 23); Herbe aux plaies, Orvale (23); Sauge écarlate (4).
Uses: Leaves and inflorescence summits stimulant, antispasmodic, anticatarrhal, tonic, emmenagogue, antiseptic. *Ref:* 23, 24, 45

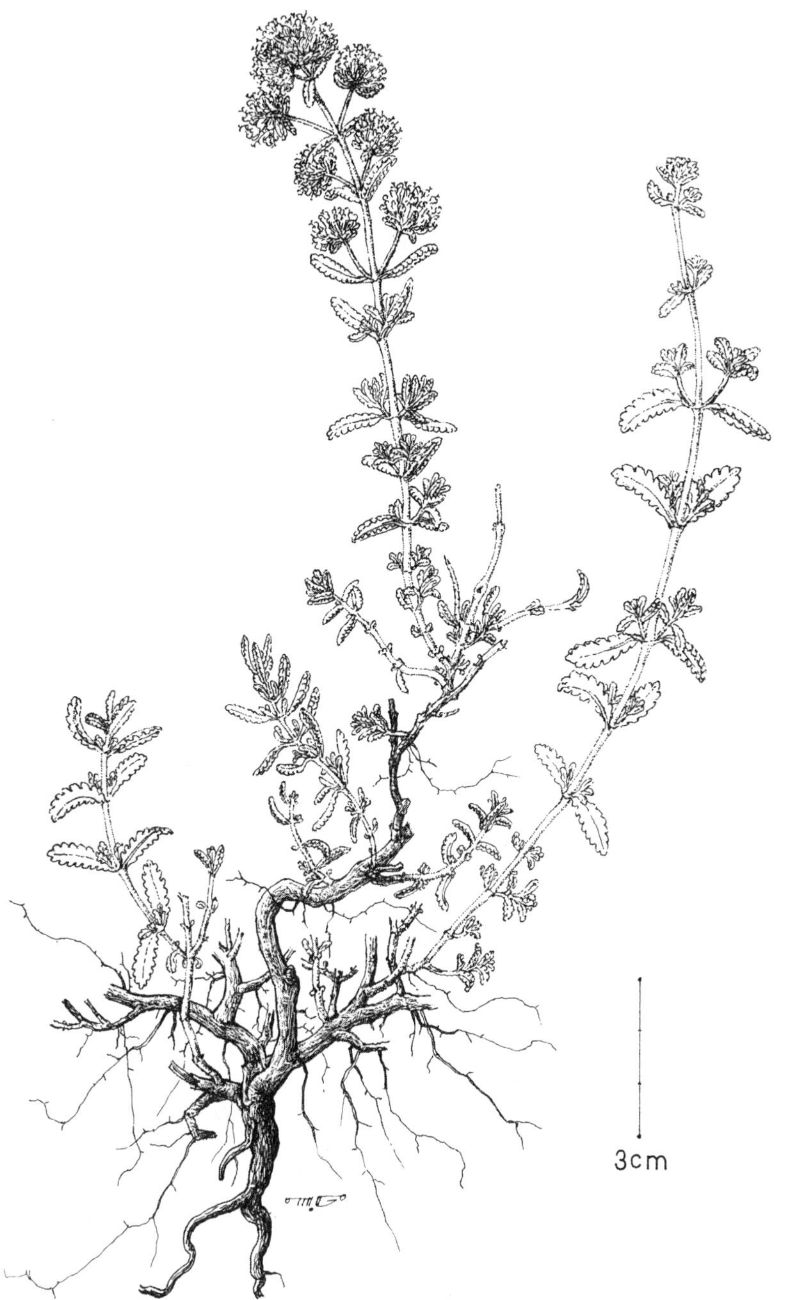

Teucrium polium

***Stachys officinalis** (L.) Trev. *Area:* Tunisia to Morocco.
Names: Arabic: Eshbet netegerfa, Eshbet el-ghorab (23); Batuniqa, Shatra (4). English: Betony, Wound-wort, Bishop's-wort (4). French: Bétonie (4, 23); Epiaire bétonie, Belle tête (4).
Uses: Entire plant stimulant, appetizer, anticatarrhal. Root slightly emetic, purgative. Flowering branches stomachic, tonic, sternutatory (sneezing powder, substitute for tobacco), vulnerary. *Ref:* 23, 24

Teucrium chamaedrys L. *Area:* Libya to Morocco.
Names: Arabic: Bellout el-ard (23, 47, 62). Berber: Akhendous (23, 62). English: Common germander, Ground oak (4). French: Petit chêne (4, 26); Germandrée (62); Germandrée officinale, Chênette (4); Chasse fièvre (23); Germandrée petit-chêne (23, 45).
Uses: Flowering branches vulnerary, bitter tonic, digestive, febrifuge. *Ref:* 23, 45

Teucrium polium L. *Area:* Egypt to Morocco.
Names: Arabic: Ja'ada (4, 5, 8, 23, 58, 62); Dja'ad (23, 37, 62); Goutiba (23, 47, 62); Haida, Felfela (23, 62); Shendgura (5); Hashishet er-rih, Misk el-gin (4). Berber: Timzourin (23, 47, 62); Timtshish (23, 62); Teqmezoutin (62). English: Mountain germander (4, 8); Cat thyme, Hulwort (4). French: Pouliot de montagne (4, 23); Germandrée en capitule (5); Polium, Germandrée tomenteuse (4); Germandrée polium (37).
Uses: Hot infusion of tender parts of plant taken for stomach and intestinal troubles. Plant used in a steam bath for colds and fevers, useful against smallpox and itch; infusion vermifuge, stimulant, depurative, for feminine sterility, colds, tonic, astringent, vulnerary. *Ref:* 5, 8, 23, 37

***Thymus algeriensis** Boiss. & Reut. *Area:* Tunisia to Morocco. Endemic to North Africa.
Names: Arabic: Djertil (23, 47, 62); Khieta, Hamriya, Mezouqesh, Hamzousha (23, 62). Berber: Rebba, Djoushshen (24, 62); Azoukni, Toushna (62). French: Thym (23).
Uses: Leaves and flowering branches condiment, stomachic, diaphoretic, antispasmodic specifically for whooping cough, stimulant for the blood circulation, aphrodisiac. *Ref:* 23

Thymus broussonettii Boiss. *Area:* Endemic to Morocco.
Names: Arabic: Ze'itra (5, 42); Za'atar el-hmir (5).
Uses: Infusion of leaves and flowering branches for colds, pains, coryzas, rheumatisms, articular pains, as a gargle for throat troubles; decoction without sugar for jaundice and other liver diseases, galactogogue, vermifuge, emmenagogue, diuretic, digestive, appetizer, general antiseptic for the intestine; used in the form of plaster on the abdomen in cases of digestive troubles. *Ref:* 5

Thymus capitatus (L.) Hoffmanns. & Link *Area:* Egypt to Morocco.
Names: Arabic: Za'atar (8, 62); Za'atar el-mediya (62); Za'atar barri, Hasha, Za'atar farsi (4). English: Headed thyme (4, 8). French: Thym de Crète (4).
Uses: Cold infusion of flowering branches tonic, for coughs; hot infusion said to be useful (by drinking) in curing some skin diseases. *Ref:* 8

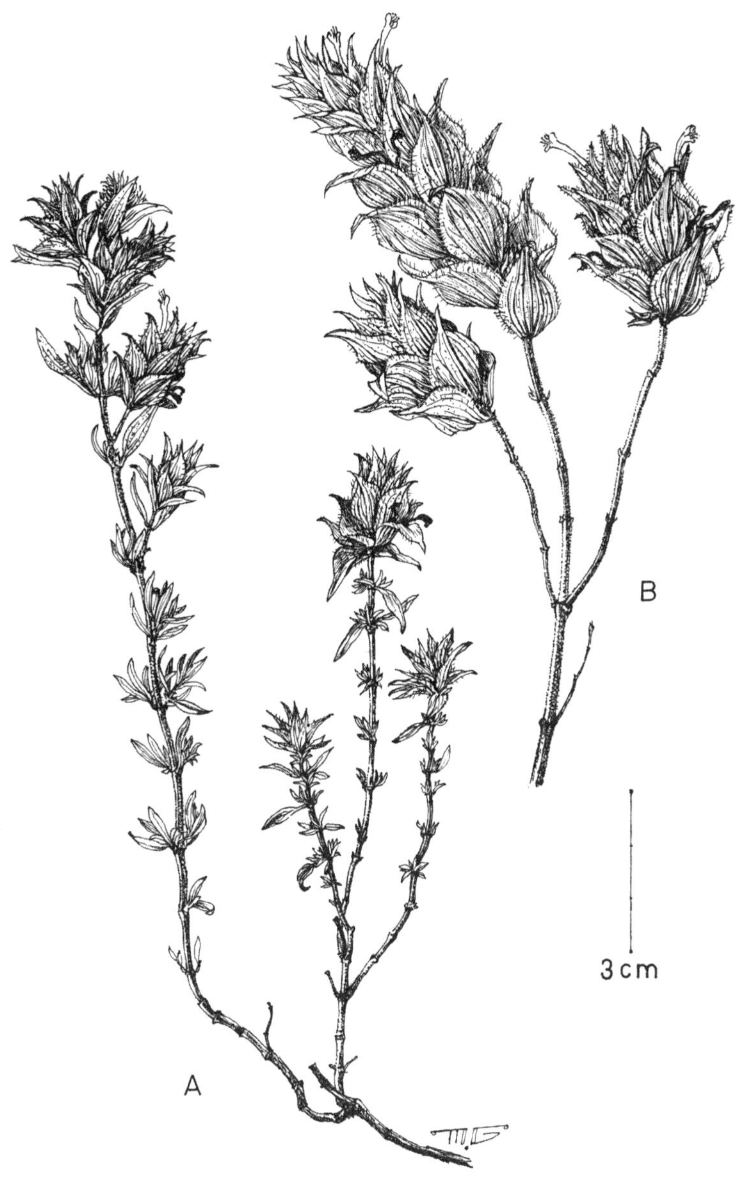

Thymus broussonettii
A. flowering branch bearing leaves
B. leafless flowering branch, a form with large bracts

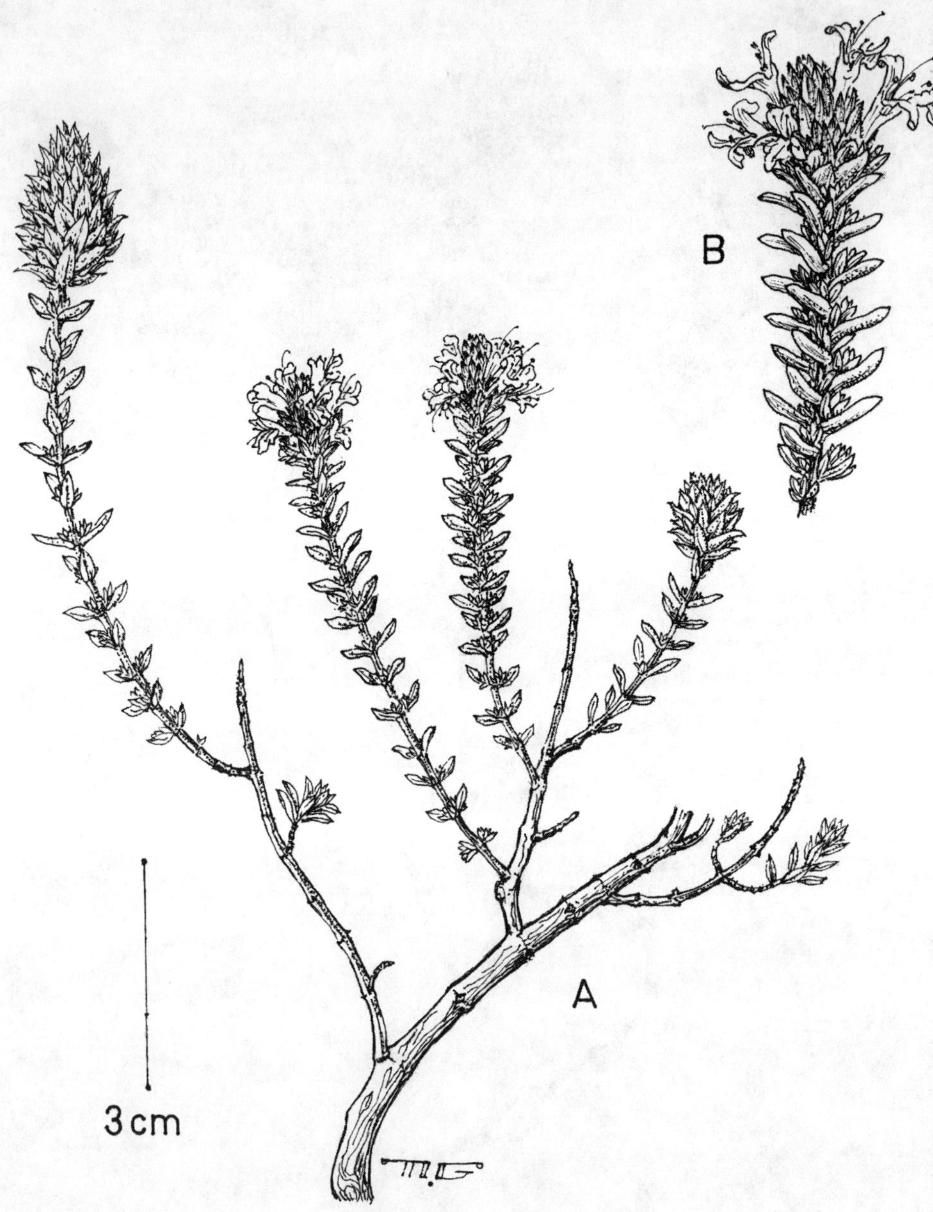

Thymus capitatus
A. flowering branch, B. flowering branchlet, enlarged

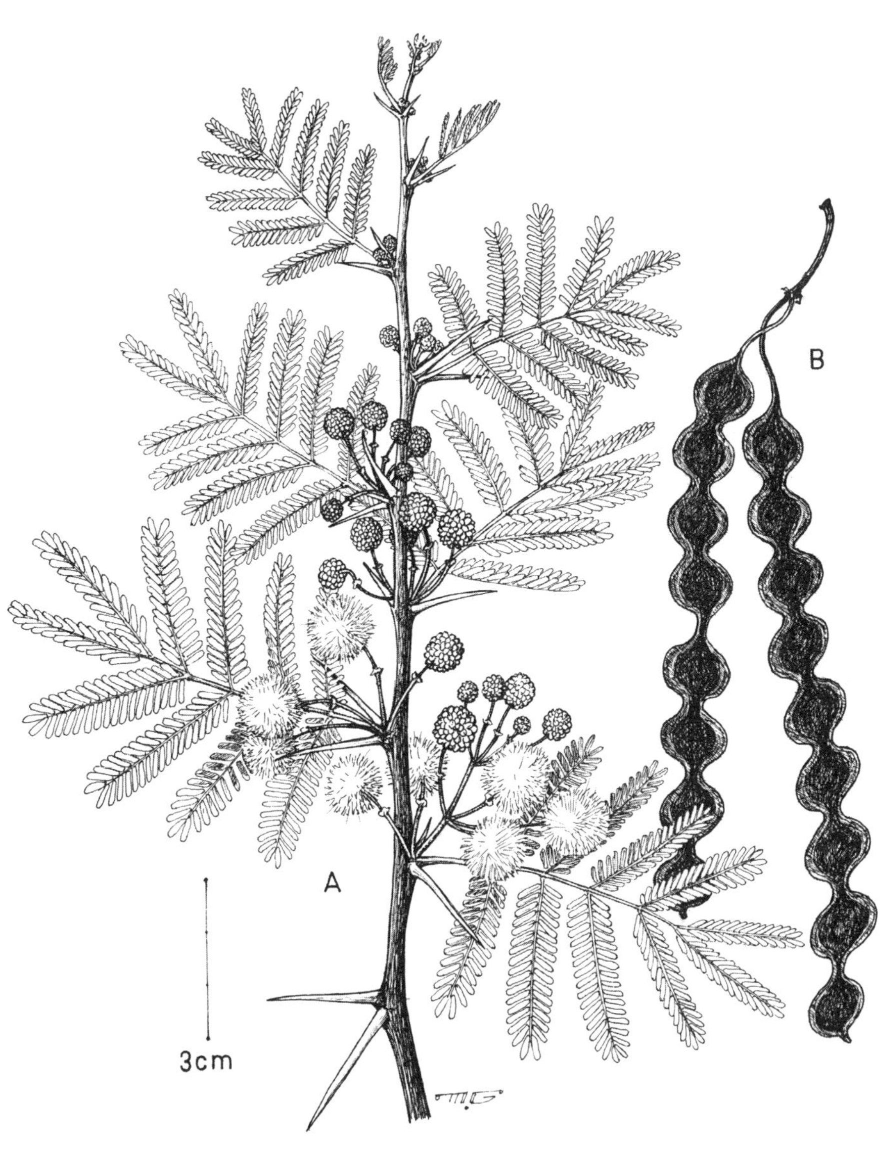

Acacia nilotica
A. flowering branch, B. fruits

In addition to the above three *Thymus* species, mostly used in folk medicine in North Africa, the following are less abundant: *T. ciliatus* (Desf.) Benth., Libya to Morocco; *T. maroccanus* Ball, endemic to Morocco; *T. serpyllum* L., *T. vulgaris* L. and *T. zygis* L. having varieties endemic to Morocco.

Lauraceae

Laurus nobilis L. *Area:* Libya to Morocco. Also cultivated.
Names: Arabic: Rand (4, 5, 23, 42, 62, Casablanca drug market); Ghar (4, 42, 62); 'Asa Musa (5); Maraget Musa (Casablanca drug market); fruit; Habb ghar (42, 62). Berber: Taset (23, 62). English: Laurel, Roman laurel, Sweet-bay (4). French: Laurier (42); Laurier commun (45); Laurier d'Apollon, Laurier sauce (23); Laurier franc, Laurier des poètes (4).
Uses: Leaves condiment, gastric stimulant, stomachic, carminative, anticatarrhal, diuretic, antispasmodic, emmenagogue; infusion sudorific. Fatty matter from berries externally used as parasiticide and for rheumatism. *Ref:* 5, 23, 24, 45

Leguminosae

Acacia albida Del. *Area:* Egypt, Libya, Algeria.
Names: Arabic: Haras (4, 62); Haraz (7, 58); 'Afrar, Telh lebiad (5); fruits: Kharrub (58). Berber: Ahates (5, 62); Ahades, Temahaq, Azawo (62). English: White acacia (4). French: Arbre blanc (4).
Uses: Decoction of bark used orally against leprosy. *Ref:* 5

***Acacia nilotica** (L.) Willd. ex Del. *Area:* Egypt.
Names: Arabic: Sant (4, 5, 17, 58); Gurti (7, 58); Shoka masrya, Shoka qibttya (17); fruit: Qarad (5, 7, 58). English: Egyptian acacia, Egyptian thorn, Gum-Arabic tree (4). French: Acacia d'Egypte, Gommier d'Egypte, Gommier rouge (4).
Uses: Gum exudates from the tree antidiarrhoeic. Stem bark extract antiamoebic, antispasmodic, hypotensive. Infusion of fruits for diarrhoea, especially for children; powdered fruits used against fevers and as a cure for sore gums and loose teeth, for diabetes by taking a teaspoonful first thing in the morning. Nubians in southern Egypt believe that diabetic patients may eat as much food rich in carbohydrates as they please without risk if they regularly take powdered pods. Mixture of powdered pods and henna (*Lawsonia inermis*) leaves made into a plaster is effective against some skin diseases and the irritated parts between toes; the applied plaster must be left to dry for a few days, then washed with cold water. *Ref:* 2, 5, 7

***Acacia raddiana** Savi *Area:* Egypt to Morocco.
Names: Arabic: Talh (5, 11, 58, 62); Sayal (11, 58, 62); Hares (62). Berber: Tamat, Tadjdjart, Abzac, Abser (62); Tihi (11). French: Gommier de Tunisie (4).
Uses: Gum from the tree is dissolved in water and used to treat occular affections, jaundice, pulmonary diseases. Dried powdered bark disinfectant, for healing wounds. Seeds, entire or powdered, taken as antidiarrhoeic. *Ref:* 5

Acacia seyal Del. *Area:* Egypt, Algeria, Morocco.
Names: Arabic: Seyal (4, 62); Talh (4, 5); gum: 'Alk (5). Berber: Tamat (5, 62); Tefi,

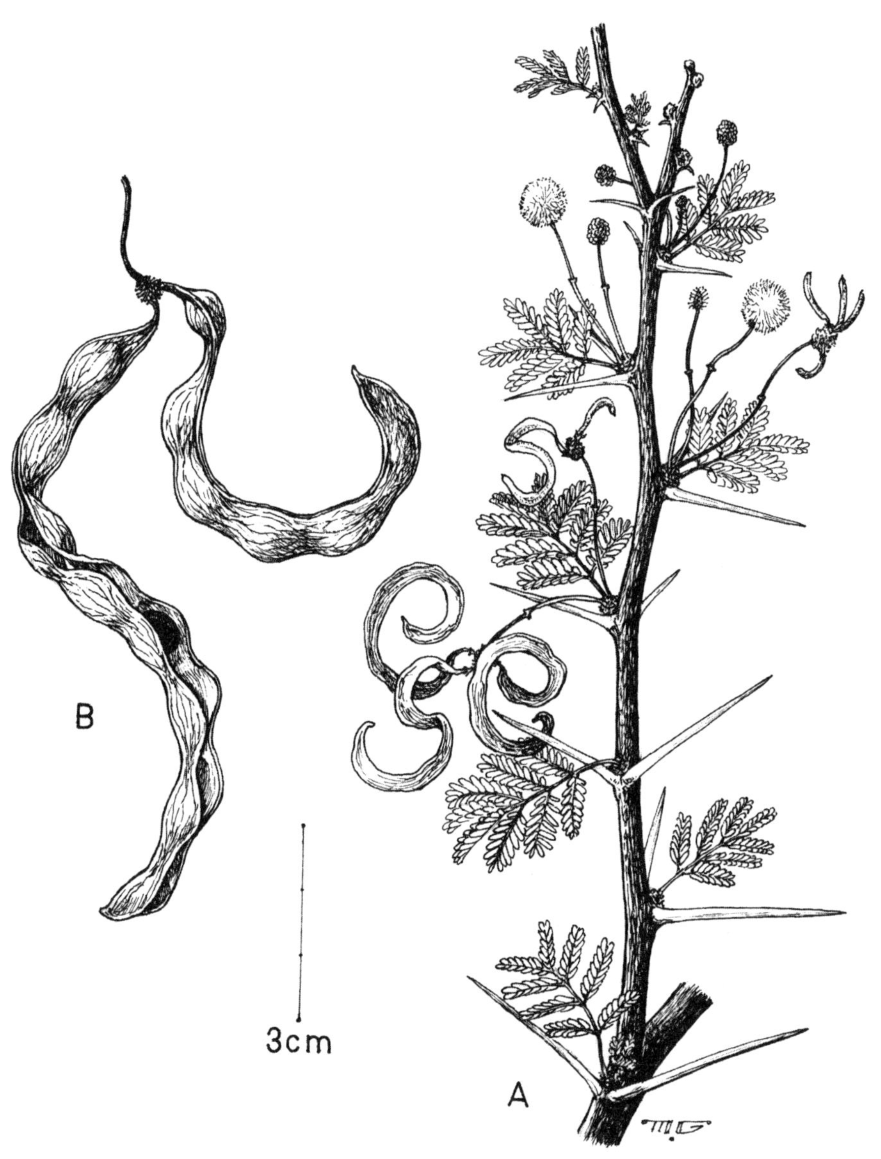

Acacia raddiana
A. flowering branch with young fruits
B. mature fruits with seeds

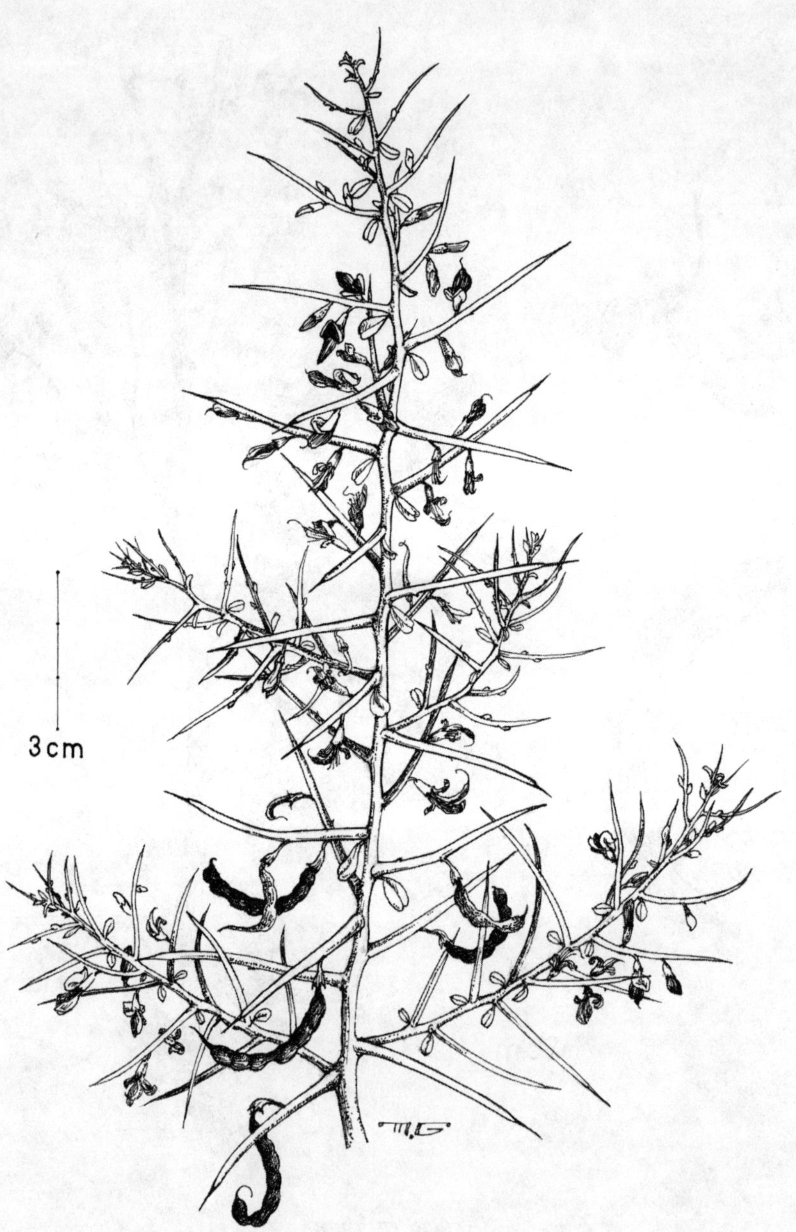

Alhagi graecorum

Talakh, Thala (62). English: Shittah tree, Shittim wood, Thirsty thorn (4). French: Arbre à gomme (4).
Uses: Wood a fumigant for rheumatic pains, to protect women against cold and fever two weeks after childbirth. Leaves and bark used in treating gastric ulcers. Gum edible, effective against rheumatism and inflammations of the respiratory system. Pods contain more than 20% proteins and are very nourishing for livestock.
Ref: 5, 7

***Alhagi graecorum** Boiss. *Area:* Egypt, Libya, Algeria.
Names: Arabic: 'Agoul (4, 7, 8, 47, 62); Shouk el-gimal (4). Berber: Lakor (62). English: Camel thorn (4,8); Hebrew manna plant (4). French: Alhagi des maures, Sainfoin agul (4).
Uses: Infusion of branches laxative, used to cure rheumatic pains and bilharziasis, vermifuge, purgative. *Ref:* 7, 8, 17

Anagyris foetida L. *Area:* Libya to Morocco.
Names: Arabic: Kharroub el-khinzir (4, 13, 17, 23, 62); Beqoul el-kelb, Kharroub el-maiz, Kharroub tourshane (13, 23, 62); seeds: Habb el-kela (13, 17, 23, 62); Umm kalb, Garrud (4, 17). Berber: Inouthoun, Afnen, Oufni, Aldhaz (62). English: Bean-clover, Stinking wood (4). French: Bois puant, Anagyre fétide (4, 13, 23, 24); Anagyris (4); Fève de loup (24).
Uses: Leaves, branches and root purgative; vermifuge in moderate doses and emetic, emmenagogue in higher doses. Powdered leaves used externally against migraine, tumors, oedema, scrofula and ulcers. Cataplasm of leaves resolvent. Fruit toxic. Seeds emmenagogue, emetic, purgative, for renal affections.
Ref: 13, 17, 23, 24, 62

Anthyllis vulneraria L. *Area:* Egypt to Morocco.
Names: Arabic: Hashishet ed-dabb (4, 23, 62); 'Arq safir (23, 62). English: Kidney-vetch, Lady's fingers, Wound-wort (4). French: Vulnéraire (4, 23, 62); Trèfle des sables (23, 62); Trèfle jaune des sables (4); Anthyllide vulnéraire, Triolet jaune (23).
Uses: Flowering branches vulnerary, astringent, depurative. Flowers mild purgative, cataplasm or lotions for contusions and wounds. *Ref:* 23, 24, 45

***Cassia italica** (Miller) F. W. Andr. *Area:* Egypt, Libya, Algeria.
Names: Arabic: Senna (5, 8, 58, 62); Ashreq (62); Senna ghanami (58); Zenina (16). Berber: Agerger (5, 47, 62); Affelajet (5, 62). English: Senna (8). French: Senné (62); Séné du Sénégal, Séné de Syrie, Séné d'Alep, Séné du Soudan (5, 16).
Uses: Leaflets and pods well-known for purgative effect. Crushed seeds used for ophthalmic diseases. *Ref:* 5, 8, 16

***Cassia senna** L. *Area:* Egypt, Libya, Algeria.
Names: Arabic: Senna mekki (42, 58, 62); Senna haram (42); Senna sa'eidi (58); Senna, Senna hindi (4). Berber: Agerger (62). English: Indian senna, Tinnevelly senna plant (4). French: Séné (42, 62); Casse trompeuse, Casse à feuilles étroites (4).
Uses: Infusion of powdered leaflets and pods a popular laxative and purgative. Infusion of leaves purgative, often mixed with leaves of roses. *Ref:* 42, 45

Ceratonia siliqua L. *Area:* Libya to Morocco. Cultivated in Egypt.
Names: Arabic: Kharroub (4, 5); Kharrouba (47, 62); Kharnub (4, 17); Ribba (62). Berber: Tikida (5, 62); Tikidit, Tisliwha (5); Tikidat, Selarwa, Ikidou, Abernid,

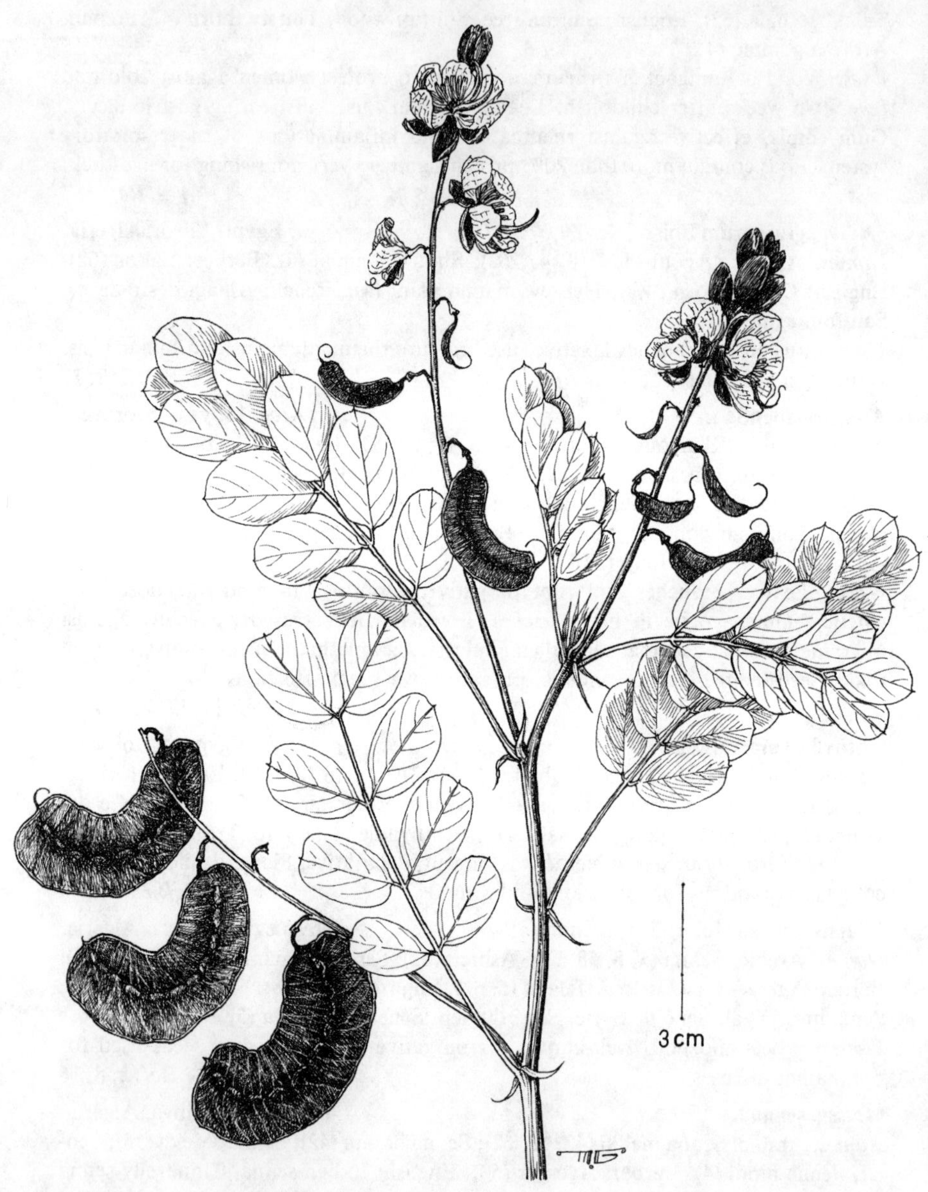

Cassia italica
flowering and fruiting branch

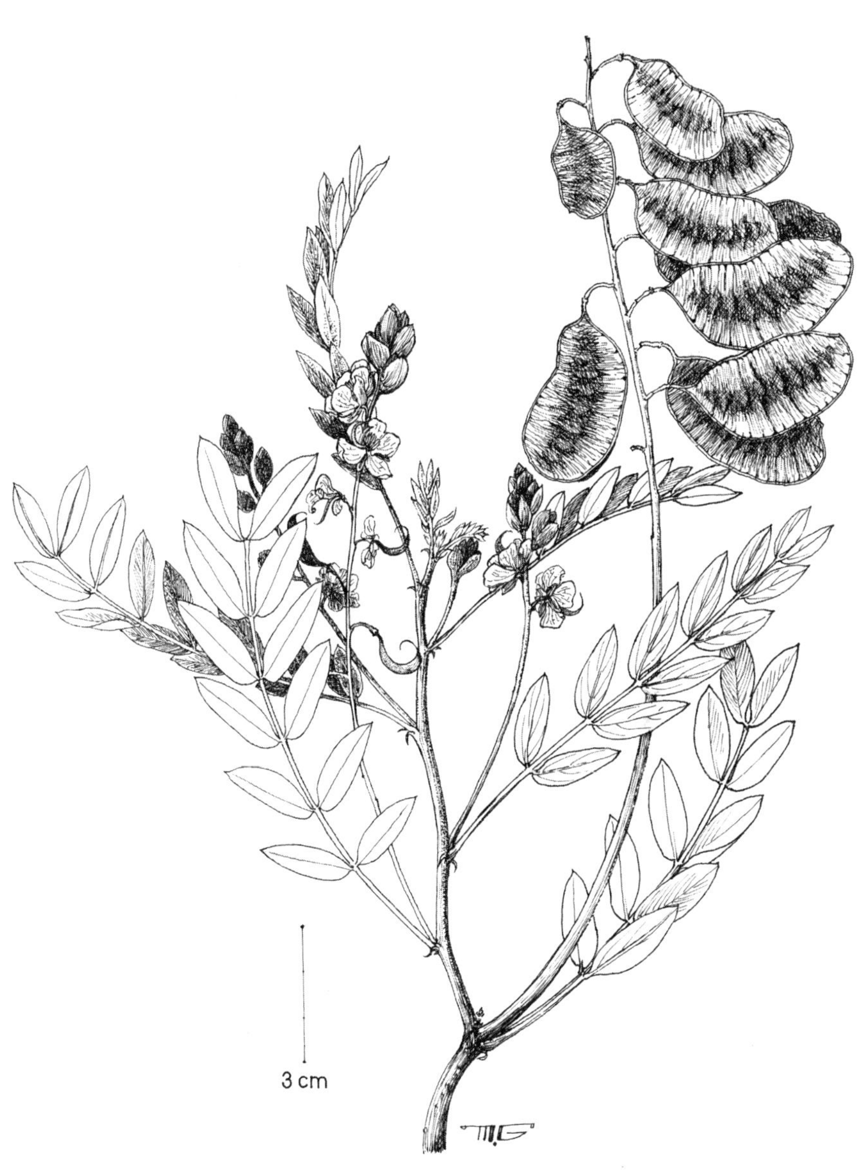

Cassia senna

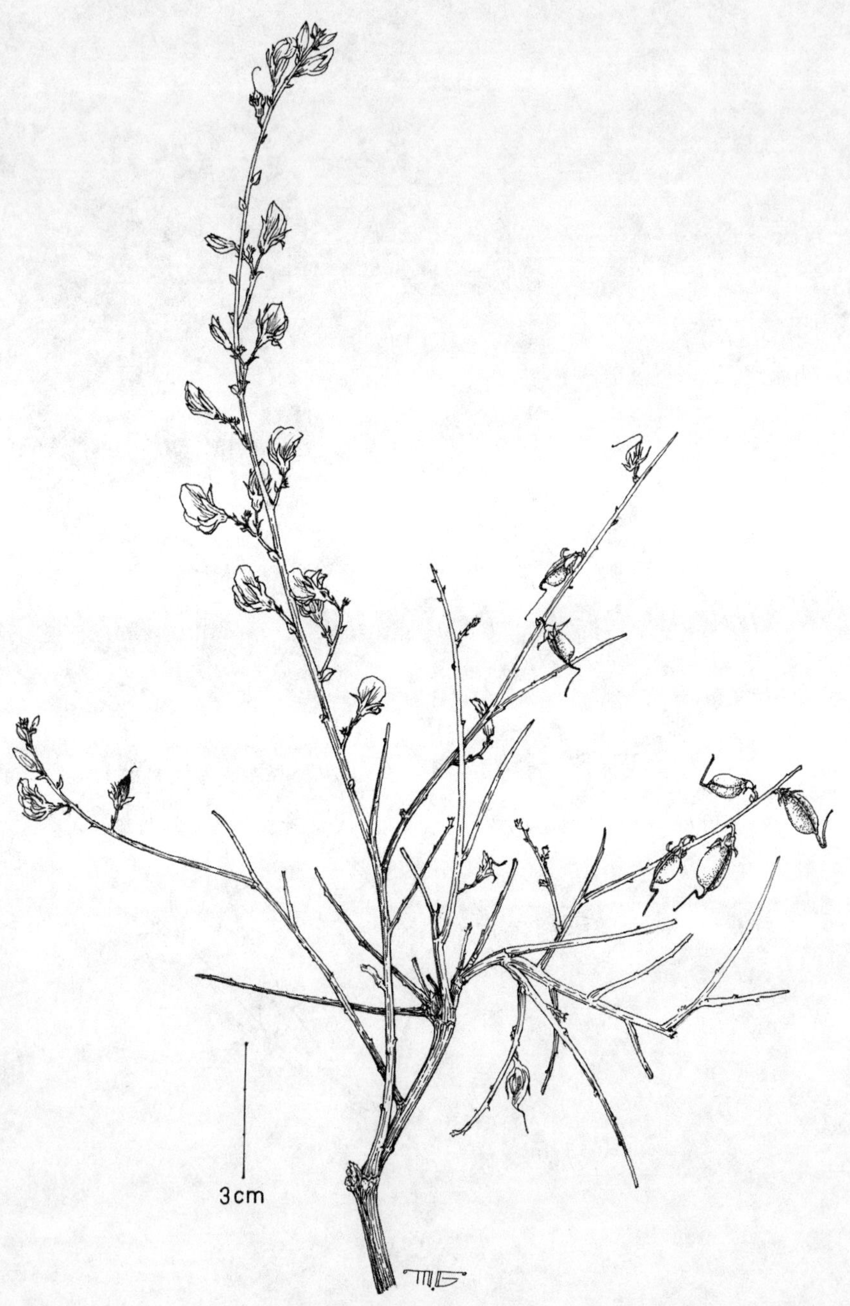

Crotalaria aegyptiaca

Tikherroubt (62). English: Carob tree, Locust tree, St. John's-bread (4). French: Caroubier (4, 5, 45, 62).
Uses: Entire pods or seeds alone used principally against diarrhoea in children and babies, also for adults. Fruit astringent, diuretic, laxative, bechic. *Ref:* 5, 17, 45

Cicer arietinum L. *Area:* Commonly cultivated in North Africa.
Names: Arabic: Hommos (4, 5, 42, 47, 62); Beiqa (62). Berber: Ikiker, Hamaz, Djelbane (62). English: Chick-pea (4). French: Pois chiche (4, 5, 42, 62); Cicérole, Gairance (4).
Uses: Seeds give nourishment and energy, reinvigorative, aphrodisiac, decoction used in a formula against itch, leprosy, healing of small pox. If inadequately cooked, seeds can cause paralysis of limbs (lathyrism), as can the ordinary pea.
Ref: 5, 42, 56

Colutea arborescens L. *Area:* Algeria, Morocco.
Names: Arabic: Qelouta (4, 23, 47, 62); Senna barri (4). English: Bladder-senna tree (4). French: Baguenaudier (4, 23, 47, 62); Faux séné (4, 23); Colutier (23); Colutéa, Séné bâtard (4).
Uses: Leaves purgative, laxative. Seeds poisonous in large doses. *Ref:* 23, 24

Coronilla scorpioides (L.) Koch *Area:* Egypt to Morocco.
Names: Arabic: Redjel el-wa'al, Qors begra, 'Akefa (23, 47, 62); Khweitmah (58). French: Coronille, Herbe de coronille (23).
Uses: Leaves purgative. Seeds cardiotonic. *Ref:* 23

Crotalaria aegyptiaca Benth. *Area:* Egypt.
Names: Arabic: Natash (4, 58). English: Rattle-box (4). French: Crotalaire (4).
Uses: Green plant grazed by camels and desert gazelles, poisonous to sheep and goats if grazed in large quantities (Bedouins, Egypt).

Glycyrrhiza foetida Desf. *Area:* Tunisia to Morocco.
Names: Arabic: 'Areq sous (23, 47, 62). French: Réglisse (23, 47).
Uses: Roots sweetening agent, used in preparation of liquorice sap and powder, pectoral pastes. Subterranean parts of plant contain the same products as *Glycyrrhiza glabra.* *Ref:* 23, 62.

Glycyrrhiza glabra L. *Area:* Cultivated and naturalized in North Africa.
Names: Arabic: 'Areq sous (4, 5, 42, 62, Rabat and Cairo drug markets); Sous (42, 62); Shagaret es-sous (4); Matak (62). Berber: Azrar azidane (62). English: Liquorice plant (4). French: Réglisse (4, 5, 42, 62); Réglisse glabre (4); Réglisse officinale (45).
Uses: Extract of root used for hoarseness of voice, cough, respiratory ailments, gastritis, abdominal pains, diuretic, febrifuge, emmenagogue, to relax uterine muscles, expectorant. Infusion of root for cough due to its emollient, depurative and sweetening properties; decoction boiled to facilitate the period due to the presence of oestrogenic hormones in appreciable quantities. Roots chewed for throat troubles and rheumatism (Rabat drug market). Refreshing drink made from root antispasmodic, for gastric ulcer. *Ref:* 5, 42, 45, 56

* **Lupinus albus** L. *Area:* Cultivated and naturalized in Egypt and Algeria, and probably elsewhere.
Names: Arabic: Termes (4, 47, 58, 62, Rabat drug market); Baqilla masri (17).

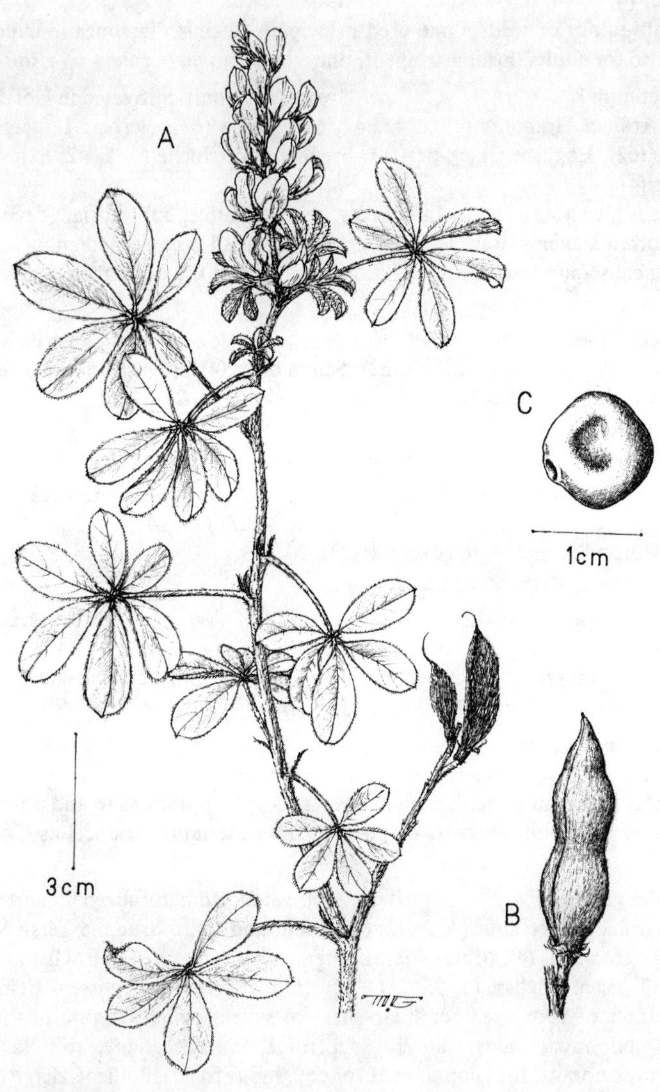

Lupinus albus
A. flowering branch with immature fruits
B. mature fruit, C. seed, enlarged

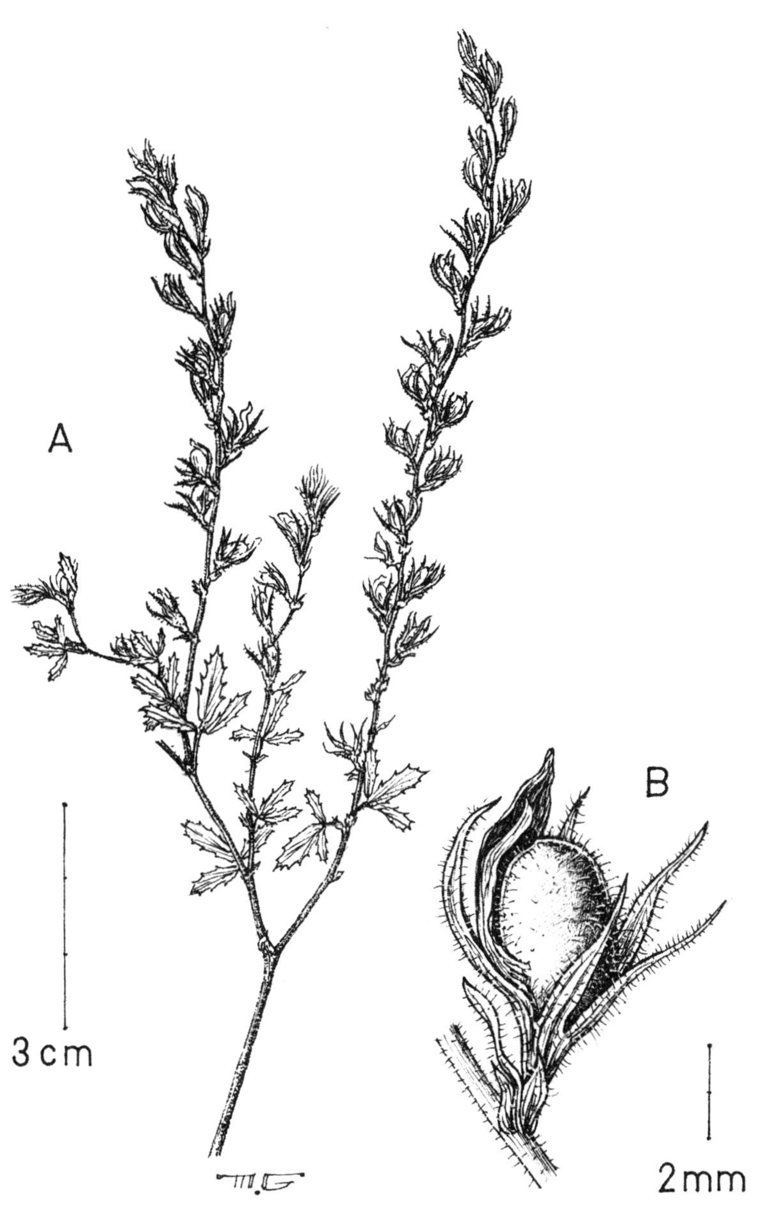

Ononis tournefortii
A. flowering and fruiting branch
B. fruit, enlarged

English: Egyptian lupin (4). French: Lupin (62); Lupin d'Egypte (4).
Uses: Seeds vermifuge, the liquid left after soaking the bitter seeds in water used as parasiticide, emollient of the skin for scurf, tinea, itch. Cataplasm of seeds emollient, resolvent; powdered dry seeds taken against diabetes (Rabat drug market). *Ref:* 17

Melilotus indica (L.) All. *Area:* Egypt to Morocco.
Names: Arabic: Handaquq murr (58, 62); Nafal (4, 42, 58); Iklil el-malek (4, 42, 62); Eshb el-malek, Reqraq, Hanini, Gourt (62); Qort (58). English: Scented trefoil (4). French: Trèfle musqué; Mélilot (42, 62).
Uses: Infusion of flowering branches emollient, antispasmodic. Seeds for diseases of genital organs of both sexes. *Ref:* 42

***Ononis spinosa** L. *Area:* Libya to Morocco.
Names: Arabic: Shirsh (4). Berber: Aoushket (62). English: Tall rest-harrow (4). French: Arrête-boeuf (4, 45).
Uses: Root diuretic. Infusion of flowers depurative; decoction of flowering branches externally used as antiseptic for eczema, infusion for kidney stones and disorders of the urinary tract. *Ref:* 24, 43, 45, 56, 62

Ononis tournefortii Cosson *Area:* Morocco.
Names: Berber: Afsdad (Rabat drug market).
Uses: Entire plant is boiled with eggs until these become hard, and patients suffering from jaundice are recommended to eat one treated egg (not the liquid) first thing in the morning for seven successive days (Rabat drug market).

Psoralea plicata Del. *Area:* Egypt, Algeria, Morocco.
Names: Arabic: Marmid (58); Djettiat, Hama (62); Qattayah, Hawmanah (4). Berber: Tareda (62). English: Bread-root, Scurfy pea (4). French: Psoralier, Pomme de prairie (4).
Uses: Infusion of leaves administered orally for respiratory and intestinal ailments. Decoction of fruits for gastric ulcers. *Ref:* 5

Retama raetam (Forssk.) Webb *Area:* Egypt to Morocco.
Names: Arabic: Retem (16, 58, 62); Retem behan (58); Besliga (62). Berber: Telit (26, 62); Alougo, Allgo (26); Tselgoust (62).
Uses: Plant used for making eye wash for eye troubles. Root used against diarrhoea. Branches febrifuge, used for treatment of wounds; powdered branches mixed with honey are emetic, given as a purgative and vermifuge, abortive in large doses. Fruits toxic. *Ref:* 12, 16, 26, 57, 62

Spartium junceum L. *Area:* Libya to Morocco. Often cultivated as an ornamental.
Names: Arabic: Tertakh, Kessaba (42, 47, 62); Bou tertakh (42, 62); Khabour, Gendoul (42); Ratam, Sitt Khadigah, Badhisqan (4). Berber: Attertag (23, 42, 62); Tegtag (23, 62); Tertag (42). English: Spanish broom, Rush broom (4). French: Genêt d'Espagne (4, 13, 23, 42, 45, 62); Spartier genêt (4).
Uses: Plant is toxic. Flowers diuretic, purgative in small doses. Seeds purgative. *Ref:* 23, 24, 42

Tamarindus indica L. *Area:* Cultivated in Egypt. Fruits sold in drug markets of North Africa are mainly imported from Sudan and tropical Africa.

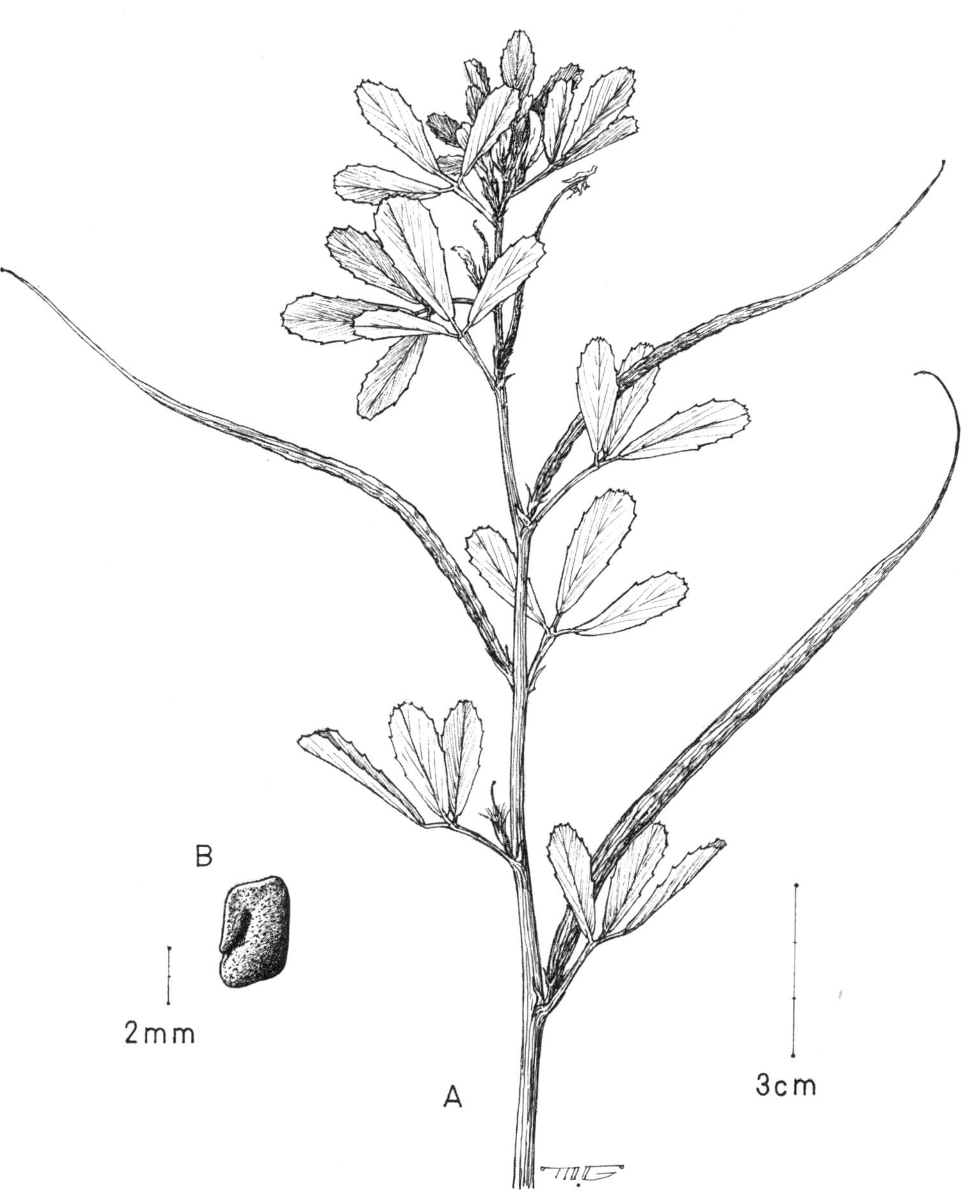

Trigonella foenum-graecum
A. flowering and fruiting branch
B. seed, enlarged

Helba

Names: Arabic: Tamr hindi (4, 5, 17); Hawmar (4, 17). Berber: Aganat (5). English: Tamarind tree (4). French: Tamarin (4, 5); Tamarnier (4).
Uses: Fruit for dysentery, coughs, fevers, sore throat, laxative; mouth wash made from fruit used against aphtha. Popular refreshing drink is prepared by soaking the pulpy fruit in water, sugar is added to taste, the drink is a mild laxative (Cairo drug market). *Ref:* 2, 5, 17

Trigonella foenum-graecum L. *Area:* Commonly cultivated in North Africa. Naturalized in several regions.
Names: Arabic: Hulba (4, 23, 42, 47, 50, 62); Helba (4, 5, 16). Berber: Tifidas (5). English: Fenugreek (4). French: Fénugrec (4, 5, 12, 16, 23, 42, 47, 50); Sénegrain (4).
Uses: Decoction of whole plant used as a seat bath for uterus affections. Seeds tonic, restorative, aphrodisiac, galactogogue, laxative, taken by women, convalescents and children to get fat, analeptic, stimulant, emollient, for gastro-intestinal troubles, anemia, broncho-pulmonary affections, febrifuge, stimulate childbirth, curative of tonsillitis and itch; cataplasm obtained by boiling the flour of seeds with vinegar and saltpeter used for swelling of spleen. *Ref:* 2, 5, 12, 16, 23, 42, 50

Vicia faba L. *Area:* Commonly cultivated in North Africa.
Names: Arabic: Foul (4, 23, 42); Baqela (4, 42); Foul hashadi (23). Berber: Djilla, Aboaun (23). English: Broad bean (4). French: Fève (4, 13, 42, 47); Fève cultivée, Fèverolle (23); Fève de marais (4).
Uses: Flowers diuretic, antispasmodic. Seeds chologogue, for hepatic and nephritic pains; two grilled beans (on a hot plate for preparing bread) nibbled first thing in the morning are considered excellent remedy for all kinds of stomach pains. *Ref:* 23, 24, 42

Vicia sativa L. *Area:* Egypt to Morocco.
Names: Arabic: Nefel, Djelban (47, 62); Douhreig (4, 58, 62); Besillet iblis, 'Eddeis (4, 58); 'Esh en-niml, Gharfala (62); Bakhr, Bakhran (58); 'Ain el-arnab (Rabat drug market). Berber: Tadjilban (62). English: Common vetch, Lints, Tare (4). French: Vesce (4, 47); Bisaille, Pasquier, Barbotte (4).
Uses: Infusion of entire plant useful for rheumatism (Rabat drug market). Seeds taken internally against smallpox and measles; cataplasm of seeds mixed with flour resolvent. *Ref:* 24

Liliaceae

Aloe perryi Baker *Area:* Drug imported from Socotra Island where the plant occurs. Popular drug in markets of North Africa.
Names: Arabic: Sabir suqutri (5, 17, 42, 60). English: Socotra aloe (60). French: Aloe (5, 42).
Uses: Dried sap of leaves (the drug) detersive, desiccative, emmenagogue, powerful purgative, improves the digestion, cathartic, insecticide, antiseptic, vermifuge, chologogue, bitter tonic. Drug is rarely used by itself (toxic in moderate doses), but usually mixed with gum Arabic, honey or sugar, tonic, stomachic, for amenorrhea, jaundice, dyspepsia. *Ref:* 2, 5, 17, 60

***Androcymbium gramineum** (Cav.) McBride *Area:* Egypt to Morocco.
Names: Arabic: Kershout (60, 62); Shge'at el-arneb (5, 62); Shge'a, Lofut (5); Te-

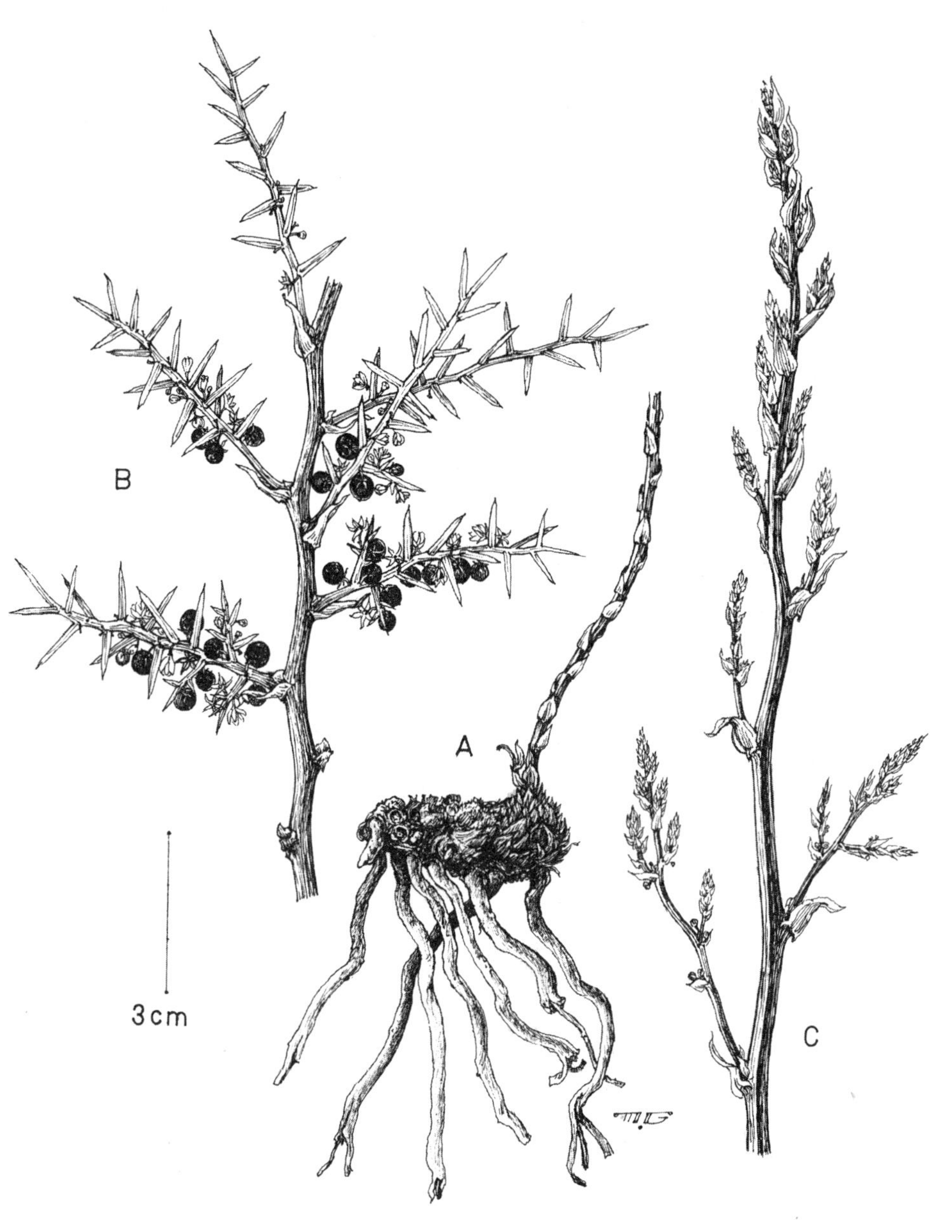

Asparagus stipularis
A. basal part with roots, B. flowering and fruiting branch
C. young shoot

qout (8); Kikout, 'Akreish, Becid (62). Berber: Afahlehlé-n-aheddan (62).
Uses: Plant is toxic to man and animals. Corms antimitotic, contain colchicine which is known to cause pain and congestion if applied to the skin; when inhaled it causes violent sneezing, internally it increases the amount of bile poured into the intestine.
Ref: 2, 5, 8, 60, 62

***Asparagus stipularis** Forssk. *Area:* Egypt to Morocco.
Names: Arabic: Shouk (47, 60, 62); Haliyun (5, 42, 47, 60, 62); Sekkoum (42, 47, 62); Shebrog, 'Aneb ed-dib (47, 62); 'Aqoul el-gabal, Serr (60). Berber: Azzou (5, 42, 62); Tazzawt (5, 62). French: Asperge (5, 42).
Uses: Roots for syphilis; infusion of tuberous roots used to remove renal stones (Bedouins, Mediterranean region, Egypt); infusion of pounded roots for headache. Decoction of whole plant diaphoretic; young tender shoots appetizer, stomachic, diuretic, for jaundice, liver ailments, rheumatism; berries, shoots and roots stomachic, appetizer; decoction of shoots and roots for the treatment of syphilis; the plant fried with eggs and camel's fat is spermatogenic, aphrodisiac, facilitates secretions and releases obstructions. Decoction of seeds for hemorrhoids.
Ref: 5, 42, 57, 60

***Asphodelus aestivus** Brot. *Area:* Egypt to Morocco.
Names: Arabic: Belwaz (62, Algiers drug market); 'Onsal, Berwaga (62); 'Onsol, Belouza, Belozet el-'onsol, Sowai (60); Berwag (5, 12, 42). Berber: Ingri (5, 62); Tiglish, Taziout, Hirri, Aouti (62). French: Asphodèle (42).
Uses: Cataplasm of leaves antirheumatic. Rubbing the body with roasted tubers and drinking the decoction of leaves and scapes is a good remedy for withering and paralysis. Dried tubers cooked in oil and poured into the ear at the opposite side where the sick tooth is; this oil also used as ear drops to treat ears discharging liquids (Algiers drug market). Powdered dried tubercles mixed with barley flour are used as dressing against ulcers and abscesses of the breast; ash of tubercles diuretic and often used as eye powder against leucoma of the cornea. Powdered dry tuberous roots are locally applied to abscesses; exposing body to fumigated dry, tuberous roots is said to help against jaundice. Fruits for treating earache and acute toothache.
Ref: 5, 12, 42, 60

Colchicum autumnale L. *Area:* Tunisia to Morocco.
Names: Arabic: Khamira (23, 37, 47, 62); Qatel el-kelb (23, 47, 62); 'Okna, Sourendjan (4, 47, 62); Hafer el-mohar (47, 62); Asabi' hermes (62); Khamal, Lahlah (4). English: Meadow saffron, Colchicum, Naked ladies, Autumn crocus, Purple crocus (4). French: Safran bâtard (4, 23); Colchique (37, 45, 62); Tue chien, Colchique d'automne, Safran d'automne (4); Bulbes de Colchique, Safran des prés (23).
Uses: Plant contains colchicine, a compound capable of preventing cell division, unfortunately too toxic to use against cancer; plant is classic treatment for acute arthritis, renal disorders, dropsy and asthma. Corms and seeds used in homeopathy; seeds for gout, arthritis, rheumatism, diuretic, purgative. *Ref:* 2, 23, 37, 45, 56

***Urginea maritima** (L.) Baker *Area:* Egypt to Morocco.
Names: Arabic: 'Onsul, 'Onsel, 'Onsal, 'Onseil (4, 5, 8, 13, 42, 47, 60, 62); Far'on (8, 23, 47, 60, 62); Basal Far'on (5, 42, 60, Algiers drug market); Basal el-far (4, 5, 13, 42, 47, 62); Silla (13, 47, 62); Buseil (40, Rabat drug market); Basul, Basal el-

kelb; 'Onsul bahari (60); Sam el-far (4). Berber: Ichkil (13, 23, 62); Isfil, Ikfilen, Lobsol bouchen, Ibsel idam (13, 62). English: Medicinal squill, Sea onion (4, 60); Squill (4). French: Scille maritime (4, 13, 47, 62); Oignon marin (4); Scille (5, 42, 45). *Uses:* Handling of all parts of plant causes irritation to the skin. Bulb is toxic to man and rats. Two varieties of bulbs are known: red and white. Red squill is mainly dried and powdered to furnish a rat poison; white squill is used in treatment of heart diseases and to prepare cough mixtures, diuretic. Fresh slimy bulbs applied to wounds and tumors for healing, expectorant in bronchitis, chronic catarrh and pneumonia; in strong doses emetic, cathartic and upsets the nerves. Fresh bulb is vesicant, rubefacient, anthelmintic, useful for rheumatism, oedema and gout; its cardiac action is like that of *Digitalis,* slowing down the pulse and increasing its strength, emmenagogue, abortive, aphrodisiac. Dried powdered bulbs made into tablets, sucked slowly in the mouth against internal tumors (Rabat drug market); infusion of dried bulb strong purgative (Algiers drug market). *Ref:* 5, 8, 13, 23, 45, 60

Linaceae

Linum usitatissimum L. *Area:* Commonly cultivated in North Africa.
Names: Arabic: Kettan (4, 13, 23, 37, 42, 62). Berber: Tifert (13, 23, 42, 62); Delkmouch (13, 23, 62). English: Common flax (4). French: Lin (23, 42, 37, 45, 62).
Uses: Seeds laxative, soothing and pain-relieving; infusion of seeds good for inflammation of digestive and urinary tracts, antidiarrhoeic, often mixed with *Althaea* flowers. Seeds used in preparation of cataplasms for their emollient properties against boils and inflammations. *Ref:* 23, 37, 42, 45, 56

Loranthaceae

Viscum cruciatum Sieber ex Boiss. *Area:* Morocco.
Names: Arabic: Bontouma (62); Lenjbar (23, 42). Berber: Taburzigt (5, 13, 42). French: Gui (5, 13, 42); Gui rouge (62).
Uses: The plant enters in preparation of plasters for bone fractures, sprains and contusions, general tonic, large doses cardiotoxic, astringent, emetic, for epilepsy, hysteria, asthma. *Ref:* 5, 13

Lythraceae

***Lawsonia inermis** L. *Area:* Commonly cultivated in North Africa.
Names: Arabic: Henna (4, 5, 13, 23, 42, 50, 62; flowers: Faghia (5, 13, 23, 62). Berber: Hamella, Rhanni, Diabé, Foudeoum, Lalle (13). English: Henna, Egyptian privet, Alcanna, Camphire (4). French: Henné (4, 5, 13, 16, 23, 42, 45, 50, 62); Alcanna (4).
Uses: Leaves astringent, antiseptic, vulnerary, for wounds and burns, used in the preparation of numerous eye lotions and antirheumatic liniments, for leprosy. Flowers insecticide. *Ref:* 5, 13, 16, 23, 42, 50

Lythrum salicaria L. *Area:* Tunisia to Morocco.
Names: Arabic: Rihanet el-maa (23, 47, 62); Sabun el-'aris (23, 62); Farandal (4).

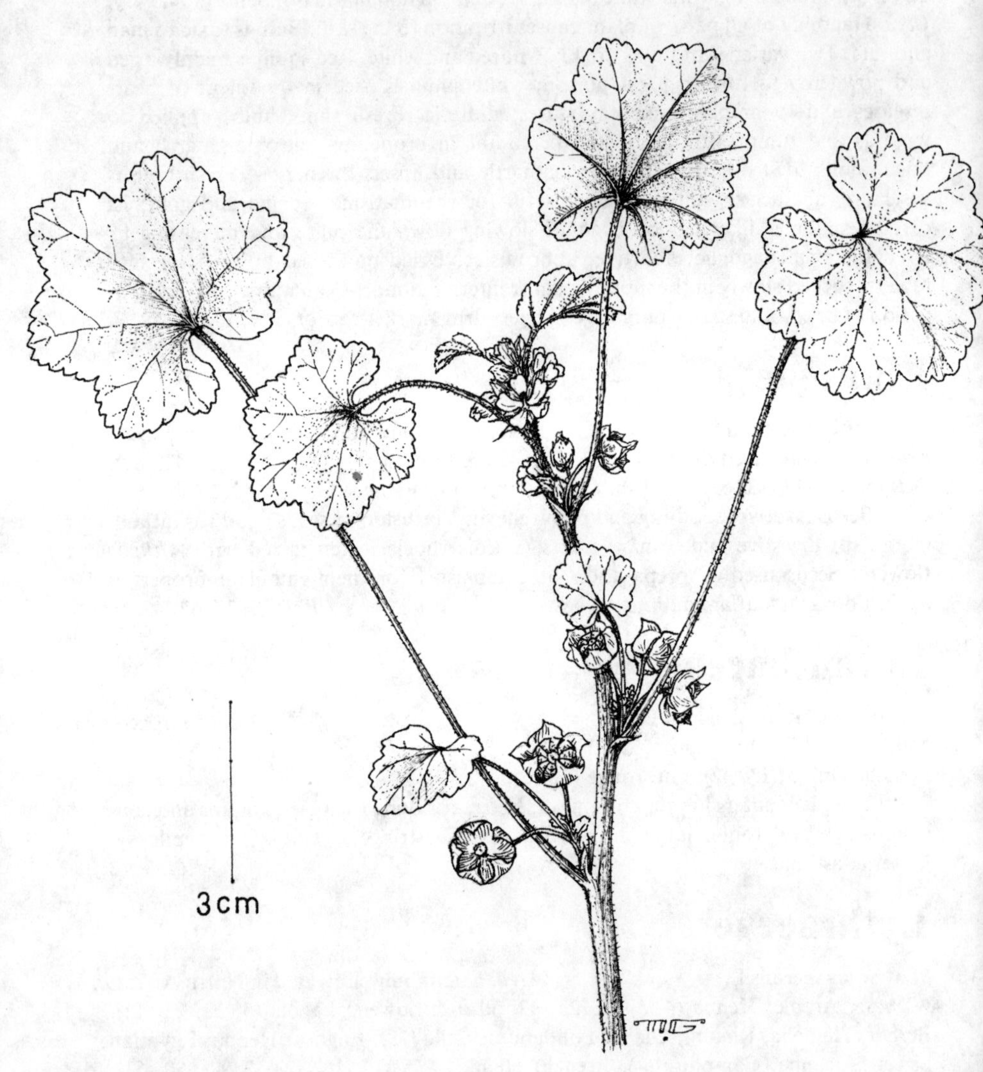

Malva parviflora

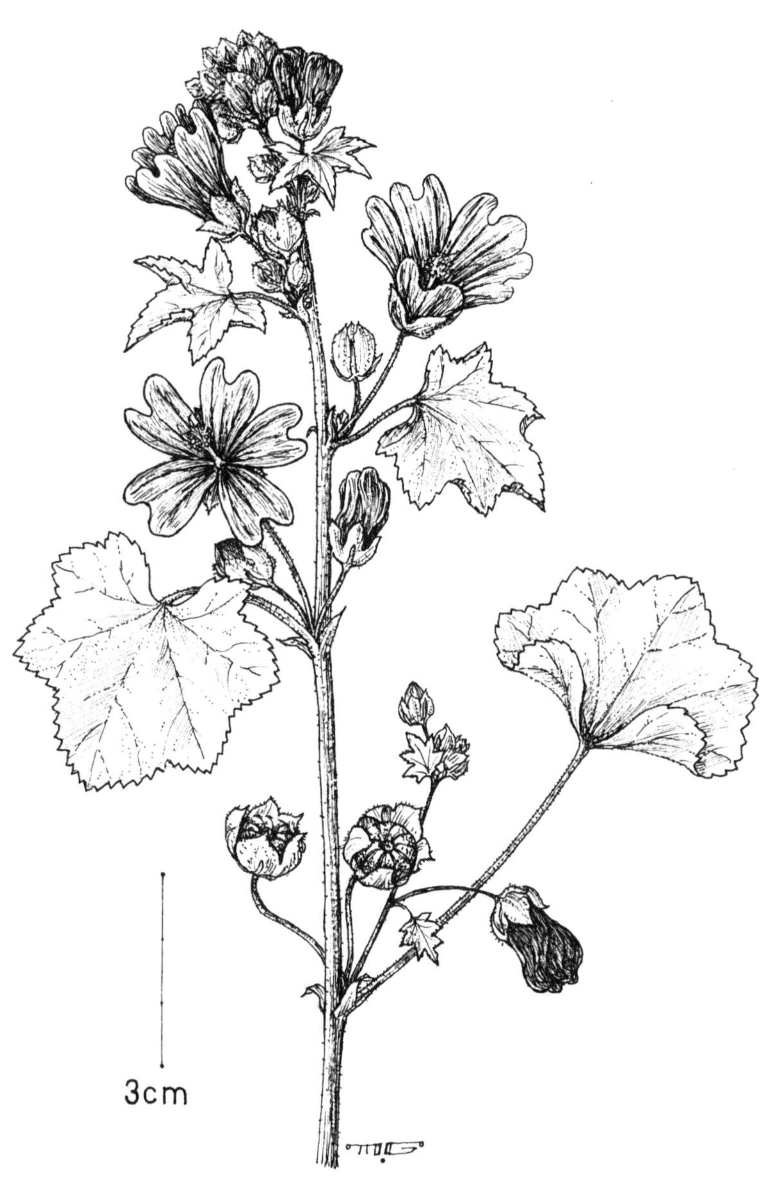

Malva sylvestris

English: Purple loosestrife, Willow weed (4). French: Salicaire (23, 45, 62); Lysimaque rouge (23); Salicaire commune, Lysimachie rouge (4).
Uses: Flowering tips antidiarrhoeic, vulnerary, astringent, hemostatic, tonic, used for dysentery especially for babies in the form of an infusion, powder or tincture. *Ref:* 23, 24, 45

Malvaceae

Althaea officinalis L. *Area:* Tunisia, Algeria.
Names: Arabic: Lamedij (5, 47, 62); Ward ez-zawan (5, 42); Khitmi (4, 5, 42); Medjir, Khobaiza, Medja el-abiad (62). Berber: Tibinsert (42, 62); Tibisrennit, Binesar (62). English: Marsh mallow, White mallow (4). French: Guimauve (5, 62); Guimauve officinale (4, 45).
Uses: Infusion of plant emollient against cough, decoction used against blennorrhagia. Root and leaves emollient. Root, leaves and seeds for bronchial and throat catarrhs, chronic coughs. Root chewed by children to reduce pains due to the appearance of first teeth, cures the incontinence of urine. Cataplasm of root for the treatment of tumor. *Ref:* 5, 42, 45

Malva parviflora L. *Area:* Egypt to Morocco.
Names: Arabic: Khobbeiza (5, 58, 62); Raqma, Raqmiya (58); Khobbeiza reziza (62); Bqula (5). Berber: Amedjir, Imejjir, Mejjir, Tibb, Ibeqqoula (62). French: Mauve (5, 62).
Uses: Root chewed or rubbed into the gums for pyorrhea. Infusion of flowering and fruiting branches used as a gargle for their astringent properties, prescribed for people on diet, for gastro-intestinal ailments, bechic, emollient. Seeds and leaves used as a cataplasm, rectal injection or gargle according to the case. *Ref:* 5, 15

Malva sylvestris L. *Area:* Egypt to Morocco.
Names: Arabic: Khobbeiza (4, 23, 42, 58, 62); Raqma, Raqmiya (58); Ad-dahma (4). Berber: Amedjir (23, 62); Mamejjirt (42); Imejjir, Mejjir, Ouabejjir, Djir, Ibeqqoula (62). English: Common mallow, Marsh mallow (4). French: Grande mauve (4, 23, 45); Fromageon (4, 23); Mauve (23, 42, 62); Fouassier (23); Mauve sauvage, Meule (4).
Uses: Leaves and flowers soothing, pectoral, mild astringent, intestinal stimulant, laxative in large doses; infusion for digestive and urinary diseases; externally used as decoction for bathing, a gargle for inflammations of the skin and mucous membranes; emollient, pectoral; used against all occular ailments; infusion for cough and diarrhoea. *Ref:* 23, 45, 56

Moraceae

Ficus carica L. *Area:* Commonly cultivated and often naturalized in North Africa.
Names: Arabic: Tine (4, 62); Karm, Kerma (42, 62); fruit: Karmus (42, 62). Berber: Tazert (42, 62); Taguerourt, Tanaglet, Tamazate, Tamehit, Azart; fruit: Bakhis, Emohi (62). English: Common fig tree (4). French: Figuier (4, 42, 45, 62); Carique (4).
Uses: Wood ash used as antipoison. Leaves for treatment of eyes: red and painful

conjunctiva are rubbed with the leaves and then subjected to a bath of rose water in which pounded bitter almonds were soaked; apparently the leaves with their villous surface perform a good cleansing of the eyelids. Dry pounded leaves mixed with honey cures white leprosy; decoction of leaves erases freckles. Fruits used in preparation of antipoisons, diuretic, emollient, laxative; fermented fruits distilled to yield strong alcoholic liquour, usually perfumed by anise, excellent tonic. *Ref:* 42, 45

Morus alba L. *Area:* Commonly cultivated in North Africa. Introduced from China.
Names: Arabic: Tout, Tout abyad (4); Touta, Tout helw, Tout el-harir (62). Berber: Tatoutet, Atoukelissa (62). English: White mulberry (4). French: Mûrier (62); Mûrier blanc (4, 5, 45);
Uses: Root bark antitussive and expectorant in asthma, bronchitis, cough; diuretic, resolvent. Leaves antipyretic; leaf febrifuge, vulnerary. Fruit considered tonic in neurasthenia, insomnia, hypertension. *Ref:* 24, 34

Myristicaceae

***Myristica fragrans** Houtt. *Area:* Imported from India to drug markets of North Africa.
Names: Arabic: seed: Gouz et-tib, Gouz bouwa (4, 5, 42); bark: Dar sini (42). English: Nutmeg (4). French: Muscadier (4, 5, 42, 45).
Uses: Bark aromatic, often used as tonic, stimulant and calefacient. Nut prescribed for bad digestion, aphrodisiac, dangerous even in moderate doses, enters in numerous prescriptions, mainly as stimulant; diminishes pains of circumcision for children. *Ref:* 5, 42, 45

Myrtaceae

Eucalyptus globulus Labill. *Area:* Commonly cultivated in North Africa.
Names: Arabic: Calibtus (42, Rabat drug market); Kafur (4). English: Eucalyptus, Blue gum tree (4). French: Eucalyptus officinal (45); Eucalyptus, Gommier bleu (4, 24).
Uses: Leaves antispasmodic, antiseptic for respiratory tracts, astringent, febrifuge, tonic, anticathartic, antiseptic; crushed dried leaves smoked as cigarettes against asthma and ailments of respiratory system. Dried leaves and flower buds mixed with henna leaves *(Lawsonia inermis)* are crushed and used as shampoo, a good hair tonic (Rabat drug market). Essential oil diaphoretic, expectorant, insecticidal, oestrogenic. *E. rostrata* Schlecht. *(E. camaldulensis* Dehnhardt) may be used in the same way as *E. globulus.* *Ref:* 2, 23, 24, 45

Myrtus communis L. *Area:* Libya to Morocco. Cultivated in Egypt.
Names: Arabic: Mersin (4, 8, 13, 62); Rihan (5, 8, 13, 23, 37, 42, 62, Rabat and Algiers drug markets); Aas (4, 5, 13, 42, 62); Shalmun (13, Algiers drug market); Halmoush (13). Berber: Tarihant (13, 23, 24, 62). English: Myrtle (4). French: Myrte (4, 5, 13, 23, 42, 45, 62).
Uses: Infusion of the whole plant stimulant, antidiarrhoeic. Roots astringent. Infu-

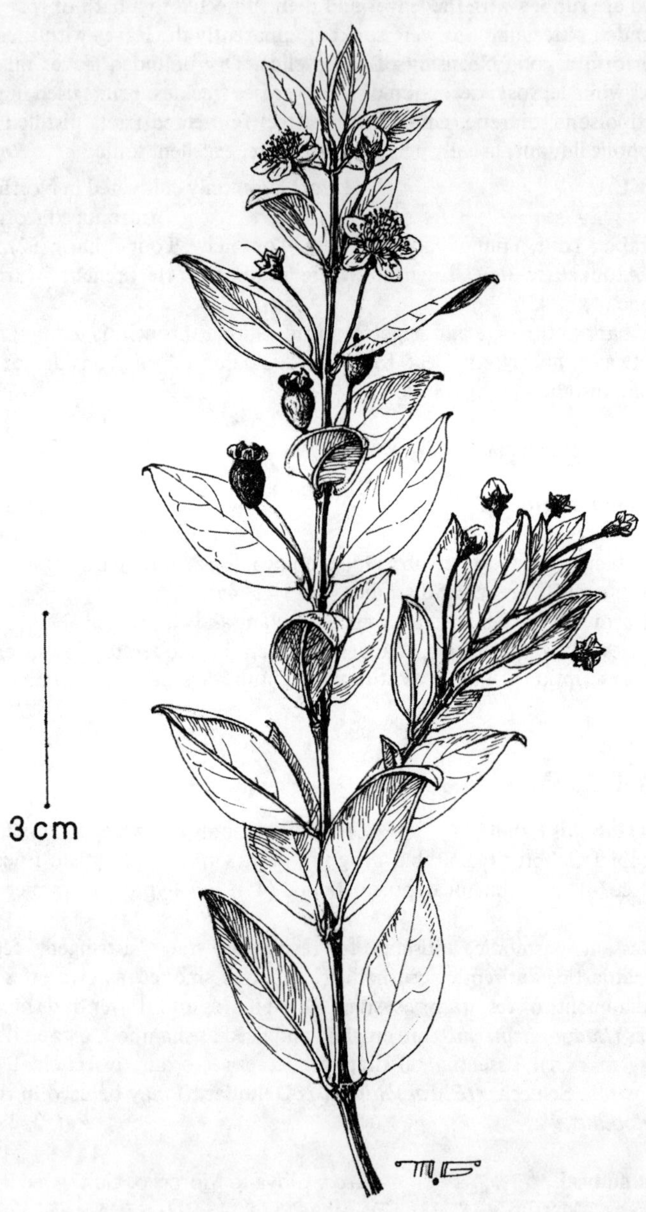

Myrtus communis

sion of leaves and young branches excellent remedy for asthma (Algiers drug market). Leaves stomachic, astringent, antiseptic for the respiratory system; infusion of leaves for respiratory ailments and as cataplasm for painful organs, antidiarrhoeic; decoction of leaves used to blacken the hair. Dry leaves and flowers mixed with other aromatic herbs used for preparing hair lotions; leaves tonic, aromatic, used for preparation of "Water of the Angle" by distillation, for the extraction of an antiseptic essence, in perfumery. Leaves fumigant or cataplasm, soothe pains of abscesses and boils; infusion of leaves used as eye lotion. Leaves mixed with shampoo to serve as hair tonic (Rabat drug market), essential oil obtained by distillation is a pulmonary antiseptic. Dry flower buds for smallpox; decoction of flowers has a beneficial regulatory action on the blood circulation. *Ref:* 5, 8, 13, 23, 42, 45

***Syzygium aromaticum** (L.) Merr. *Area:* Imported to markets of North Africa.
Names: Arabic: Qoronfel (4, 5, 42); Qoronfel abiad (4); 'Oud en-nuwwar (5, 42). English: Clove tree (4); dried flower buds: Cloves (64). French: Giroflier (4, 5); Girofle (42); flower buds: Clous de girofle (5, 42).
Uses: Dried flower buds (cloves) diuretic, odontalgic, stomachic, tonicardiac; aromatic condiment, condiment with carminative and stimulant properties.
Ref: 5, 42

Nyctaginaceae

***Boerhavia repens** L. *Area:* Egypt, Libya, Algeria, Morocco.
Names: Arabic: Moddeid, Meddad (58); Kharad (62). Berber: Ailelé (62); Amwashar, Tamoshalet (5).
Uses: Entire plant is purgative, emetic, antisyphilitic. *Ref:* 5

Oleaceae

***Fraxinus angustifolia** Vahl *Area:* Tunisia to Morocco.
Names: Arabic: Dardar (23, 37, 42, 62); Sella, Messharwan; fruit: Lesan el-'asfour (23, 62); Lesan et-teir (62). Berber: Asseln, Taslent, Islène, Taboushisht (23, 62); Islel, Asel, Sell (62); Azlen, Touzzelt (42). French: Frêne de kabylie (23, 42, 62).
Uses: Decoction of bark febrifuge. Leaves antirheumatic, laxative, febrifuge, purgative, diuretic; infusion of leaves useful for cough (Rabat drug market). Fruits used as condiment; infusion of fruits has an agreeable taste, tonic and aphrodisiac.
Ref: 3, 37, 42

Olea europaea L. *Area:* Many cultivars are known in North Africa. The wild var. *sylvestris* Brot. occurs from Libya to Morocco.
Names: Arabic: cultivated varieties: Zaytun (4, 5, 23, 42, 62); Amourgha (23, 62); wild variety: Zebboudj (5, 23, 42, 62); Zebbour (23, 62). Berber: cultivated varieties: Azemmour (5, 23, 62); Zzit, Tzetta (23, 62); Thatimt, Amil (62); wild variety: Azeboudj, Tazbboujt (23, 62). English: cultivated: Olive tree (4); wild: Wild olive tree (4). French: cultivated: Olivier (4, 5, 23, 42, 45, 62); wild: Olivier sauvage (4).
Uses: Decoction of olive wood used as remedy for mouth ailments such as aphtha, stomatitis, etc.; the same decoction if applied on the abdomen has the curious effect of stopping diarrhoea. Decoction of leaves for cough. Leaves astringent, hypoten-

sive, antidiabetic, chologogue; extracts of leaves hypoglycemic, diuretic, antibacterial. Olive oil chologogue, for hepatic ailments, chronic constipation, asthenia, bad appetite; oil from wild fruits used as antidote against all poisons, hair tonic. Olive oil is an excellent purgative with no side effects; mixed with flour, it is used as a plaster for boils and abscesses. *Ref: 2, 5, 23, 37,42, 45*

Orchidaceae

Aceras anthropophorum (L.) Ait.fil. *Area:* Tunisia to Morocco.
Names: Arabic: Faham (23, 42, 62). French: Homme pendu (32, 62); Faham d'Algérie, Pantine, Ophrys homme (23).
Uses: Leaves sedative, aromatic, diaphoretic; infusion tonic, stimulant, aphrodisiac. *Ref:* 23, 42

Orobanchaceae

***Cistanche phelypaea** (L.) Coutinho *Area:* Egypt to Morocco.
Names: Arabic: Danun (4, 5, 12, 42, 58, 62); Turfas (4, 58); Zob el-ard (42, 58); Zob en-nasrani (26, 42); Tartut, 'Asi rebbo (42); Danun el-gin (4); Zob ed-dib (58); Tartut el-kelb, Zob el qa'a (62); Zob er-roumi (12). Berber: Deris (26, 42, 62); Zimzellil, Temzelit, Aboushel-n-tekkouk (62); Idergis (26); Barru (11).
Uses: Aspect of plant gives the reputation of being aphrodisiac; diuretic. Thick lower part of plant dried and powdered for use against diarrhoea; aphrodisiac and tonic in speratorrhea impotence. Dried powdered plant mixed with camel's milk is employed as cataplasm against contusions. *Ref:* 12, 26, 34, 42, 62

Paeoniaceae

***Paeonia coriacea** Boiss. *Area:* Algeria, Morocco.
Names: Arabic: Fawaniya, 'Oud es-salib (42, 62); Ward ez-zawan (42). Berber: Telfa-giddaoun (42, 62). French: Pivoine (42, 62).
Uses: Roots, flowers and seeds, in decoction with honey, absorbed as antispasmodic, to act against the convulsions of infants or epilepsy attacks, to calm rebellious coughs. Decoction of flowers facilitates contractions of the uterus which is useful during childbirth, also used as abortive. *Ref:* 42

Palmae

Hyphaene thebaica (L.) Mart. *Area:* Egypt, Libya.
Names: Arabic: Doum (4, 5, 58, 59, 62); Shagaret el-muql (4, 59); Toufi (62); resin: Muql makki (59); El-hashal (5). Berber: Tazait, Soubou, Faraoun (62); Zgallem, Zglem (5). English: Doum palm, Ginger bread tree (4, 59). French: Doum, Palmier doum (4); Doum oriental, Doum d'Egypte (5).
Uses: Thick roots used for treatment of bilharziasis. Resin from tree diuretic, diaphoretic, recommended for tapeworm; resin used against bites of poisonous animals. Fruit astringent. *Ref:* 5, 59

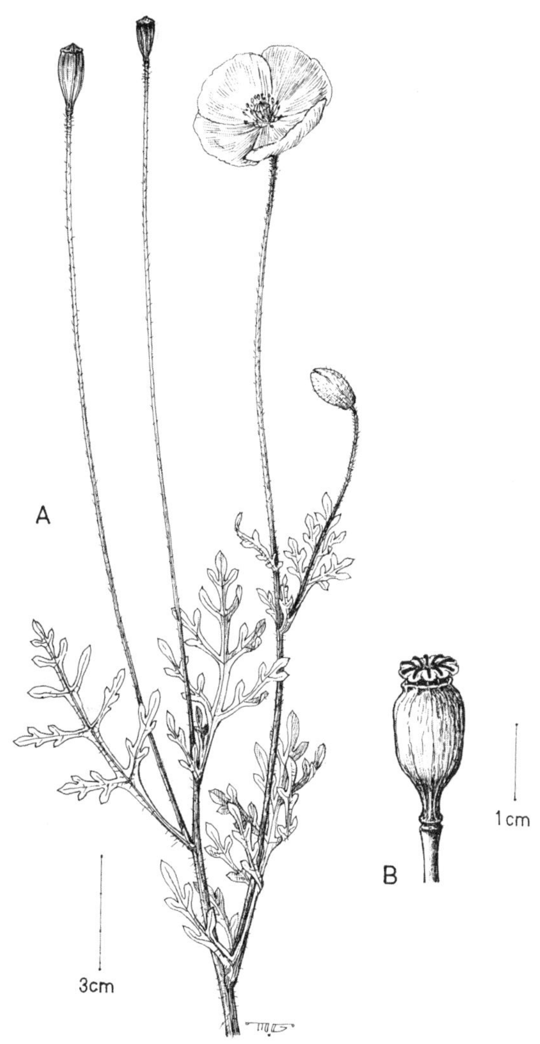

Papaver dubium
A. flowering and fruiting branch
B. ripe fruit, enlarged

Phoenix dactylifera L. *Area:* Egypt to Morocco. Cultivated and subspontaneous. *Names:* Arabic: Nakhl (4, 59); Nekhla (5, 42, 62); El-nakheil (59); fruit: Balah, Tamr (59); Blah, Ttmer (5); numerous names also given to different varieties and different parts of the tree, for details see 5, 59, 62. Berber: Tanekht, Tazdait, Tafinaout, Isgaren, Hazdacht (62); Agjjuf, Tayniyut (5); fruit: Tiyni (5). English: Date palm (4, 59). French: Dattier (62); Palmier-dattier (5, 42).
Uses: Date palm wood is used as toothbrush. Terminal bud "djoummar" for intestinal hemorrhage, diarrhoea, jaundice. Dates were used internally in medications designed to purge, to clear the enigmatic, or to regulate the urine; in vaginal pessaries, with other ingredients, they enhance fertility; relieve cough and are flesh-forming; juice of boiled dates is given to invalids to restore their strength and to assuage thirst. Green dates reputed as aphrodisiac and tonic. Kernels of dates made into cataplasm used against ulcers of genital organs; ash of kernels used to prepare an eye lotion against blepharitis. *Ref:* 5, 12, 15

Papaveraceae

Papaver dubium L. *Area:* Egypt to Morocco.
Names: Arabic: Belna'aman (62, Rabat drug market). Berber: Tadjira, Adekkoush (62).
Uses: Infusion of capsules given to children suffering from measles (Rabat drug market).

Papaver rhoeas L. *Area:* Egypt to Morocco.
Names: Arabic: Ben na'aman (13, 23, 42, 62); Zaghlil (4, 13, 58, 62); Khushkhash manthur (4, 13, 62); Deydahan (4); Qebaboush (42, 62). Berber: Tadjibout (13, 23, 62); Taloubat, Tadjira, Flilou (13). English: Corn poppy, Field poppy (4). French: Coquelicot (4, 13, 23, 24, 42, 45, 62); Ponceau, Pavot des moissons (4).
Uses: Capsules (often mixed with those of *Papaver somniferum*) used as soporific for babies and act against cardiac affections. Flowers and grains pectoral, calmative, emollient, slightly narcotic, sudorific, expectorant. Syrup produced from the flower used as sedative to soothe coughs. *Ref:* 13, 23, 24, 42, 45, 56

Papaver somniferum L. *Area:* Cultivation prohibited by law in North Africa. Naturalized in some regions from old garden plants.
Names: Arabic: Bou en-noum (13, 23, 24, 47, 62); Abou en-noum (4, 17); Khashkhash aswad (4, 5); Boundi (47); Boudi (23, 62); Harir igran (23, 62); Kheshkhash (13, 62); the drug: Afioun (5, 13, 42, 62). Berber: Tilidout (13, 42). English: Opium poppy, Poppy (4). French: Pavot (4, 23, 42, 47, 62).
Uses: Opium, the dried latex from capsules, analgesic, narcotic. Capsules used for intestinal disorders, chest ailments, cough, diarrhoea, all sorts of pains, soporific for babies, mild sedative, external and internal stimulant, antispasmodic, emmenagogue, calmative, for genital ailments of women. Capsules used in preparation of beverage against cough, especially for babies, other components are a decoction of *Lavandula angustifolia, Cuminum cyminum* and *Mentha pulegium*.
Ref: 2, 5, 17, 23, 42, 45

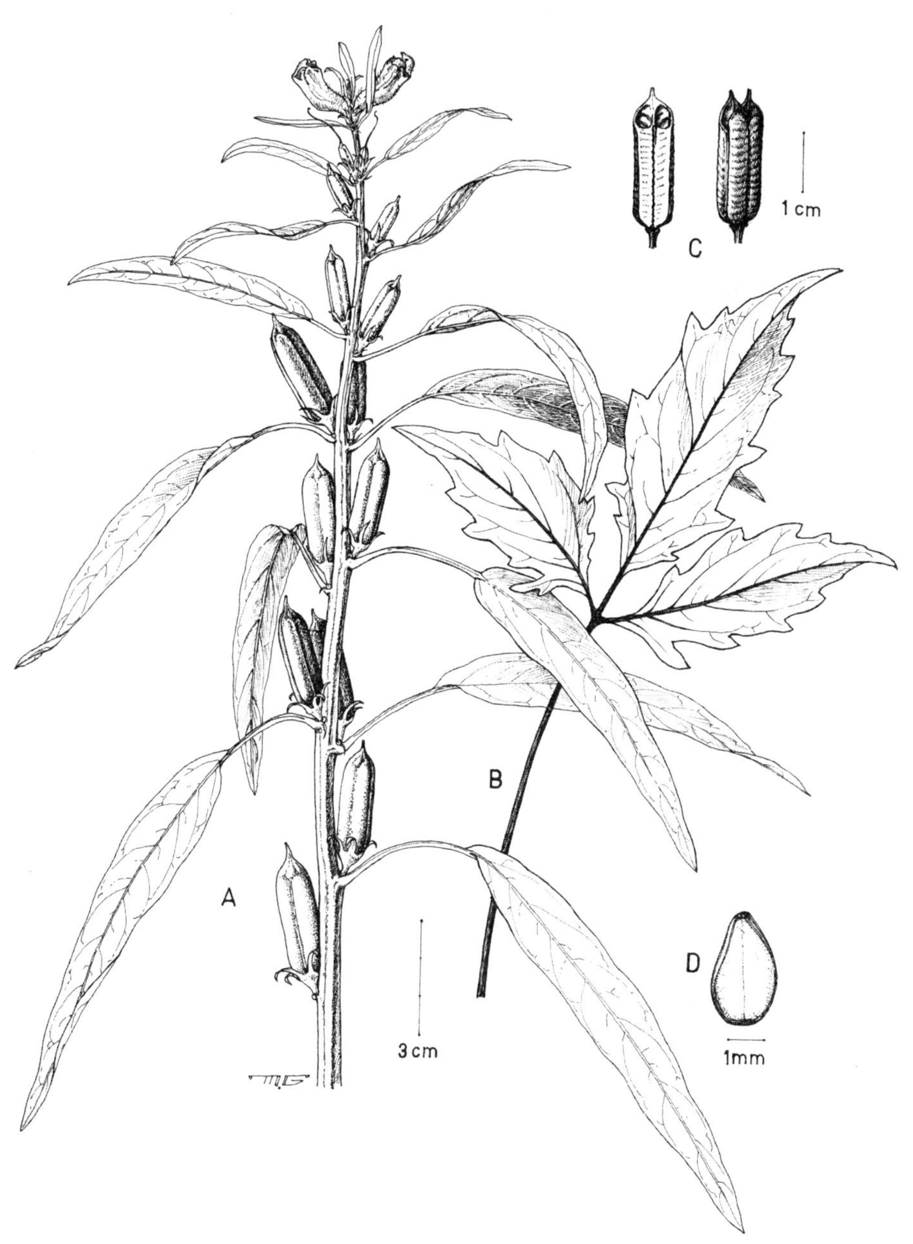

Sesamum indicum
A. flowering and fruiting branch, B. basal leaf
C. ripe fruits, D. seed, enlarged

Pedaliaceae

***Sesamum indicum** L. *Area:* Frequently cultivated in North Africa. Subspontaneous in Morocco.
Names: Arabic: Simsim (4, 5, 17, 42, 62); Jeljlan (5, 42, 62); Hall (5, 42). English: Sesame, Gingelly, Gingil (4). French: Sésame (4, 5, 17, 62); Sésame de l'Inde (42).
Uses: Seeds prescribed as lenitive in scybalous constipation, nutrient tonic in degenerative neuritis, neuroparalysis. Oily seeds known for their nutritive value, roasted seeds prescribed to convalescents and to mothers after childbirth to increase the secretion of milk. Roasted seeds emmenagogue, abortive, pulmonary affections, stomach inflammations; oil softens the skin, used against itching cracks of the skin.
Ref: 5, 17, 34

Pinaceae

Cedrus atlantica (Endl.) Carrière *Area:* Endemic to Algeria and Morocco.
Names: Arabic: Meddad (42, 47, 62); Erz, Lerz (42, 62). Berber: Beguoun (47); Igdil (42); Inguel, Iguengen, Idgel, Iblez, Edgeish, Abawal, Arzaq, Larisq (62). English: Atlas cedar, Atlantic cedar (4). French: Cèdre de l'Atlas (4, 42, 47); Cèdre (62).
Uses: Tar produced by dry distillation of wood used for dermatitis, especially in veterinary medicine. Oil produced from wood used against liver affections.
Ref: 42, 62

Pinus halepensis Miller *Area:* Libya to Morocco. Cultivated in Egypt.
Names: Arabic: Senouber (62); Sanawbar (4); Sanoubar (42); Snouber (42, 47); seeds: Zgougou (42, 62). Berbcr: Taida (42, 47, 62); Amelzi (42); resin: Ouazouri (42, 62); seeds: Igengen (42). English: Aleppo pine, Jerusalem pine (4). French: Pin d'Alep (4, 42, 47, 62); Pin de Jérusalem, Pin blanc (4).
Uses: Powdered bark externally applied to wounds for its astringent properties. Tar produced by dry distillation of wood used as antiseptic for treatment of wounds and the skin. Seeds mixed with honey (taken first thing in the morning) spermatogenic.
Ref: 42

Piperaceae

Piper cubeba L. fil. *Area:* Imported to the drug markets of North Africa.
Names: Arabic: Kababah, Habb el-'arous (4, 42); Kebbaba (5, 62); Kababa hindiya, Kababa tchini (42); Kababa sini (Cairo drug market). English: Cubeb pepper, West African black pepper (4). French: Cubèbe (4, 5, 42); Poivre cubèbe (62); Poivre à queue (4).
Uses: Fruits condiment, tonic, stimulant, aphrodisiac; mixed with honey, it is used to cure blennorrhagia and urinogenital disorders. Fruits disinfectant for the urinary tract, especially for chronic catarrh of the bladder. *Ref:* 5, 17, 42

Piper nigrum L. *Area:* Imported to the drug markets of North Africa.
Names: Arabic: Felfel aswad (4, 5, 42); Felfel akhal (5, 42). Berber: Lyebzar (5). English: Black pepper (4). French: Poivre noir (4, 42); Poivre (5, 42); Poivrier commun (45).

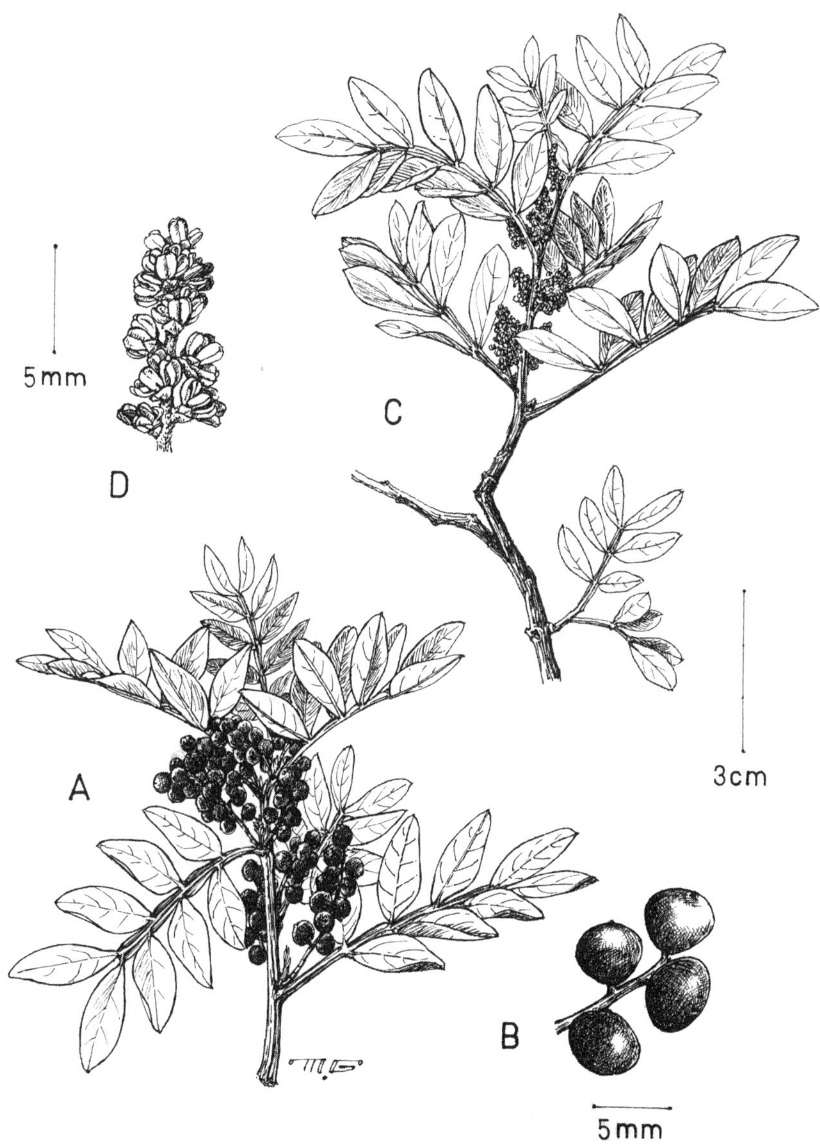

Pistacia lentiscus
A. fruiting branch of female plant
B. branchlet of female inflorescence, enlarged
C. flowering branch of male plant
D. branchlet of male inflorescence, enlarged

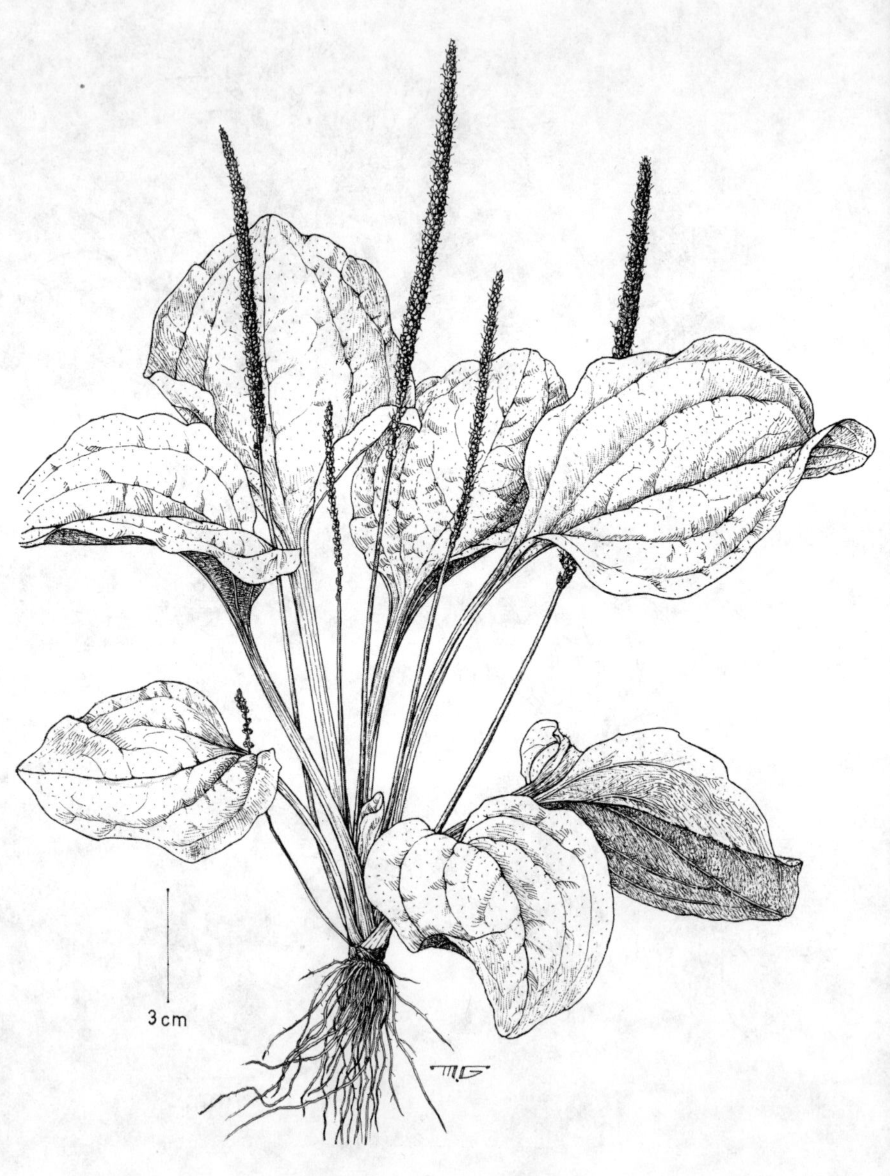

Plantago major

Uses: Fruits condiment, aphrodisiac, carminative, stomachic, diuretic, galactogogue, emmenagogue, odontalgic, for cough; mixed with oil it is used by rubbing in the treatment of acne, freckles, melanoderma and leprosy; fruits tonic, stimulant for digestive functions. *Ref:* 5, 42, 45

Pistaciaceae

***Pistacia atlantica** Desf. *Area:* Egypt to Morocco.
Names: Arabic: Botoum (5, 42, 47, 62); fruit: Hawdja, Khathiri, Gatouf (62); resin: 'Alk el-anbat (42, 62). Berber: Lggt (5, 62); Iggt (47); Idj, Iqq, Tecemlall; fruit: Gueddain; galls: Liez-ou-illeg (62). English: Atlantic pistacio (9). French: Pistachier de l'Atlas (5); Betoum (62).
Uses: Leaves used as plaster for scrofula. Fruits, with a slightly acidic taste, used to season dates. Kernel often used in pastry. Galls for tanning. *Ref:* 5, 9, 42

Pistacia lentiscus L. *Area:* Egypt to Morocco.
Names: Arabic: Derw (23, 62, Rabat and Algiers drug markets); Dirw (23, 62); Dro, Darw (5, 42); Fustuq sharqi, Shagar el-mastika (4); Battoum (9). Berber: Tidekt (5, 42); Tidekst, Tadist, Imidek (23, 62); Fethies, Fadhiss (62); fruits: Gueddain (23, 62); Goudhim, Goudhoum (62); bark: Dhou (42). English: Lentisk, Mastic tree (4, 9). French: Lentisque (4, 5, 23, 42, 62).
Uses: Resinous exudation of the tree is known as "mastic" and employed as analgesic and sedative in gastralgia, cardiodynia, mastitis, peptic ulcer, boils, carbuncles, also as antitussive and expectorant. Resin prescribed as a nervous calmative (infusion in tea) and emmenagogue, chewed to purify the breath, enters in cosmetic products and in depilatory creams. Resin boiled with milk is used for throat troubles; for ulcers, a teaspoonful of mastic pounded and mixed with an equal amount of honey is taken first thing in the morning for three weeks. Decoction of root for cough (Algiers drug market). Dried and fumigated bark of the trunk and branches is locally applied to facilitate childbirth. Infusion of leaves diuretic, astringent, emmenagogue. Peeled nuts yield an oil by hot extraction which is effective against itch and by rubbing for treating rheumatism. *Ref:* 5, 12, 34, 42

Plantaginaceae

***Plantago afra** L. *Area:* Egypt to Morocco.
Names: Arabic: 'Asloudj (23, 42, 62); Merwash, Harmola (23, 62); Zarqottouna (5, 23, 62); Umm rwis (62); Hashishet el-baraghit (4); seeds: Bizr qotuna (4, 17, 42, 58); Bezer (42, 62); Berghousti (23, 62); Lisan el-hamal (42). English: Flea-wort (4). French: Herbe aux puces (4, 23, 62); Psyllium (4, 5, 23, 42, 62); Pucière (23).
Uses: Leaves and roots have the same uses as those of *Plantago coronopus.* Seeds, previously mixed with milk overnight, are used against all sorts of dysentery, gastroduodenal ulcers, diarrhoea, chronic constipation. Seeds emollient, mechanic purgative; decoction of seeds or seeds soaked in water used as emollient and cooling agent for renal and urinary affections and inflammations, as well as in cases of internal hemorrhoids. *Ref:* 5, 17, 23, 42

Plantago coronopus L. *Area:* Egypt to Morocco.
Names: Arabic: Wideina (4, 58); Rjel el-ghorab (5, 62); Lsan el-hamal, Lsan el-begri, Lmeshasha (5); Bou djenah, Gern el-ail, Derhis (62). Berber: Tawalment (62). English: Buck's-horn plantain, Star of the earth (4). French: Plantain (5); Plantain corne de cerf, Corn de cerf, Coronope (4).
Uses: Roots used for hemorrhoids, malaria and fevers. Powdered leaves are locally applied to all sorts of wounds, burns, abscesses, bites, inflammations; leaves astringent, hemostatic, vulnerary, immediate analgesic. *Ref:* 5

Plantago major L. *Area:* Egypt to Morocco.
Names: Arabic: Lisan el-hamal, Massasah, Lisan hamad (4, 58); Mesaisa, Seif el-maa, Uzeina (23, 62); Weden el-djedd, Berraq (62); Warraq saboun (58). Berber: Agoucin bourioul (23, 62). English: Waybread, Greater plantain (4). French: Grand plantain (4, 23, 62); Plantain majeur, Plantain des oiseaux (4).
Uses: A decoction, a syrup and an aqueous extract are made from entire plant to treat bronchial catarrh, bronchitis, asthma and pulmonary tuberculosis. Roots, leaves and seeds astringent, depurative, calmative, emollient. Leaves used externally to heal wounds, varicose, ulcers; as a gargle it soothes sore throats. Leaves mild astringent, used as eye drops against conjunctivitis and blepharitis. Seeds diuretic, expectorant. *Ref:* 23, 24, 34, 56

Plumbaginaceae

Plumbago europaea L. *Area:* Tunisia to Morocco.
Names: Arabic: Swak er-ra'ian (23, 42, 62); Djouz er-ra'ian, Tefel el-djouza (23, 62); Shitaradj (42); Hashishet el-asnan (4). English: Toothwort, Lead-wort (4). French: Dentelaire (4, 23, 24, 42, 62); Plombagine, Malherbe (4).
Uses: Root used for mouth care, gives a good color to the gums and whitens the teeth, dried powdered roots used for cutaneous affections and wounds; roots vesicant, odontalgic. *Ref:* 23, 42

Polygonaceae

Polygonum aviculare L. *Area:* Egypt to Morocco.
Names: Arabic: Gerda (23, 37, 62); 'Assa er-ra'i (4, 62); El-betbat, Bou'aggad (5); Qordab, Qoddab, (58). Berber: Mesenzer mazir (23, 62). English: Knot-grass, Centinode, Knot-weed, Armstrong (4). French: Centinode, Trainasse (4, 23); Renouée des oiseaux (4, 5, 23, 37, 45); Herbe à cochon (4).
Uses: Plant astringent, vulnerary, hemostatic. Decoction of entire plant recommended for enteritis, diarrhoea, dysentery, bronchitis. Leaves and stems diuretic, anthelmintic, antidiarrhoeic; externally employed as emollient, astringent for hemorrhoids, pruritus, chancroid. *Ref:* 5, 13, 23, 34, 37, 45, 56

Polygonum maritimum L. *Area:* Egypt to Morocco.
Names: Arabic: Zaita (42, 50); Qordab (58). French: Renouée maritime (42).
Uses: Infusion of leaves and roots astringent and antidiarrhoeic, decoction or cataplasm used to reduce swellings and soothe burns. *Ref:* 42, 50

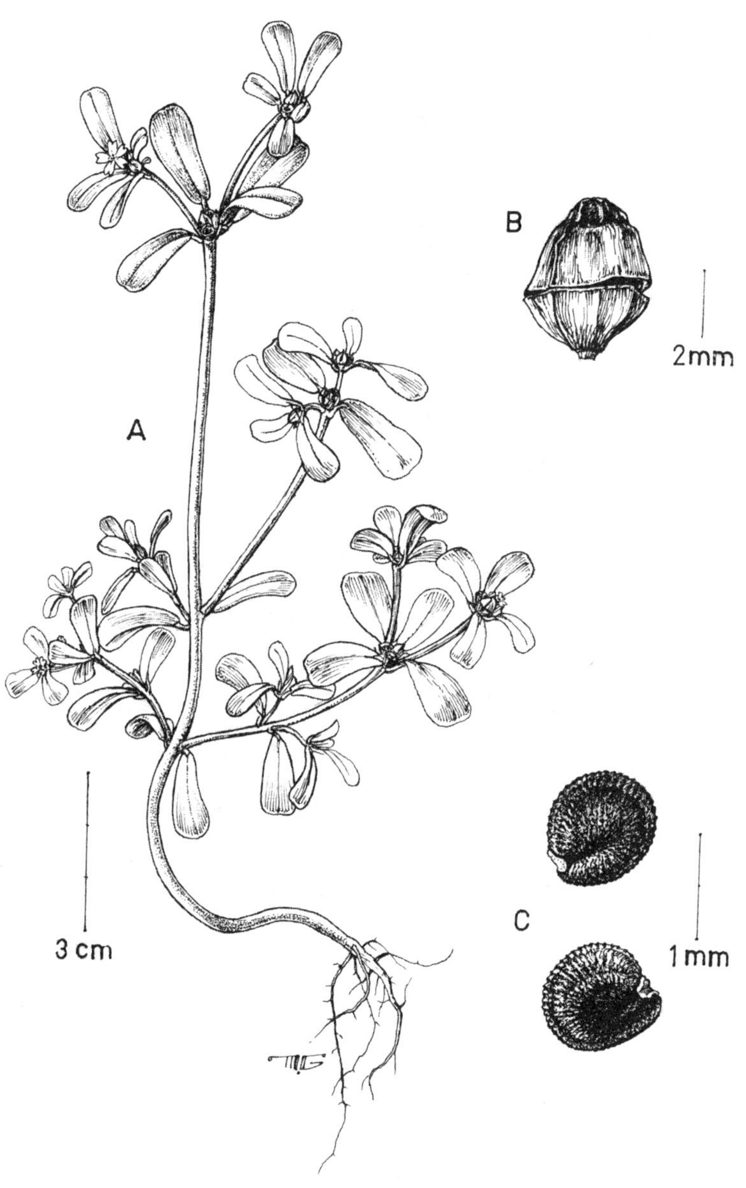

Portulaca oleracea
A. flowering and fruiting plant
B. ripe capsule, enlarged, C. seeds, enlarged

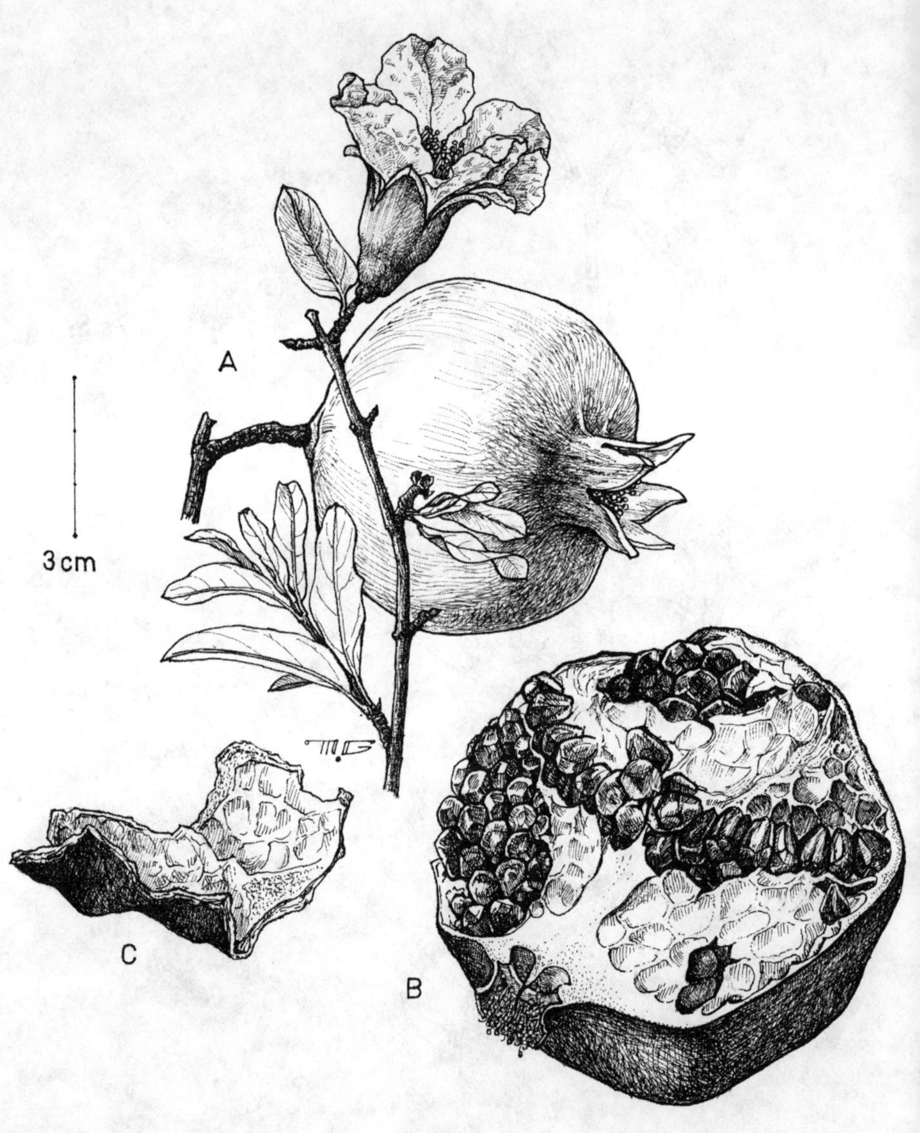

Punica granatum
A. flowering and fruiting branches
B. open fruit exposing the berries
C. dry leathery fruit coat after removing the berries

***Rumex vesicarius** L. *Area:* Egypt to Morocco.
Names: Arabic: Hommad (4, 5, 58, 62); Hanbeit (4, 58, 62); Qorissa (5, 62); Goulglam (62). Berber: Brisemmou (62); Tasemmumt (5). English: Sorrel, Bladder-dock (4). French: Oseille sauvage (5); Oseille d'Amérique (4).
Uses: Plant is eaten fresh against jaundice, hepatic conditions, constipation, calculus, bad digestion. *Ref:* 5

Polypodiaceae

Polypodium vulgare L. *Area:* Tunisia to Morocco.
Names: Arabic: Basbayedj (4, 62); Adras el-kelb (4, 42, 62); Ma'as (42, 62); Basfayedj (42); Thaqib el-hajar (62); Tashtiwan (4). Berber: Achtouan, Ishhouane (42, 62); Tastiwan (42); Shtiwal (62). English: Common polypody, Polypody wall fern, Golden locks (4). French: Polypode (42, 62); Polypode commun, Polypode de chêne (4).
Uses: Rhizome constitutes the drug; decoction is laxative, for indigestion and pains of rheumatic origin, expectorant, mild astringent, chologogue. *Ref:* 24, 42

Portulacaceae

Portulaca oleracea L. *Area:* Egypt to Morocco.
Names: Arabic: Rigla (4, 5, 42, 58, 62); Rashad (58); Hurfa (4); Baqlet el-hamqa, Baqlet el-mubareka (5, 62); Farfah (5); Dhou el-keffin, Aben drag, Brabra, Ornoba, Bou el-kazit, Berdougala, Bleibsha (62). Berber: Tafrita (42, 62); Rejla, Arhilem, Bouguel, Benderakesh (62). English: Purslane, Garden purslain (4). French: Pourpier (4, 5, 42, 62); Pourcellaine, Pourpie potager (4).
Uses: Whole plant is antiphlogistic and bactericide in bacillary dysentery, diarrhoea, hemorrhoids, enterorrhagia; enters into prescriptions as antidiabetic; externally used as cataplasm of fresh leaves for maturing of abscesses; whole plant anaphrodisiac, emollient, calmative, diuretic, refreshing agent, antiscorbutic, vermifuge. Seeds calmative and slake thirst. *Ref:* 5, 24, 34, 42

Punicaceae

Punica granatum L. *Area:* Commonly cultivated in North Africa.
Names: Arabic: Romman (4, 5, 13, 23, 42, 62, Cairo, Algiers and Rabat drug markets); flowers: Djolanar (23, 42, 62). Berber: Taroumant, Armoun (13, 23, 24, 62); Tarmint, Aroumane (13, 62). English: Pomegranate (4). French: Grenadier (5, 23, 42, 45, 62).
Uses: Root bark antihelmintic. Bark of the tree vermifuge. Bark and root astringent, vermifuge if taken as decoction. Peel of the fruit excellent astringent (Cairo drug market), dried powdered peel used for ulcers of the digestive tract, antidiarrhoeic, astringent, hemostatic, for cleansing the teeth and to strengthen the gum (Rabat drug market), its decoction is used as a vaginal plug for treating leukorrhea. Entire fruit is bechic and for pectoral troubles, acidic fruits astringent and diuretic, effective against diseases resulting from air infection and against plague; sweet fruits for affections of the digestive tract; leaves and fruit peels strong astringent, antidiarrhoeic

as infusions. Flower buds mild astringent. Seed oil shows uterine relaxant activity and oestrogenic effects. *Ref:* 2, 5, 13, 15, 23, 42

Ranunculaceae

Adonis aestivalis L. *Area:* Libya to Morocco.
Names: Arabic: Nab el-djemel (26, 42, 62); 'Ain el-hadjla (23, 42 62); Soufrat el-molouk (13, 42); Ben en-na'aman (13). Berber: Ouqil boulrhoun (13, 42, 62); Taynanast (13, 42); Tit-n-tacekourt (13, 62). English: Summer adonis, Tall adonis, Summer pheasant's eye (4). French: Adonis goutte de sang (42); Adonide estivale, Oeil de perdrix, Adonide d'été (4).
Uses: Entire plant is emmenagogue; infusions diuretic, febrifuge, cardiotonic for certain heart diseases. *Ref:* 26, 42, 45

***Adonis annua** L. *Area:* Tunisia to Morocco.
Names: Arabic: Nab el-djemel (4, 23, 62); Ben na'aman, 'Ain el-hadjla, 'Ain el-bouma, Shoubbetan, Nettin, Bougraouna, Zaghlil (23, 62). Berber: Ouqil boulrhoun (23, 62). English: Pheasant's eye, Autumn adonis (4). French: Adonis goutte de sang (23); Goutte de sang, Adonide automnale (4).
Uses: Entire plant tonicardiac and diuretic like *Digitalis,* used against hydropsy and gout. *Ref:* 23, 24

Clematis flammula L. *Area:* Libya to Morocco.
Names: Arabic: 'Ansara (4, 13, 42, 62); Nar berd (42, 62); Sebenq (13, 62); Qamis bent-el-malek (4, 62). Berber: Touzimt, Azenzou (13, 42, 62). English: Sweet virgin's-bower (4). French: Clématite brûlante (42); Clématite (62); Clématite flammette, Clématite odorante (4, 13).
Uses: Plant used externally for its revulsive and vesicatory properties against fall in body temperature and for treating itch; internally used as hydrogogue and strong purgative, diaphoretic, diuretic, for scabies and cancer. *Ref:* 13, 24, 42

Delphinium staphisagria L. *Area:* Tunisia to Morocco.
Names: Arabic: Ashasha (23, 62); Zbib el-jbel (4, 5, 17, 42); Zbib barri (4, 17); seeds: Habb er-ras (5, 17, 23, 42, 62). English: Stavesacre, Lousewort (4). French: Staphysaigre (4, 5, 23, 42, 62); Herbe aux poux, Dauphinelle staphisaigre (4).
Uses: Pulverized seeds poisonous, externally used as a parasiticide to kill head lice; infusion or decoction of seeds prescribed against neuralgia and as aphrodisiac; decoction or powdered seeds externally used for itch and skin diseases, emetic. *Ref:* 5, 17, 23, 42, 45

Nigella sativa L. *Area:* Commonly cultivated in North Africa. Subspontaneous in Algeria, Morocco.
Names: Arabic: Kammun aswad (4, 5, 17, 23, 42, 62); Sanoudj (5, 17, 23, 42, 62); Habba souda (4, 5, 17, 42, 62); Habbet el-barakah (4, 17, 42); Kammun el-akhal (16). Berber: Zerara (5, 23, 42, 62); Tikammin (5, 42, 62). English: Black cumin, Common fennel flower (4). French: Nigelle (4, 5, 23, 42); Cumin noir (4, 23); Toute épice, Quatre épice, Araignée (4).
Uses: Seeds poisonous to man in high doses, mixed with honey and taken first thing in the morning to stimulate appetite; seeds remedy for toothache, headache, in-

testinal parasites, abortive, antipoison, tenicide, resolvent, also take part in the treatment of influenza, migraine, sinusitis, asthma, respiratory affections, paralysis, hemorrhoids, leprosy, general antidote for poisonous bites. Seed oil popular remedy for cough and bronchial asthma; seeds used for delayed menses, flatulence, respiratory oppression, obtundent in toothaches, diuretic, emmenagogue, carminative, vermifuge, galactogogue, antispasmodic. *Ref:* 5, 17, 39, 45, 56

***Ranunculus macrophyllus** Desf. *Area:* Libya to Morocco.
Names: Arabic: Keff el-djerana (47, 62); Kaff el-hirr, Kaff ed-dabb; Kaff as-sabu', Nowar el-mdilla; root: Ouden el-hallouf (42). Berber: Telbaout (26, 42, 62). French: Renoncule (26, 42).
Uses: Root crushed and mixed with honey makes an appreciated purgative, emetic, antipoison. *Ref:* 42

Ranunculus sceleratus L. *Area:* Egypt, Tunisia to Morocco.
Names: Arabic: Zaghlil (4, 13, 62); Zaghalanta (4, 58). English: Marsh crowfoot, Celery-leaved crowfoot, Water celery (4). French: Renoncule scélérate (4, 13, 24).
Uses: Tincture from fresh plant used in treatment of skin conditions such as herpes, eczema, erysipelas, pruritus, and rheumatic conditions such as sciatica, arthritis, rhinitis. Plant appetizer, tonic, useful for asthma, gonorrhoea, ulcers. *Ref:* 13, 56

Resedaceae

Reseda luteola L. *Area:* Egypt to Morocco.
Names: Arabic: Bliha (4, 58, 62); Liroun (5, 42, 62); Asfar (42, 62); Tefshoun, Bekkem (58, 62); Islih, Bou sreira, Eimim (5); Khozama (58). Berber: Fezmir (42, 62); Tefchoune (42); Tellemt izimer (62). English: Dyer's weed, Weld, Yellow weed, Dyer's rocket (4). French: Gaude (4, 45, 62); Faux réséda de teinturiers (4).
Uses: Infusion of entire plant used for stomachache and diarrhoea. Infusion of leaves antidiarrhoeic. *Ref:* 5, 42

Rhamnaceae

Rhamnus alaternus L. *Area:* Libya to Morocco.
Names: Arabic: Qased, 'Oud el-kheir (13, 23, 62); Zafrin (4); Mlila (37). Berber: Ajrourj (13, 23, 62); Khalis-n-imidkh, Mlila, Meliles, Amlilis (62). English: Alaternus, Barren privet (4). French: Alaterne (4, 23, 24, 37, 62); Bourg-épine (4).
Uses: Bark emctocathartic. Leaves and root rich in tannin, astringent. Berries mild purgative, laxative. *Ref:* 2, 23, 24, 37

Ziziphus lotus (L.) Lam. *Area:* Egypt to Morocco.
Names: Arabic: Sedra (5, 26, 42, 62); Sidr (5, 8, 42); Sidr barri (4); fruit: Nabq (5, 42, 62); Dall (4, 62); Gheshwa (62); wood stock: Maraq es-sedra (62). Berber: Hozouggart, Tazoura, Azarkur, Azar, Tazouggert, Amzmem, Bazezour, Ouari; fruit: Tabakat (62); Azarem (26). English: Lotus jujube (4, 8); Lotus tree, Wild jujube (4). French: Jujubier sauvage (4, 42, 62); Lotus des anciens, Jujubier des totophages (4).
Uses: Fruits used for making pectoral cough drops and for preparing a tonic, febrifuge, tonic, prescribed for convalescents, active against furuncles, measles and

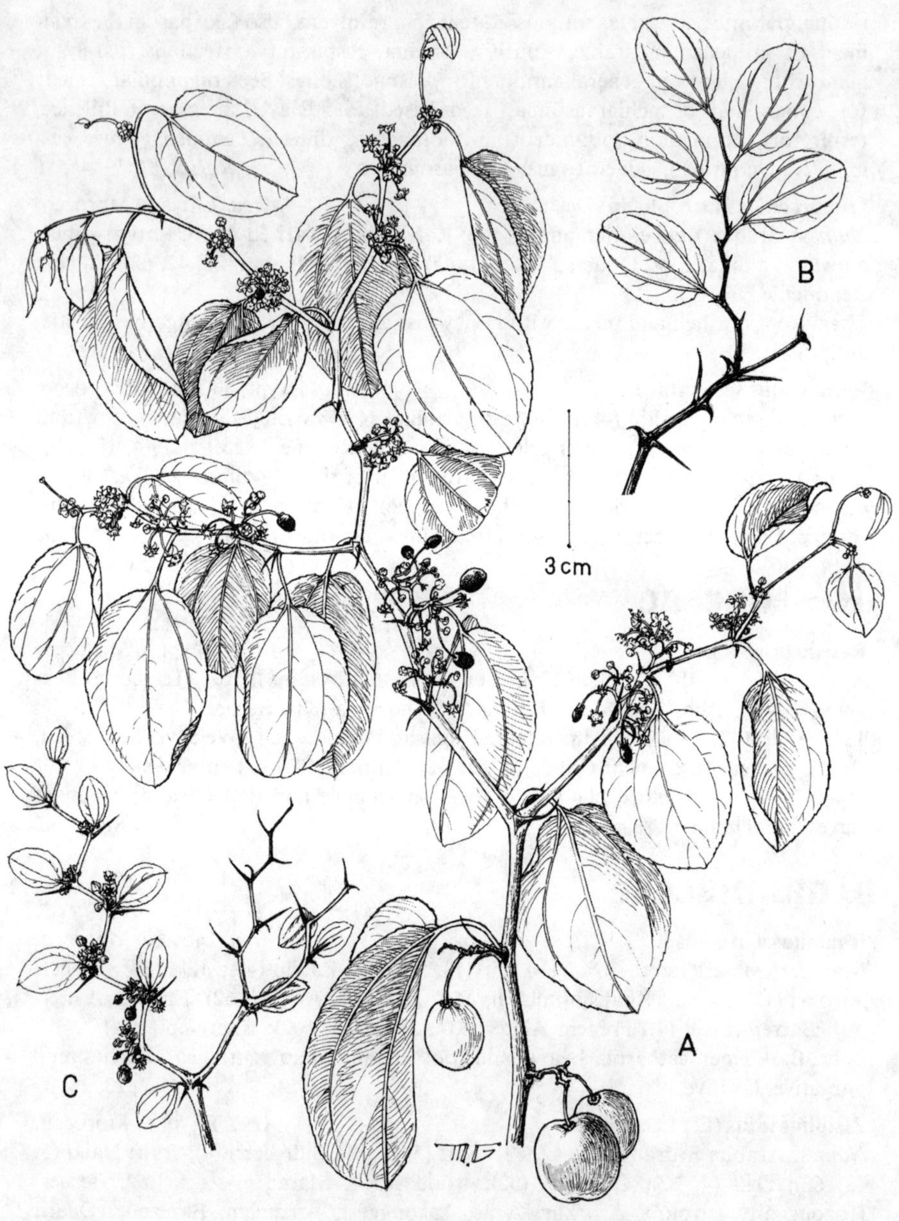

Ziziphus spina-christi
A. flowering and fruiting branch of a cultivated tree
B. vegetative branch of a wild tree
C. *Ziziphus lotus*

smallpox, emollient, tonic. *Ref:* 2, 5, 8

Ziziphus spina-christi (L.) Willd. *Area:* Egypt to Morocco. Also cultivated.
Names: Arabic: Zegzeg (42, 62); Zefzouf, Ardj, Ourdj, Ghassel (62); Sidr (4, 58, 62); fruit: Nabq (4, 58, 62). Berber: Abaqua (42, 62); Korna (62). English: Christ's thorn, Nabk tree (4). French: Nabca, Epine du Christ (4).
Uses: Ash of the wood, mixed with vinegar, is prescribed for local applications in the treatment of serpent bites. Infusion of leaves astringent, anthelmintic, antidiarrhoeic. Cataplasm of leaves for abscesses and furuncles; cataplasm of fresh green leaves is put on swollen eyes (probably due to certain inflammations) before going to bed (Bedouins, Egypt). Fruits enter in infusions used as febrifuges, emollients and laxatives; infusion of fruits is a reputed remedy of measles. *Ref:* 42

***Ziziphus zizyphus** (L.) Meikle *Area:* Frequently cultivated in North Africa. Subspontaneous in some regions.
Names: Arabic: Zefzouf, Zfeizef, Hridj (23, 62); fruit: 'Unnab (4, 23, 42, 62). Berber: Tabakath; fruits: Bazegzour (23, 62). English: Jujube tree, Indian jujube (4). French: Jujubier (4, 23, 24, 37, 45, 62); Gingeolier (4); fruits: Jujubes (23).
Uses: Leaves anthelmintic, antidiarrhoeic. Fruits bechic, for pectoral ailments, emollient, calmative, anticatarrhal, slightly diuretic. *Ref:* 12, 23, 24, 37, 45

Rosaceae

Agrimonia eupatoria L. *Area:* Tunisia to Morocco.
Names: Arabic: Ghafith (4, 23, 62); Terfaq, Garmoulya (23, 62). Berber: Abolask (23, 62). English: Agrimony, Cockle bur, Liverwort (4). French: Aigremoine (4, 23, 45, 62); Eupatoire, Soubeirette (4); Herbe de Saint-Guillaume (23).
Uses: Flowering branches astringent, diuretic, slightly emmenagogue and anthelmintic, used for chronic liver diseases, vulnerary, for diarrhoea, affections of liver and kidneys. *Ref:* 23, 24, 45

***Crataegus monogyna** Jacq. *Area:* Tunisia to Morocco.
Names: Arabic: Bou mekherri (23, 37, 62); Baba adjina (42, 62); Za'rur al-awdiyah, Ash-shawka al-haddah (4); Zu'rur, Tuffah el-muzzah (42). Berber: Admam (23, 42, 62); Atemen, Idmine (23, 62); Izmine, Demamai (62). English: Hawthorn, White thorn, May-bush (4). French: Aubépine (4, 23, 24, 37, 42, 45, 62); Epine blanche (4, 23); Epine de mai (23); Noble épine, Senelles (4).
Uses: Flowers antispasmodic, tonicardiac; infusion of flowers for chronic diarrhoea, hypotensive, for insomnia and palpitation, nerve sedative. *Ref:* 23, 24, 37, 42, 45

Fragaria vesca L. *Area:* Frequently cultivated in North Africa. Probably spontaneous in Algeria.
Names: Arabic: Tout el-ard (23, 37, 62); Tout el-qa'a, Tout en-nasara (23, 62); Shlayk, Frawlah (4). English: Common strawberry (4). French: Fraisier sauvage (24, 47); Fraisier des bois (4); Fraisier (4, 37, 45, 62).
Uses: Rhizome astringent, antidiarrhoeic. Leaves and rhizome diuretic. Fruits slightly laxative, appetizer, refreshing agent, calmative. *Ref:* 23, 24, 37, 45

Geum urbanum L. *Area:* Tunisia to Morocco.
Names: Arabic: Hashishet el-mabrouka (23, 62); Hashishet el-mubarek (4). English:

Wood avens, Herb-bennet, Avens (4). French: Bénoîte (4, 23, 45, 62); Herbe de Saint-Benoît (23); rhizome: Racine giroflée (23).
Uses: Rhizome tonic, astringent, febrifuge, stimulant. *Ref:* 23, 24, 25

Potentilla reptans L *Area:* Tunisia to Morocco.
Names: Arabic: Ben tabis (23, 62); Bentalis (37). English: Cinquefoil, Five finger grass, Five leaf (4). French: Quintefeuille (4, 23, 24, 37, 45); Potentille rampante (4).
Uses: Rhizome astringent, febrifuge, depurative, antidiarrhoeic, stomachic, antiscorbutic, febrifuge. *Ref:* 23, 24, 37

Rosa canina L. *Area:* Tunisia to Morocco.
Names: Arabic: Ward ez-zeroub, Nab el-kelb (23, 62); Ward es-sini, Ward es-siyag, Ward barri (4); Nisrin, Nesri (42); fruit: Bou soufa (23, 62). Berber: fruit: Achdirt, Tigourma (23, 62); Tafrha, Azenzou (62). English: Dog rose, Heprose, Canker flower, Dog briar (4). French: Eglantier (4, 23, 37, 62); Rosier des chiens, Rosier sauvage (23); Rose sauvage, Eglantine (4).
Uses: Fruit astringent, antidiarrhoeic, diuretic, antiscorbutic. *Ref:* 23, 37, 42, 62

Rosa damascena Miller *Area:* Cultivated in North Africa. Naturalized in Morocco.
Names: Arabic: Ward djouri (4, 62); Ward (5, 26, 42, 62, Rabat drug market); dry flower buds: Sekoura (62); Zirr el-ward (Cairo drug market), Entifa, Glaoua, Skoura, Daddès, Filaly (26). Berber: Taaferd (26, 42). English: Damask rose (4). French: Rose de Damas (4, 42, 62); Rose de quatre saisons (4).
Uses: Dried flower buds are used for stomach pains and toothache; distilled water from the roses takes part, by aspersion or local application, in the treatment of fevers, migraine, dizziness, nausea, otitis, irritability and anxiety; distilled water from the roses is used as eye lotion for red and painful eyes, mixed with vinegar it has a calmative action on the cephalics. Petals are hemostatic; powdered and mixed with oil, they are used in the treatment of nasal, auricular and blennorrhagial affections. Dried flower buds are mixed with leaves of *Lawsonia inermis* and *Myrtus communis* for use as hair tonic (Rabat drug market). *Ref:* 5, 42

Rubus ulmifolius Schott *Area:* Libya to Morocco.
Names: Arabic: ’Allaiq, Lendj; fruit: Tout el-khela (23, 62). Berber: Anjjil; fruit: Tabga (23). French: Ronce (23, 62); Murier des haies (23).
Uses: Leaves astringent. *Ref:* 23

Rubiaceae

***Galium odoratum** (L.) Scop. *Area:* Algeria.
Names: Arabic: Fuwwa regiga (23, 62). Berber: Aoudmi (23, 62). English: Sweet woodruff, Mugwet, Sweet grass (4). French: Aspérule odorante, Petit muguet (4, 23); Reine des bois (4).
Uses: Entire plant is diuretic, stimulant, vulnerary, tonic. *Ref:* 23

Rubia peregrina L. *Area:* Libya to Morocco.
Names: Arabic: Fuwwa (42, 62). Berber: Tariouba (42, 62). French: Garance voyageuse (42); Garance (62).
Uses: Decoction of roots diuretic, emmenagogue, abortive, mixed with oil for rubbing against sciatica and rheumatism; root chologogue, laxative, slightly tonic and

astringent. Infusion of flowers reputed as aphrodisiac and antidiarrhoeic.
Ref: 23, 24, 42

Rubia tinctorum L. *Area:* Libya to Morocco. Cultivated and subspontaneous.
Names: Arabic: Fowwa (4, 5, 17, 23, 42, 62, Rabat drug market); 'Ourouq homor, 'Oroug sabbaghin (17, 23, 62); Fuwwat as-sabbaghin (4, 17, 42); Alizari (62). Berber: Taroubia (5, 23, 62); Tariouba (23); Taroubent, Aroubian (62). English: Madder, Dyer's madder (4). French: Garance (4, 5, 12, 23, 45, 62); Garance des teinturiers (4, 42).
Uses: Decoction of entire plant for anemia and all blood diseases (Rabat drug market), aphrodisiac, its decoction is given to babies as antidiarrrhoeic, aqueous extract or powdered plant used as a tonic, appetizer, emmenagogue, diuretic, externally used for dressing contusions, wounds, ulcers for their healing, dessication and maturing, and internally as expectorant. Powdered plant made into suppositories, used as abortive. Roots boiled in oil and the oil used for sciatica by rubbing, root tonic, vermifuge, emmenagogue; decoction of root diuretic. Stem and leaves for hypertension. *Ref:* 5, 12, 17, 23, 42, 45

Ruscaceae

Ruscus aculeatus L. *Area:* Tunisia to Morocco.
Names: Arabic: Khizana (23, 62); Aas barri (4, 62); Senesaq, Meurdjel (62); 'Unnąb barri, Shurrabet er-ra'i (4); Sobhane khallaku (37). Berber: Redradj (23, 62); Atkizounn (62). English: Butcher's broom, Knee holly, Box-holly (4). French: Fragon (62); Fragon piquant (4); Petit houx (23, 37, 45, 62); Houx frêlon, Bois pointu (4).
Uses: Rhizome diuretic, for hemorrhoids, varix, venous tonic, sudorific, appetizer. Infusion of leaves febrifuge. *Ref:* 23, 24, 37, 45

Rutaceae

***Citrus aurantium** L. *Area:* Commonly cultivated in North Africa.
Names: Arabic: Narendj (4, 23, 24, 62); Arendj (23, 62); Lareng (42); water distilled from flowers: Mazahr (Cairo drug market). English: Sour orange, Seville orange, Bitter orange (4). French: Bigaradier (4, 23, 45, 62); Orangier amer (4, 23, 62); Orangier de Séville (23, 62).
Uses: Bark infusion for stomach pains and dysentery; bark tonic, stomachic, carminative. Infusion of leaves digestive, antispasmodic, diaphoretic, mild sedative. Infusion of dried flowers nerve sedative, antispasmodic (hysteria, spasms, hiccup); water distilled from flowers given to babies to calm their agitations and to help them to sleep; mixed with *Carum carvi* seeds, is given to adults for aerophagy. Infusion of flowers stimulant, antidiarrhoeic. *Ref:* 3, 5, 42, 45

Haplophyllum tuberculatum (Forssk.) A. Juss. *Area:* Egypt to Morocco.
Names: Arabic: Fijel (16, 62); Shagaret er-rih, Mejennin (58, 62); Shagaret el-ghazal (58).
Uses: Flowering and fruiting branches febrifuge, local antipoison, for vomiting, nausea, constipation, malaria, difficult childbirth, anemia, rheumatism, gastric

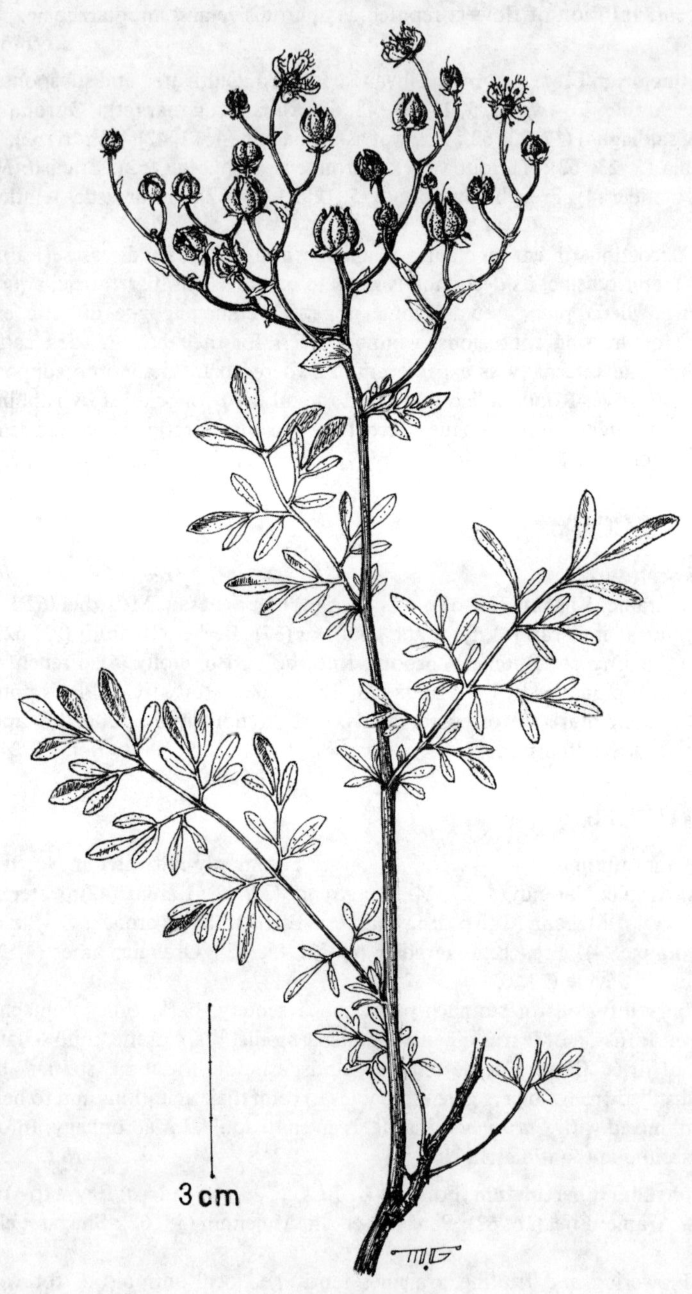

Ruta chalepensis

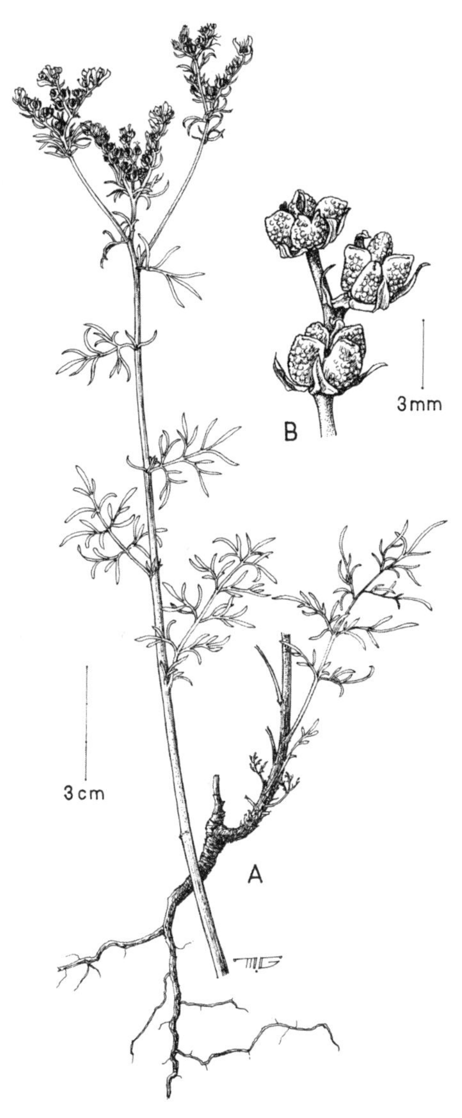

Ruta montana
A. flowering and fruiting plant
B. branchlet of a fruiting inflorescence, enlarged

pains, intestinal worms, eye and ear troubles, aphrodisiac; decoction for rheumatic pains. *Ref:* 7, 16

Ruta chalepensis L. *Area:* Libya to Morocco.
Names: Arabic: Fidjel (8, 13, 23, 37, 62); Fidjla (13, 23, 62, Algiers drug market); Sadhab (4, 13, 23, 62); Bou ghans, Rutsa (13, 62); Ruta (Rabat drug market). Berber: Aourmi (13, 23, 62); Issin, Zent, Issel (13, 62); Djell (62). English: Aleppo rue, Syrian rue (4); Rue (8). French: Rue d'Alep (4, 13, 42); Rue (37, 62).
Uses: Fresh plant scorpion repellant due to its strong smell; leaves and seeds boiled in oil and the oil is rubbed for rheumatic pains and swellings. Infusion of entire plant for colds, intestinal troubles and earaches; hot infusion of plant is cooled and used as ear drops for earaches. Plant boiled in milk and taken against nervousness (Rabat drug market); dried plant used as snuff for nasal diseases, its infusion as nose drops against vomiting and fevers of children and babies (Algiers drug market); same uses as for *Ruta montana.* Flowering branches vulnerary, emmenagogue, spasmodic. *Ref:* 8, 23, 24, 37

Ruta montana (L.) L. *Area:* Tunisia to Morocco.
Names: Arabic: Fidjla el-djebeli, Sadhab el-djebeli (23, 62); Fidjel (5, 13, 42, Rabat and Algiers drug markets); Ruta, El-sedab el-jebli (13, 42); Sadhab el-barr (4). Berber: Aourmi (13, 23, 24, 62), Awermi (5); Aourma (13, 42). English: Mountain rue, Wild rue (4). French: Rue des montagnes (4, 13, 42); Rue sauvage (4, 5).
Uses: Plant emmenagogue, diuretic, a general antipoison, antidote against snake bites, appetizer, abortive, despite the danger of its use as a decoction or by vaginal injection. Cataplasm of fresh plant for headaches due to its revulsive effect; plant steeped in oil, then filtered, is applied to the ear for its beneficial action on otitis and bourdonnement of the ears; infusion of dried plant for stomach pains, aphrodisiac. Juice of leaves used as eye drops to fortify the sight. Flowering branches for migraine, epilepsy, affections of the respiratory system, gout, oedema, paralysis, antispasmodic, rubefacient, the powder escharotic. *Ref:* 5, 13, 23, 42

Salicaceae

Populus nigra L. *Area:* Tunisia to Morocco.
Names: Arabic: Safsaf (23, 62); Baqs, Hour aswad (4). Berber: Arig, Asafsaf (23, 62); Erg, Ouisd (62). English: Black poplar, Italian poplar (4). French: Peuplier noir (23, 45, 62); Peuplier suisse, Peuplier franc (4).
Uses: Charcoal of wood absorbent, intestinal antiseptic. Vegetative buds resolvent, calmative, local sedative especially for hemorrhoids. *Ref:* 23, 45

Salix alba L. *Area:* Libya, Algeria, Morocco.
Names: Arabic: Khilaf (23, 42); 'Oud el-maa (62); Safsaf abiad (4). Berber: Talezzast amellal (23, 62). English: White willow, Swallow-tailed willow (4). French: Saule blanc (4, 23, 45, 62); Osier blanc (4, 23, 24).
Uses: Bark febrifuge, for rheumatism, tonic, astringent, antiseptic, vulnerary. Leaves calmative, antispasmodic, genital sedative. *Ref:* 23, 45, 62

Salvadoraceae

Salvadora persica L. *Area:* Egypt, Libya, Algeria.

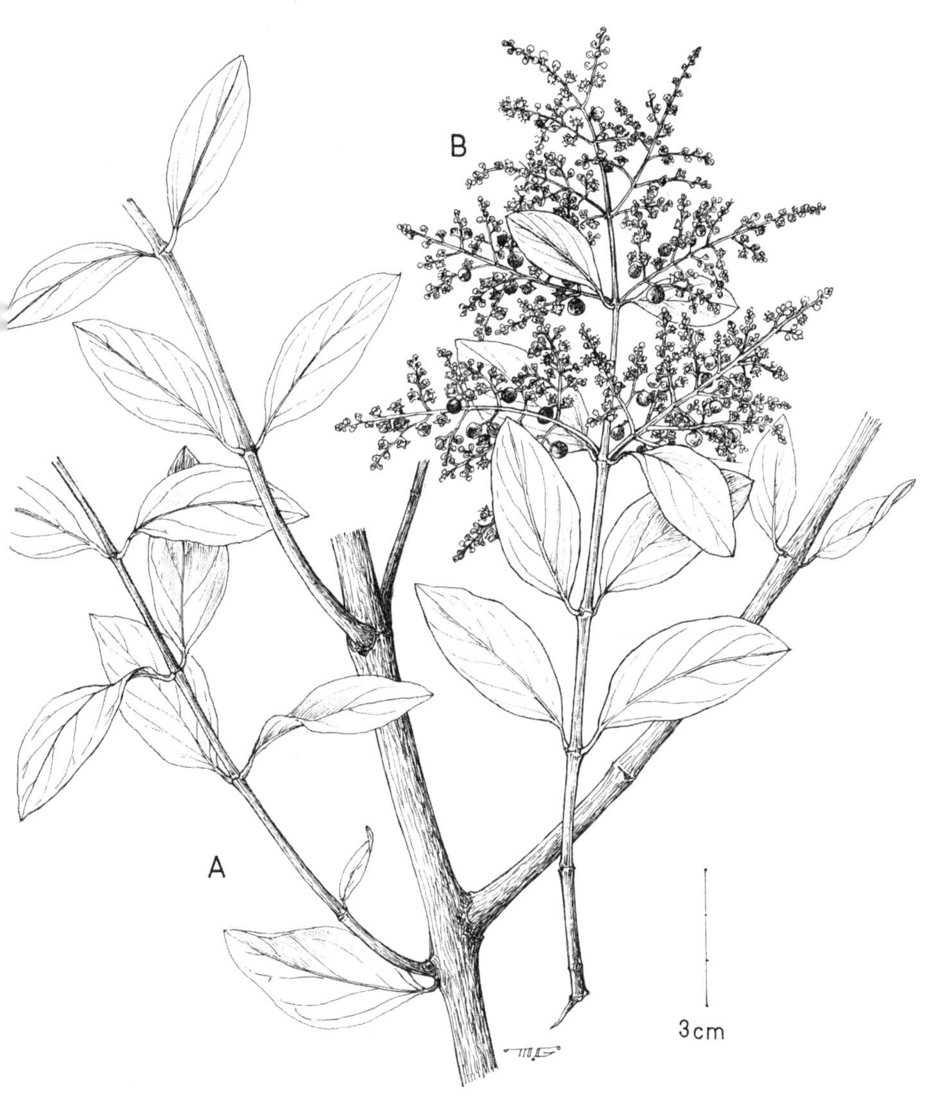

Salvadora persica
A. vegetative branch
B. flowering and fruiting branch

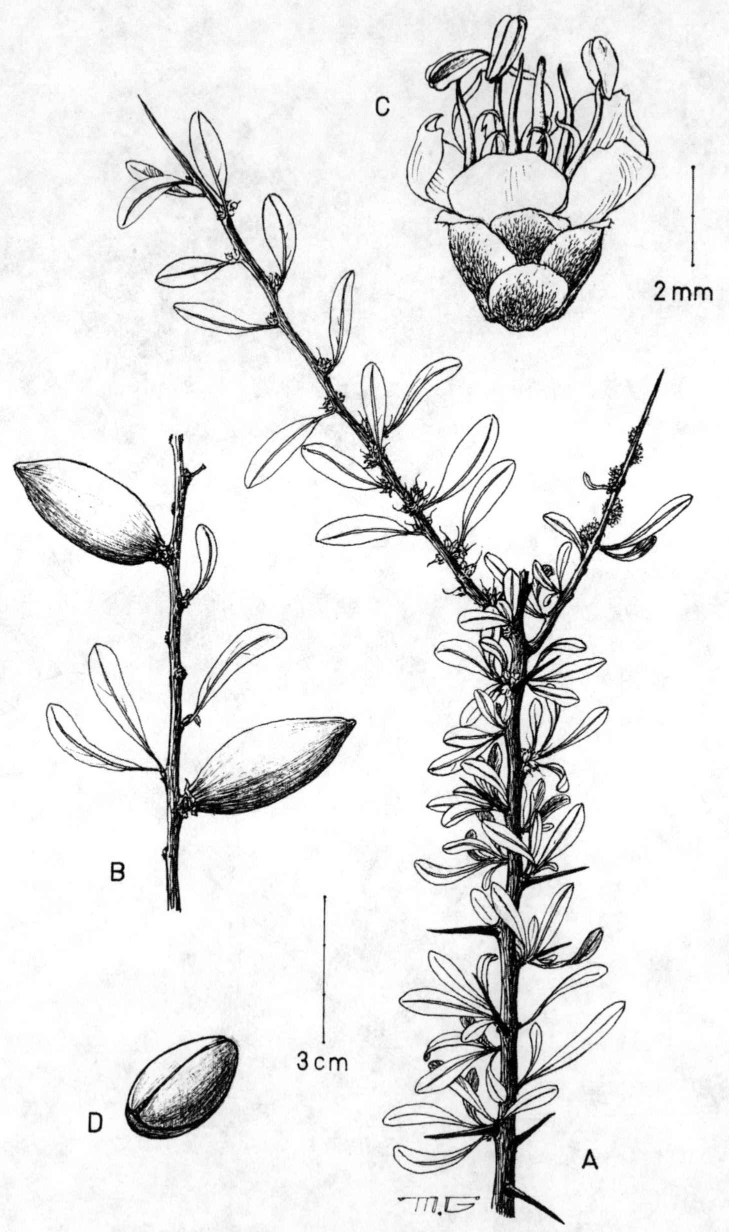

Argania spinosa
A. flowering branch, B. fruiting branchlet
C. flower, enlarged, D. seed

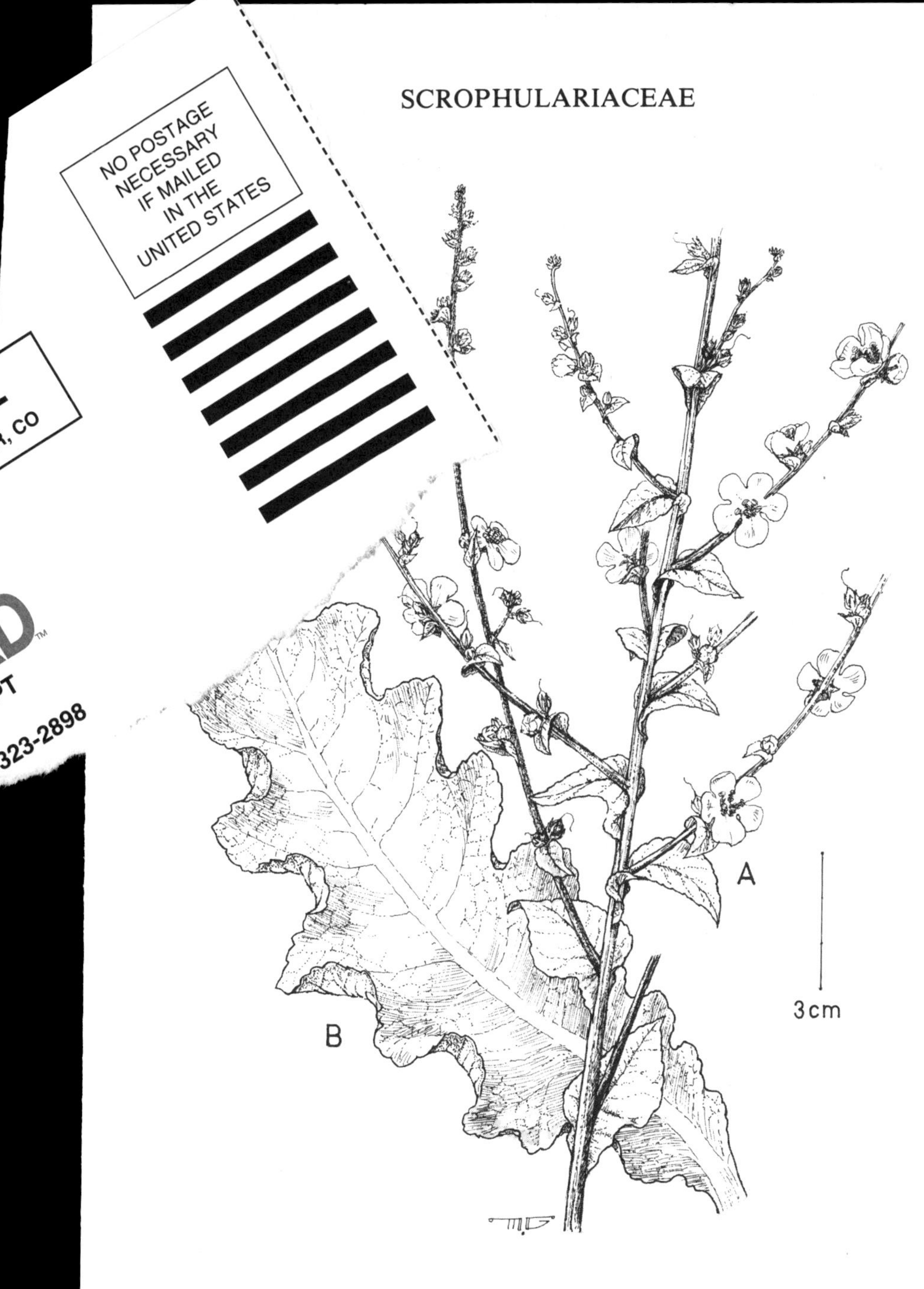

Verbascum sinuatum
A. flowering and fruiting branch
B. basal leaf

Names: Arabic: Arak (4, 5, 12, 17, 58, 62); Miswak (58, 62); Siwak (4, 5, 17, 62); fruit: Kabats (17, 62). Berber: Tidjat (5, 62); Adjou, Abisga, Babul (62). English: Toothbrush tree (4). French: Arac, Mésuak (4).
Uses: Plant used for gonorrhoea, spleen, boils, sores, gum disease, stomachache. Wood boiled in oil constitutes a liniment against contusions. Bark tonic, powdered bark used for bites of poisonous animals. Leaves, roots, bark and flowers contain oil, diuretic. Powdered leaves mixed with millet flour and honey are made into small balls and taken every morning for 40 days as antisyphilitic. Fruits edible, stomachic, carminative, febrifuge, fortify the stomach and bring good appetite.
Ref: 2, 5, 12, 17, 62, 66

Sapotaceae

Argania spinosa (L.) Skeels *Area:* Endemic to Morocco.
Names: Arabic: Argan (4, 5); fruit: Louz el-berber (4, 62). Berber: Argan, Ardjan; fruit: Tiznint (62); Feyyasha, Afiyyash, Tafiyyasht, Zekmuna, Tazgemmut, Iglim (5). English: Argan tree (4). French: Arganier (4, 5, 62).
Uses: Kernel of the fruit yields an oil which is recommended to reinvigorate the body and as an aphrodisiac. *Ref:* 5

Scrophulariaceae

Verbascum sinuatum L. *Area:* Egypt to Morocco.
Names: Arabic: Muslih al-andar (5, 26, 42, 62, Rabat drug market); Bousira (37, 42, 62); Bousir (5); Tsalal el-antar, Ouden el-homar (62); 'Awarwar, Kharma (58); Birhoum (26); Bousir aswad-el-waraq (4). Berber: Tisseraw (26, 62); Touffelt (62); Meslah (26, 42). English: Black-leaved mullein (4). French: Molène noire (4); Molène (42).
Uses: Roots and leaves popular drug for the hygiene of eyes, having the reputation of ameliorating the sight, for inflammations, antipoison. Dried powdered plant for all eye diseases by putting the powder under eyelids; plant burnt, powdered and mixed with alcohol, then applied to the eyes in small doses for weakness of the sight, probably cataract (Rabat drug market). Leaves emollient. *Ref:* 5, 26, 37, 42

Smilacaceae

Smilax aspera L. *Area:* Libya to Morocco.
Names: Arabic: Zeqresh (23, 62); 'Ulliq (5, 62); 'Ushba rumiya, 'Ushba (42, 62); 'Ushba maghrabiya (4). Berber: Sigarsou (23, 62); Tanesfalt (42). English: Rough bindweed, Prickly ivy (4). French: Salsepareille (4, 5, 42); Salsepareille indigène, Salsipareille d'Italie (23); Liseron épineux, Smilax rude (4).
Uses: Root sudorific, depurative, diaphoretic, diuretic, antisyphilitic, for hydropsy, gout, inflammatory conditions; decoction of root for skin diseases, rheumatism.
Ref: 5, 23, 24, 42

Solanaceae

Atropa bella-donna L. *Area:* Algeria, Morocco.

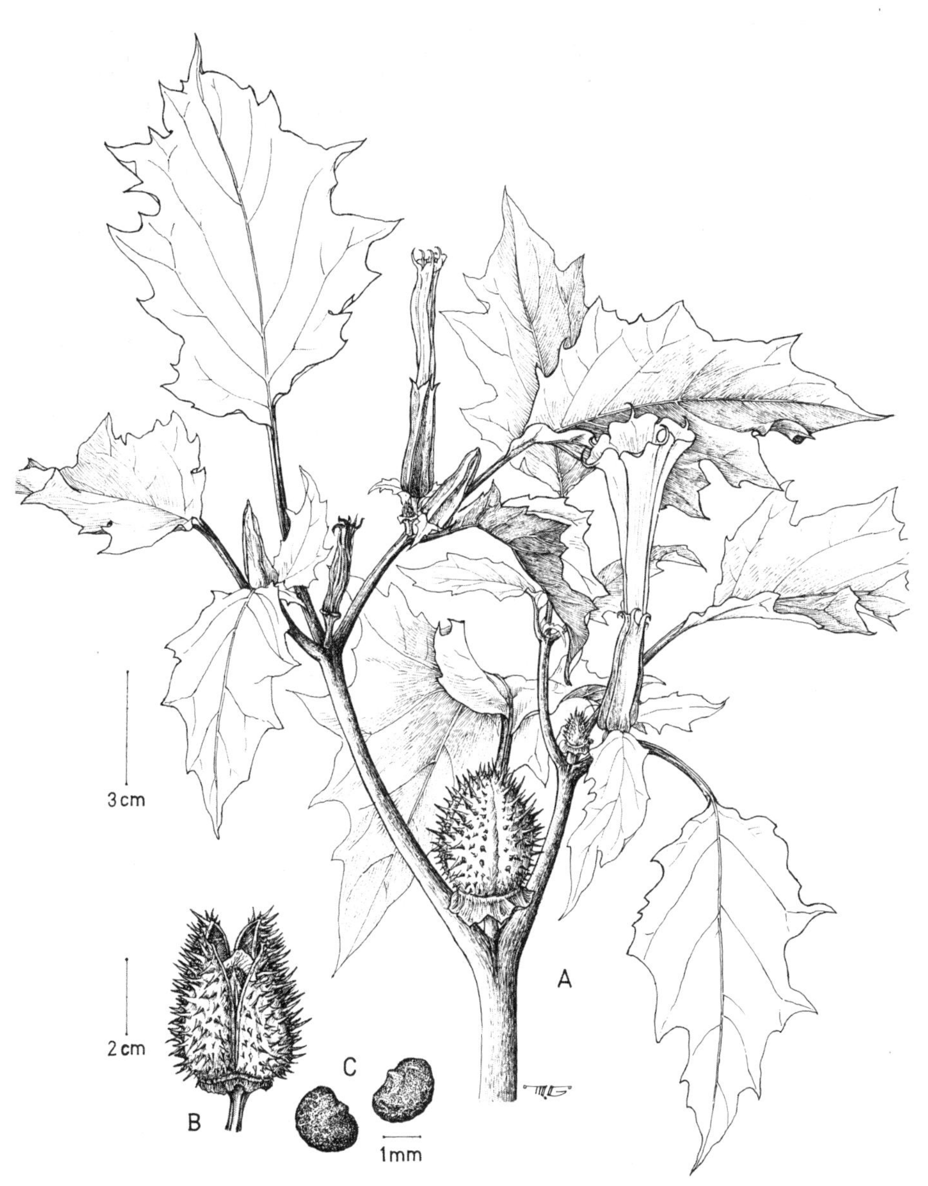

Datura stramonium
A. flowering and fruiting branch
B. ripe opened fruit capsule
C. seeds

Names: Arabic: Bou rendjouf, Bou qini (13, 23, 62); Belaidour (13, 23, 24, 62); dried berries: Zbib el-laidour (13, 42). Berber: Adil-ououchchn (13, 23, 42, 62); Mledor (62); Bubqini (42). English: Deadly nightshade, Dwale, Banewort (4). French: Belladone (4, 23, 24, 45, 62); Atrope, Bouton noir (4); Guigne de cote, Belle-dame, Morelle furieuse (23).
Uses: Berries antiseptic, mydriatic, sedative, toxic. Although known to be toxic, berries used as aphrodisiac, to stimulate intelligence and to develop the memory. In order to benefit from the effects without getting its toxicity, the berries are mixed with the diet of a chicken for one week, then the bird is slaughtered and its flesh is eaten for three days; another method is to drink regularly for several days the milk of a goat which has already been fed with the berries. Extracts of the plant are classical parasympatholytic agents. *Ref:* 2, 13, 23, 42

Capsicum annuum L. *Area:* Commonly cultivated in North Africa.
Names: Arabic: Felfel ahmar (4, 23, 62); Felfel rumi (4, 42); Felfel haar, Felfel helw (23, 37, 62); Felfel torshi, Felfila (62). Berber: Ifelfel (23, 62); Chilla (62). English: Capsicum, Red pepper, Guinea pepper (4). French: Piment des jardins (23, 42); Piment cultivé (62); Poivre de Guinée (4, 23); Corail des jardins, Poivre d'Inde (23); Piment, Capsique, Poivrier long, Poivron (4).
Uses: Fruit a condiment, stomachic, diuretic, stimulant, revulsive, tonic, aphrodisiac, externally used as rubefacient, anthihemorrhoidal in small doses. *Ref:* 23, 24, 37, 42, 45

Capsicum frutescens L. *Area:* Commonly cultivated in North Africa.
Names: Arabic: Dar felfel (4, 62); Felfel glib-el-ttir (62); Felfel merrakshi (5, 42); Felfel haar, Sudaniya (5). English: Bird pepper, Goat pepper, Spur pepper (4). French: Piment enragé (4, 5, 42); Piment d'oiseau (4); Piment de Cayenne (5, 62).
Uses: Fruit used mainly as a condiment, tonic, appetizer, revulsive in aqueous solution, stimulant for gastric secretion, aphrodisiac; cataplasm revulsive, stomachic, antihemorrhoid. *Ref:* 5, 37, 42

Datura stramonium L. *Area:* Egypt to Morocco. Naturalized.
Names: Arabic: Shedjret el-janna (13, 23, 24, 62); Tatura (4, 8, 42, 58, 62); Nefir (4, 58); Datura, Semm el-far (58); Djahnama, Messekra (23, 62); Shedjret el-jemel (42); fruit: Djouza matel; seeds: Habb el-foua (23, 62). Berber: Tabourzigt (13, 23, 62); Tidilla (5). English: Thorn-apple (4, 8); Devil's apple, Devil's trumpet (4). French: Datura (23, 42); Stramoine (23, 26); Pomme épineuse (4, 23); Herbe aux sorcières (23); Pomme du diable, Endormie (4).
Uses: Tincture of leaves prescribed for spasmodic coughs, chronic laryngitis and asthma; leaves used in fumigations and in cigarettes to ease asthma attacks. Dried leaves smoked as cigarettes for the treatment of asthma, sedative, anesthetic, antiasthmatic; also smoked as cigarettes, alone or mixed with *Atropa* and *Hyoscyamus,* to act as antispasmodic, antiasthmatic, sedative, for coughs and violent headaches. Fresh or dry seeds enter in aphrodisiac mixtures, similar to *Atropa* in action and toxicity. *Ref:* 2, 5, 8, 42, 56

Hyoscyamus albus L. *Area:* Egypt to Morocco.
Names: Arabic: Houbbail (13, 23, 24, 62); Bou rendjouf (13, 23, 62); Bing (4, 13, 58); Gengeit (8, 13); Sikran (42). Berber: Tesker (13, 23, 24, 62); Bounerdjoul (13,

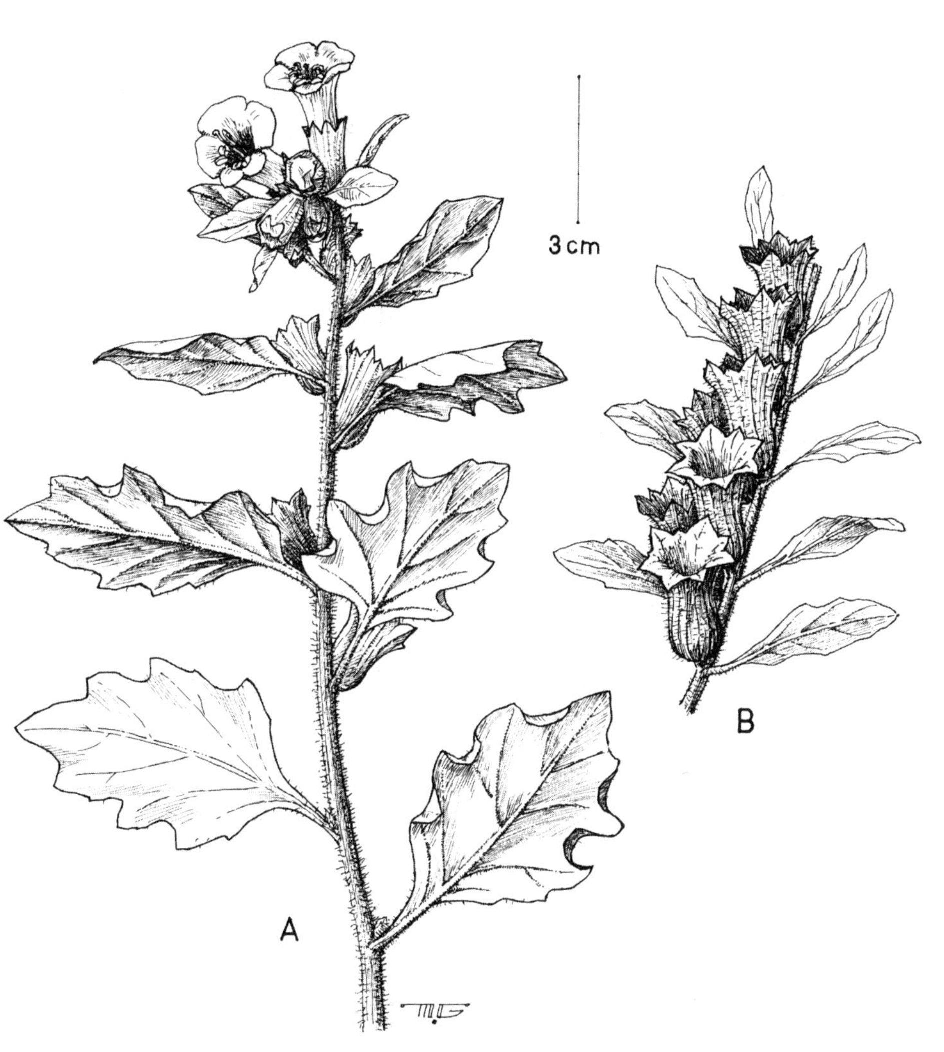

Hyoscyamus albus
A. flowering branch, B. fruiting branch

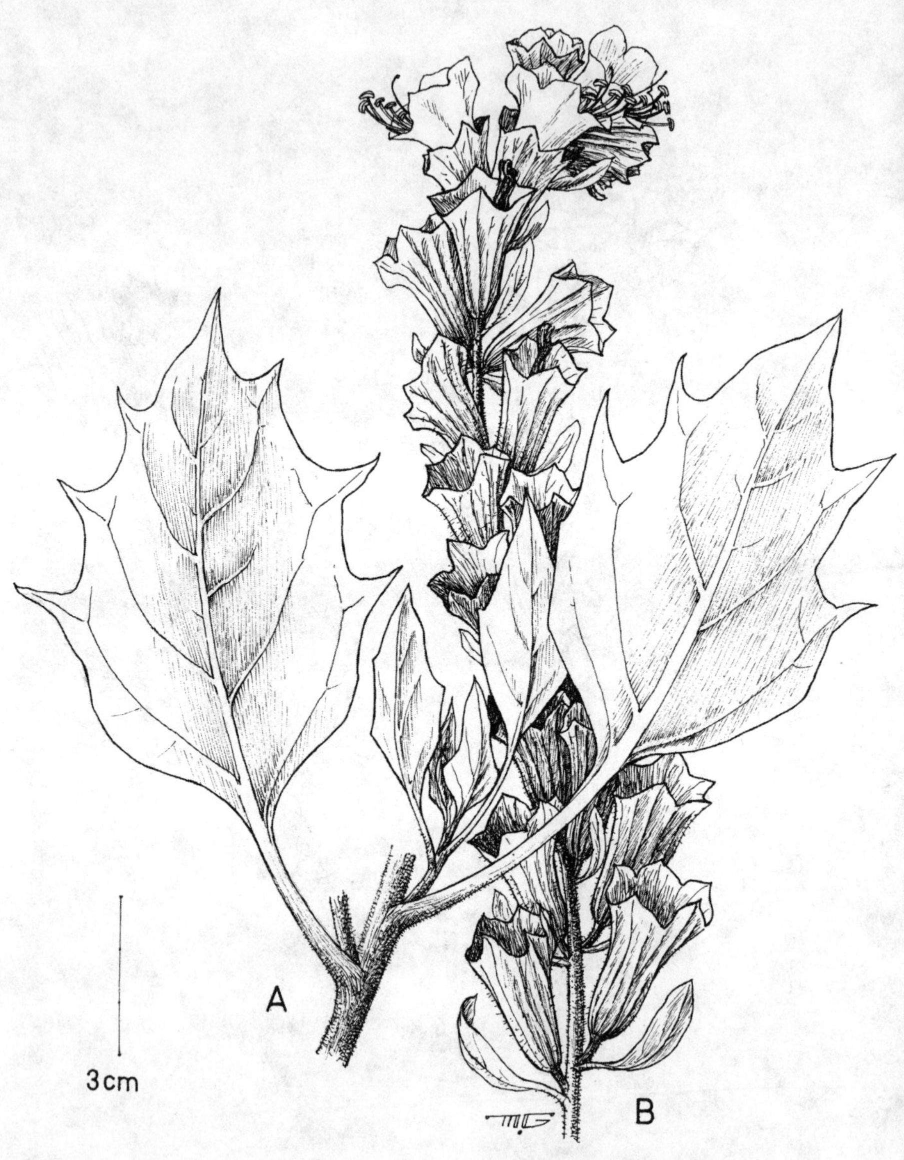

Hyoscyamus muticus
A. vegetative branch, B. flowering and fruiting branch

23, 62); Hillou (42). English: White henbane (4, 8). French: Jusquiame blanche (4, 13, 42, 62); Jusquiame, Henebane, Porcelet, Mort aux poules (23).
Uses: Plant provides relief from painful spasmodic conditions, alleviates nervous irritation such as various forms of hysteria and irritable cough; plant soporific, anesthetic, calmative for pains due to snake and scorpion bites. Leaves heated and applied over the eyes as a compress to reduce pain. *Ref:* 8, 42

***Hyoscyamus faleslez** Coss. *Area:* Algeria, Morocco.
Names: Arabic: Betina (5, 13, 42, 62); Falezlez (13, 42, 62); Goungat (13, 62). Berber: Gengi (42, 62); Afalehlé (13, 42, 62). French: Jusquiame flaeslez (13, 42); Jusquiame du désert (5).
Uses: Toxicity of this species is greater than other *Hyoscyamus* species, but it has the same properties. Plant is extremely poisonous and was used as a war poison in the Sahara as well as for criminal purposes; strong sedative, anesthetic, aphrodisiac, hallucinogenic. Seeds used by women to gain weight. *Ref:* 5, 42

Hyoscyamus muticus L. *Area:* Egypt.
Names: Arabic: Sakaran (7, 58). English: Egyptian henbane (14). French: Jusquiame d'Egypte (23).
Uses: Similar to *Hyoscyamus albus*. Plant provides relief from painful spasmodic conditions of the non-striated muscles, characteristic of lead colic and irritation of the bladder; also used to allay nervous irritation of hysteria and irritable cough. Cataplasm of fresh leaves used to allay pain; dried leaves smoked as cigarettes against asthma. *Ref:* 7, 14

Lycium intricatum Boiss. *Area:* Algeria, Morocco.
Names: Arabic: 'Awsaj, Ghardeq (5, 62). Berber: Inzzriki, Ossis (62); berries: Tabenenna, Tamenunnait, Timmuma (5). French: Lyciet (62).
Uses: Juice of leaves used as eye lotion for albugo and other ophthalmic diseases, possesses properties which act against tuberculosis, antirabic by rubbing the bitten area. Decoction of leaves for fall of hair and to give a brown-red color to the hair. Red berries are edible, antidiarrhoeic, and possess properties more or less similar to the leaves. *Ref:* 5

Mandragora autumnalis Bertol. *Area:* Tunisia to Morocco.
Names: Arabic: Beid el-ghoul (13, 42, 50, 62, Rabat drug market); Yabruh, Lufah (13, 42, 62); Lufa el-djin (62). Berber: Taryala (13, 42, 62). French: Mandragore (42, 50, 62).
Uses: Root soporific. Dried roots pounded into a powder of large particles termed "taryala" and sprinkled over pellets of "ibelba" bread, then taken by women despite their high toxicity in order to get fat; taryala is also used as a narcotic, sedative and calmative of pains. Fumigated dry leaves possess beneficial action against cough, bronchitis, throat pains, diseases of genital organs by local action. *Ref:* 13, 42, 50, 62

Nicotiana rustica L. *Area:* Frequently cultivated from Libya to Morocco. Cultivation in Egypt prohibited by law.
Names: Arabic: Dokhan akhdar (4, 62); Dokhan (42); Dokhan soufi (62); Dokhan barri (4). Berber: Taba (11, 42, 62); Tabga, Tabera (62). English: Wild tobacco, Brazilian tobacco (4). French: Tabac rustique (4, 62); Tabac du Brézil (4); Tabac (42).

Uses: Leaves vermifuge, parasiticide, mixed with *Thymus* and *Origanum* and smoked for throat pains and toothache; taken as snuff for beneficial action on eye pains; powdered leaves put on wounds as antiseptic and for their healing effect. *Ref:* 42, 45

Physalis alkekengi L. *Area:* Cultivated and frequently naturalized in Algeria and Morocco.
Names: Arabic: Kakenedj, 'Inab at-ta'leb (42); Kakang, Karaz el-quds (4); berries: Habb el-lahw (42). Berber: Lahw (42). English: Winter cherry, Alkekeng, Bladder herb (4). French: Alkékenge (4, 23, 42, 45); Coqueret (23, 24); Cerise de Juif (4).
Uses: Green plant vermifuge. Cataplasm of leaves emollient, calmative. Berries diuretic, for rheumatic and nephritic colics, laxative, for gout and conditions of urinary bladder. *Ref:* 23, 24, 42, 45

Solanum dulcamara L. *Area:* Algeria, Morocco.
Names: Arabic: Hulwa murra (4, 13, 23, 42, 62); Yasmin el-khela (13, 62); Orizia, 'Anab ed-dib (13, 42); Thulthulan (4). Berber: Sekigigeren, Aourizi (13, 23, 24, 62). English: Bitter-sweet, Woody nightshade, Felon-wort (4). French: Douce-amère (4, 23, 24, 42, 45, 62); Morelle grimpante (4, 23); Vigne de Judée (4).
Uses: Extracts of plant show antitumor activity, antisyphilitic. Berries aphrodisiac, diuretic, antirheumatic, depurative, diaphoretic, laxative, stimulant, sudorific, expectorant, slightly narcotic and revulsive. *Ref:* 2, 13, 23, 24, 42

Solanum nigrum L. *Area:* Egypt to Morocco.
Names: Arabic: 'Enab ed-dib, 'Inab ed-dib, 'Anab ed-dib (4, 5, 13, 42, 58, 62); 'Enab et-ta'leb (4, 5, 13, 42); Meghnenou, Messila, Bou Meknina (13, 23, 62); Bou qnina, Mu-qnina (5, 23); Baqnin, Baqninou (42). Berber: Touchanina (13, 23, 42, 62); Tiourmi (13, 23, 62); Azouri imouchene (42, 62). English: Black nightshade, Hound's-berry (4). French: Morelle noire (4, 5, 13, 23, 42, 45, 62); Crève chien (23, 62).
Uses: Plant toxic. Cataplasm of entire plant calmative, emollient for burns, dermal affections; decoction of plant used as wash for burnt parts and vaginal injection. Diluted infusion of berries used as mydriatic eye lotion, ear drops and emollient for external use. Berries narcotic, analgesic if used externally, sedative. Seeds aphrodisiac (mixed with food). *Ref:* 5, 23, 42, 45

Withania somnifera (L.) Dunal *Area:* Egypt to Morocco.
Names: Arabic: Ben nour, Abeb, Semm el-far, Ferkai (13, 62); Sekran (5, 42, 58); 'Inab el-ta'leb (5); 'Aneb ed-dib (13, 42, 50); Semm el-firakh, Foqqish, Sharma (58); Zafwa (62); Foulet el-kalb (8); fruit: Morgan (42, 58, 62). Berber: Terroumt (23, 62); Faraorao (62); Bousidan (42); Lahu, Bellehu (5). English: Rennet (8). French: Coqueret somnifère (13, 42).
Uses: Plant narcotic, employed against women's sterility, anti-epileptic, hypotonic, for stomachache, ulcers, colds, rashes, gonorrhoea. Roots used for treatment of rheumatic pains, hypotonic, calmative; dried powdered roots taken in small doses by women for sterility. Leaves and fruits febrifuge, diuretic, antirheumatic. Berries mild laxative; seeds toxic, emetic, diuretic, anesthetic. *Ref:* 2, 5, 8, 23, 36, 42, 50, 62

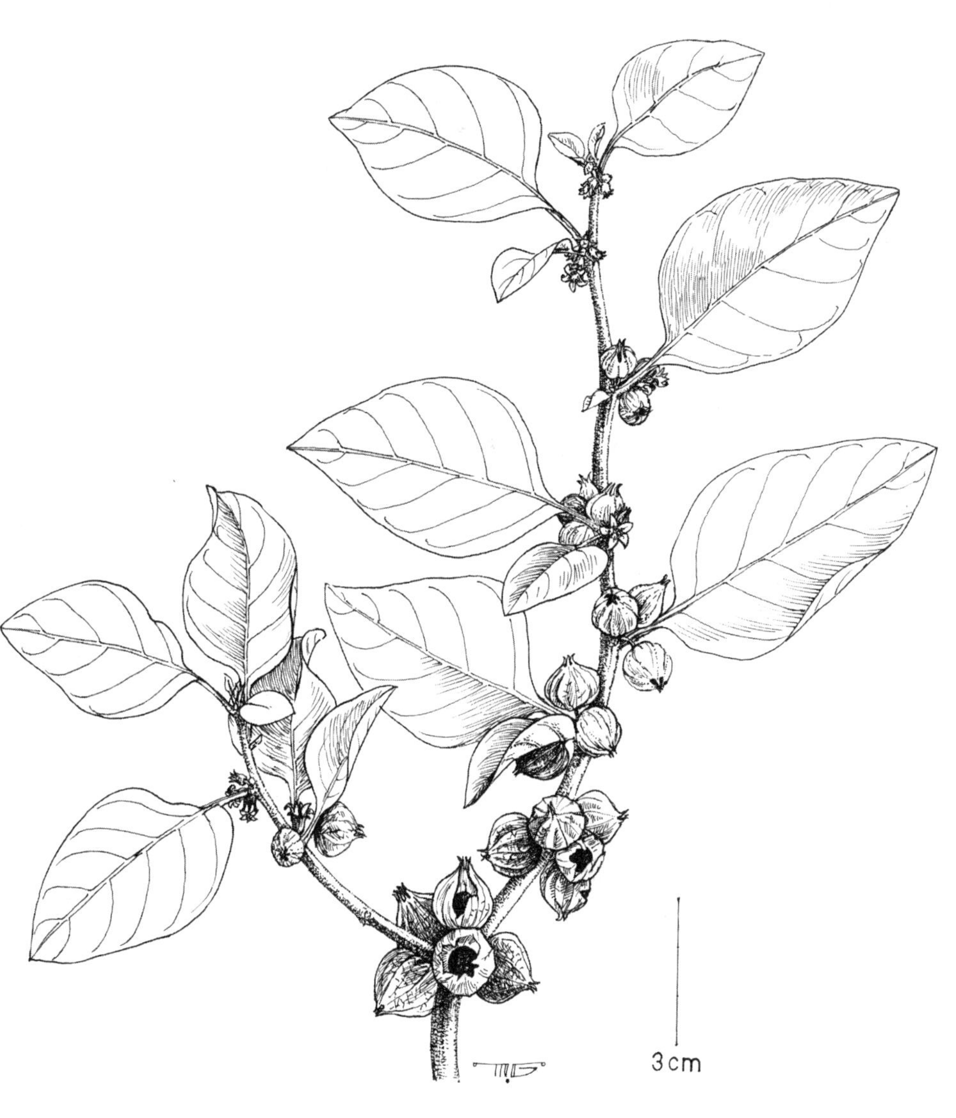

Withania somnifera

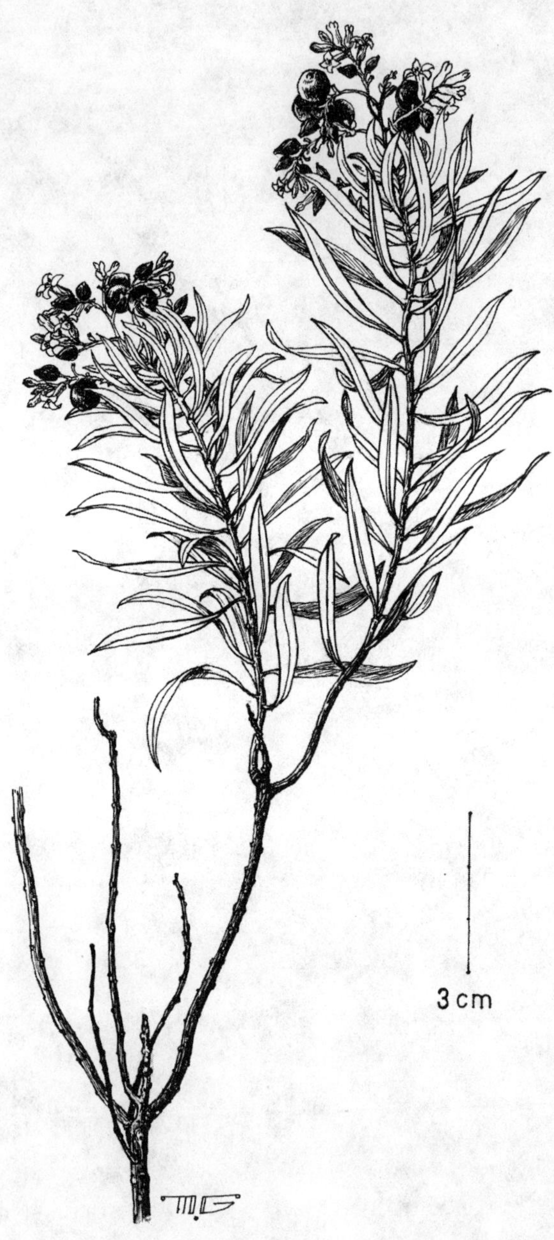

Daphne gnidium

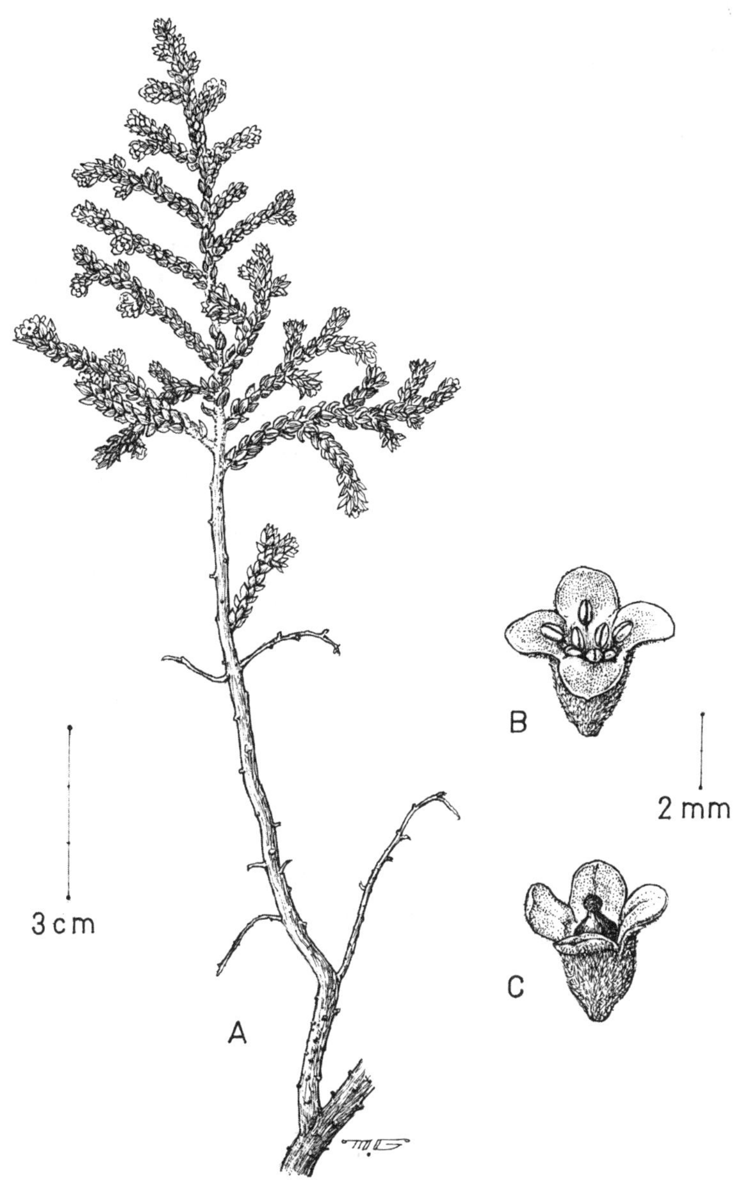

Thymelaea hirsuta
A. flowering branch, B. male flower, enlarged
C. female flower, enlarged

Tamaricaceae

***Tamarix aphylla** L. *Area:* Egypt, Libya, Algeria, Morocco.
Names: Arabic: Etel (12, 26); galls: Takaout (26). Berber: Tabrakat (26). French: Tamarix à galle (26).
Uses: Decoction of leaves and young branches for oedema of spleen; same decoction mixed with ginger for uterus affections. Bark of large branches, boiled in water with vinegar, is used as lotion against lice. Infusion of galls astringent, used for enteritis and gastralgia. *Ref:* 12, 26

Thymelaeaceae

Daphne gnidium L. *Area:* Tunisia to Morocco.
Names: Arabic: Lezzaz (5, 13, 23, 42, 62, Rabat drug market); Djouzet er-ra'iane (13, 62). Berber: Sebbarh (13, 23, 42, 62); Init (13, 42, 62); Alezzaz (13, 42). English: Gnidium, Spurge flax (4). French: Garou (4, 13, 23, 24, 26, 42, 45); Sain-bois (4, 23); Saint-bois, Daphné paniculé, Ecorce de garou commun (23).
Uses: Stem bark revulsive, abortive, vesicant, rubefacient. Syphilitic lesions disappear if treated with the powdered bark; bark aphrodisiac, used for venereal and dermal diseases. Bark, seeds, and leaves purgative, for itch. Cataplasm of dried powdered leaves rubbed into the hair and scalp, left for 24 hours, then hair washed, helping against loss of hair and dandruff (Rabat drug market). Leaves have the same role as "henna", being used for dyeing the hair black and for cutaneous affections. Red berries toxic. *Ref:* 5, 13, 23, 24, 42, 45, 62

Thymelaea hirsuta (L.) Endl. *Area:* Egypt to Morocco.
Names: Arabic: Methnan (58, 62, Algiers drug market); Metnan (47, 55, 58); Methnan akhdar (62). French: Passerine (62).
Uses: Leaves efficient anthelmintic, powerful hydragogue, cathartic and expectorant; decoction of leaves used as hair shampoo for dandruff (Algiers drug market). *Ref:* 55

Typhaceae

***Typha domingensis** (Pers.) Steud. *Area:* Egypt to Morocco.
Names: Arabic: Bardi (4, 5, 58, 62); Berdi (58, 62); Deis (58); Bout (4). Berber: Tabuda (5, 62); Taheli, Akaioud (62); Ugin (11). English: Reed-mace, Small bulrush, Cat tail (4). French: Massette (4, 62); Roseau (5); Massette des étangs, Massette à feuilles étroites (4).
Uses: Ash of rhizomes is applied to wounds as hemostatic. *Ref:* 5

Ulmaceae

Ulmus campestris L. *Area:* Tunisia to Morocco.
Names: Arabic: Neshem (23, 62); Gharghar (4). Berber: Oulmou (23, 62). English: Elm, English elm (4). French: Orme (4, 62); Orme campêtre (23, 24, 45); Orme pyramidale (23).

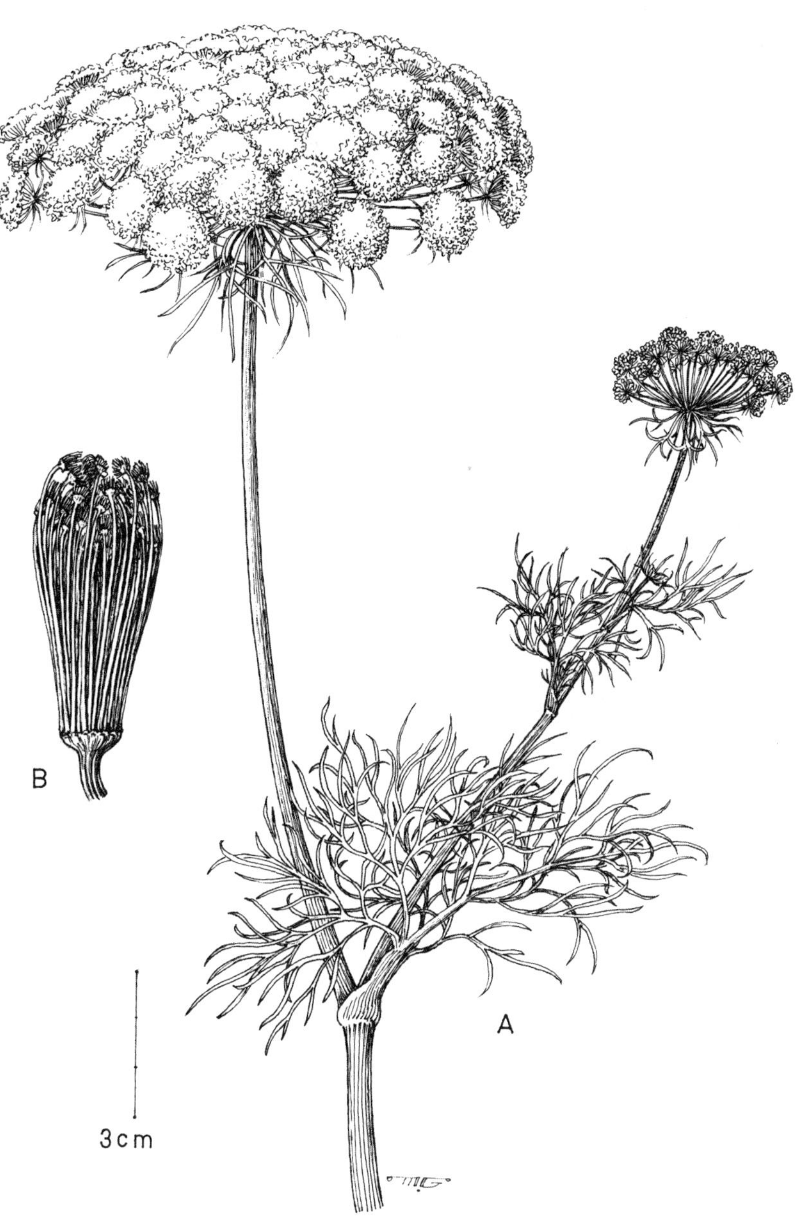

Ammi visnaga
A. flowering branch, B. mature inflorescence

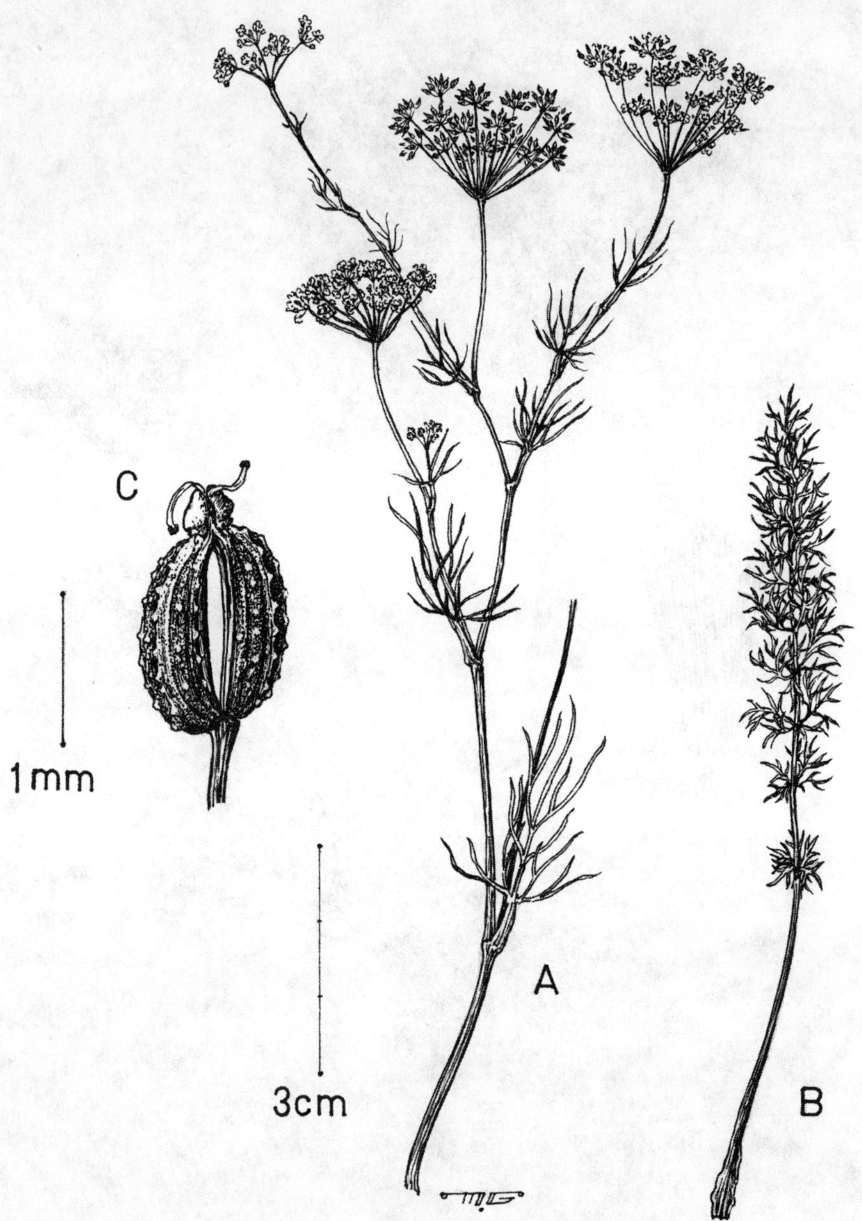

Ammoides pusilla
A. flowering branch, B. basal leaf
C. ripe fruit, enlarged

Uses: Bark astringent, stimulant, sudorific, diuretic, resolvent, emollient.
Ref: 23, 24, 45

Umbelliferae

Ammi majus L. *Area:* Egypt to Morocco.
Names: Arabic: Khilla, Khilla sheitani (4, 58); Qseiba, Nounkha, Zfenari el-ma'iz (62). Berber: Afhrilal, Therilal, Thalilen, Lattilel, Akhella (62). English: Bishop's weed (24, 25, 58). French: Ammi commun (24, 58); Ammi officinal, Ammi inodore (24).
Uses: Seeds diuretic, carminative, tonic, digestive, stomachic, for angina pectoris and asthma. *Ref:* 24, 25

Ammi visnaga L. *Area:* Egypt, Tunisia to Morocco.
Names: Arabic: Swak En-Nebi, Khelal, Khell, Kemmoun habashi (23, 62); Besnikha (42, Rabat drug market); Shoukail, Khoudab, Khebab, Qinawa, Dafs, Sennairya, Tamk, Khobz el-fara'na (62); Khilla (4, 17, 58); Khilla baladi (Cairo drug market); Gazar shaytani (4). Berber: Tabellaout (23, 62). English: Pick-tooth (4, 24,); Tooth pick (4). French: Herbe aux cure-dents (4, 23, 24); Cure dents du Prophète (23, 62).
Uses: Seeds diuretic, appetizer, carminative, stimulant, emmenagogue, lithontriptic, vasodilator, antispasmodic, relieve congestion of prostate gland, emetic, purgative, for urinary disorders, angina pectoris, asthma, gastric ulcers. Infusion of seeds releases renal stones (come out with urine), used as a gargle for toothache (Rabat drug market). *Ref:* 17, 23, 24, 25, 27, 42, 45

Ammodaucus leucotrichus Coss. & Dur. *Area:* Egypt to Morocco.
Names: Arabic: Kemmoun soufi (62, Algiers drug market); Kemmoun bou-tofa (26, 42, 62); Kemmoun el-ibel, Umm ed-driga (62); Kemmoun lemsewuf (5). Berber: Akamen (62); Sanug (42). French: Cumin du Sahara (62); Cumin laineux (5); Cumin à laine (26, 42).
Uses: Leaves for chest complaints. Fruit used in the same way as cumin. Seeds excellent aromatic spice, carminative, for gastric troubles and stomach pains (Algiers drug market), digestive troubles due to fear. *Ref:* 5, 16, 25, 42

***Ammoides pusilla** (Brot.) Breistr. *Area:* Libya to Morocco.
Names: Arabic: Nanoukha (62, Rabat drug market); Nabta (62); Rigl el-ghorab, Gazar esh-sheytan (4). English: Cerfolium (4). French: Cerfeuil (4).
Uses: Infusion of the entire plant digestive; edible snails are boiled in water to which branches of the plant are added (Rabat drug market).

Anethum graveolens L. *Area:* Widely cultivated in North Africa. Often naturalized.
Names: Arabic: Shibit (4, 23, 42, 62); Shamar (23, 62); Shebet, Tebs (42). English: Dill, Anet, Dill-seed (4). French: Aneth (4, 23, 42, 45, 62); Fenouil puant, Fenouil bâtard (4).
Uses: Fruits condiment, aromatic, stimulant, carminative, stomachic, digestive, diuretic, antispasmodic, antiemetic, sedative, galactogogue; externally emollient, resolvent; infusion calmative of stomach pains; decoction antipoison.
Ref: 23, 24, 25, 42

Apium graveolens L. *Area:* Cultivated and naturalized in North Africa.

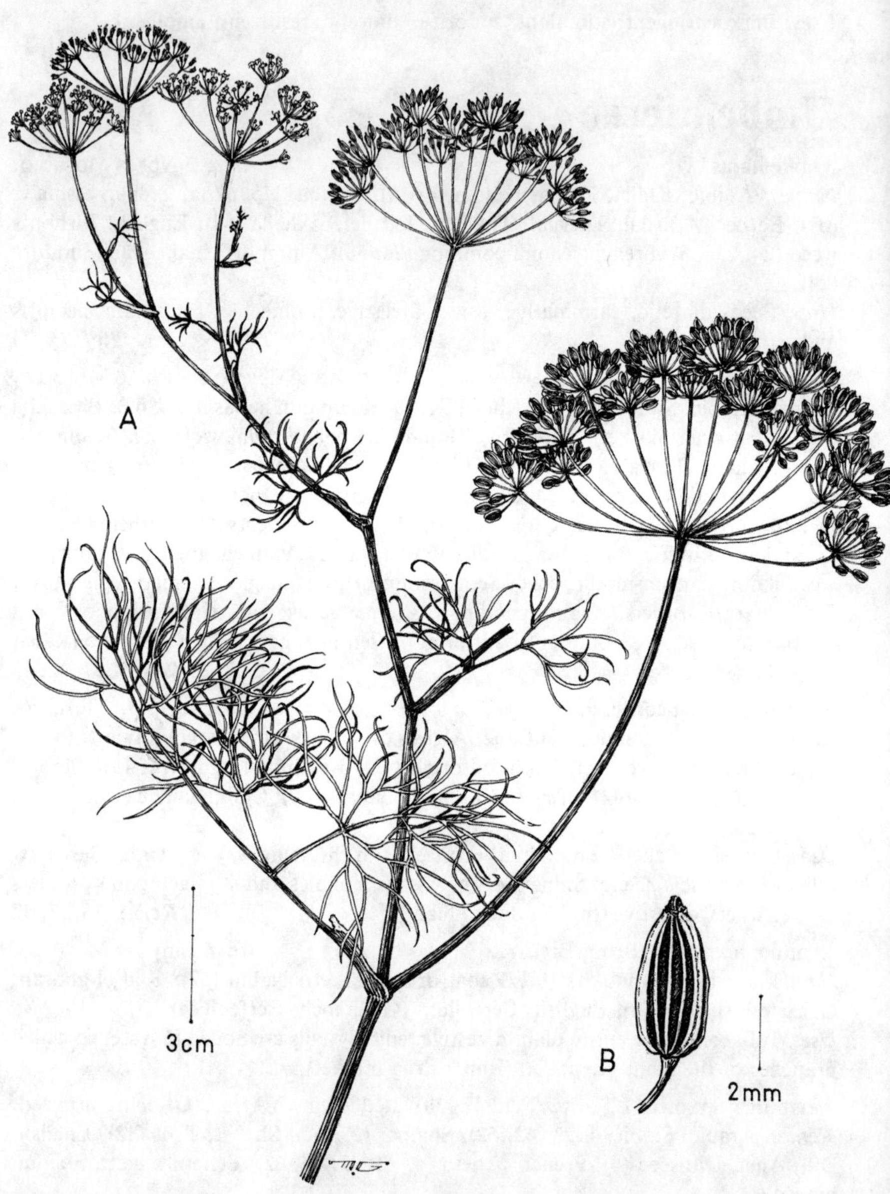

Anethum graveolens
A. flowering and fruiting branch, B. ripe seed, enlarged

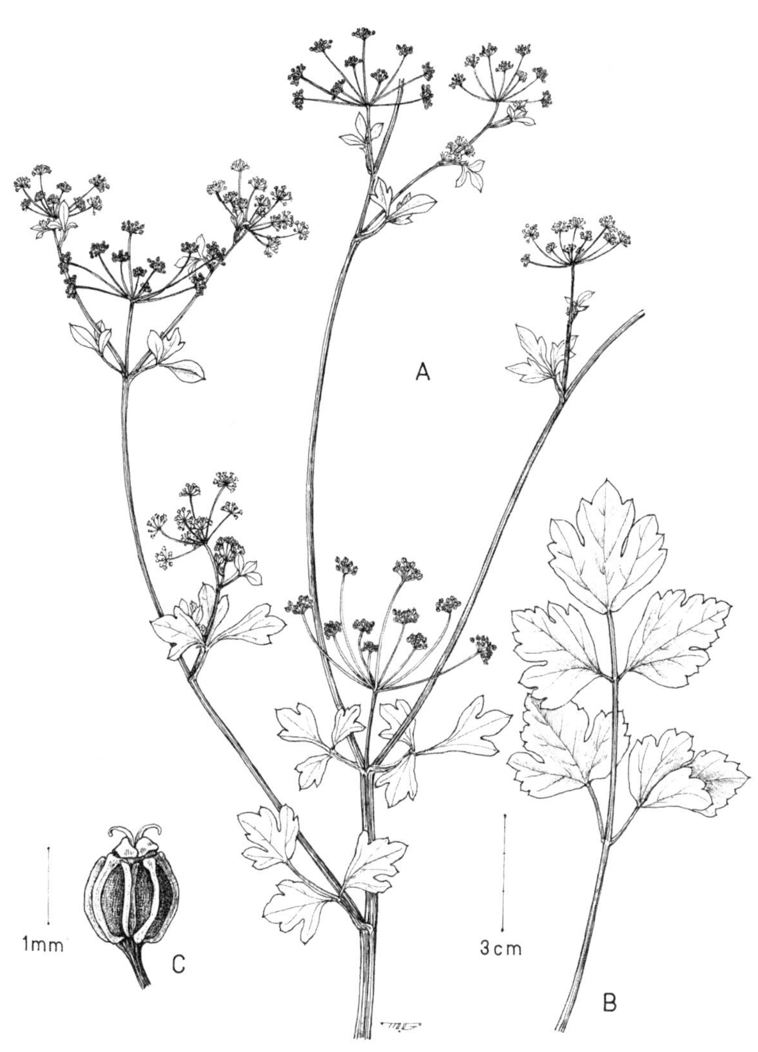

Apium graveolens
A. flowering and fruiting branch, B. basal leaf
C. ripe seed, enlarged

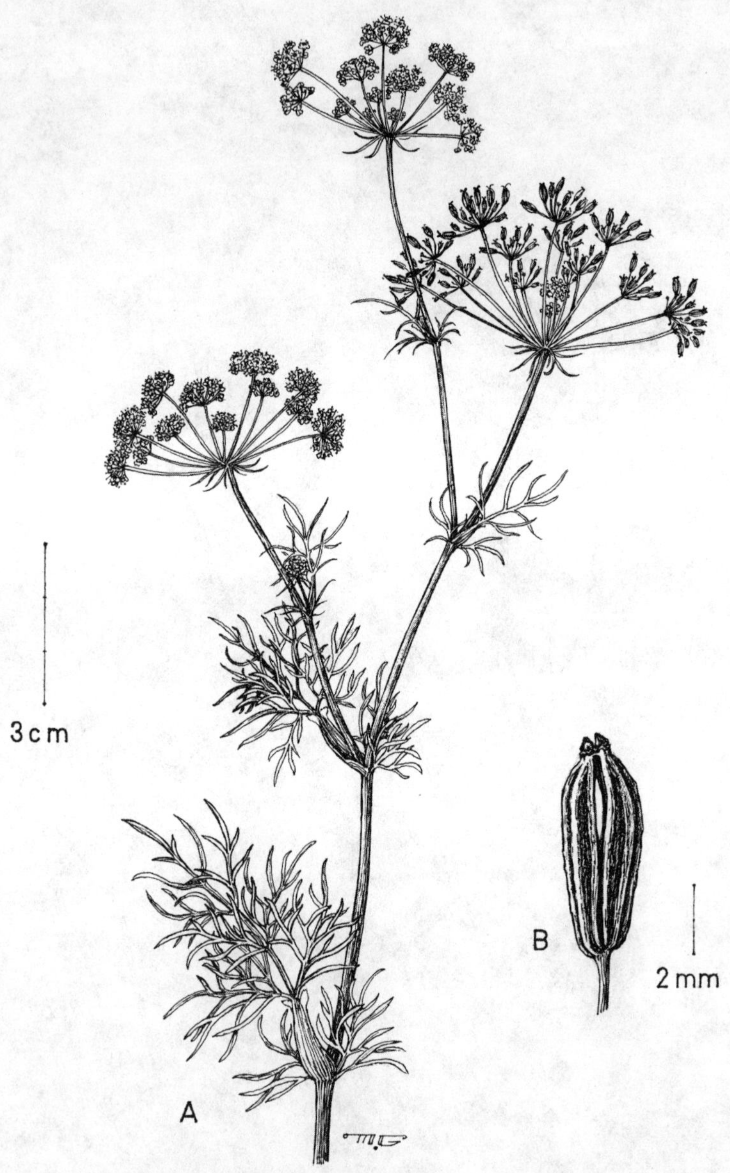

Carum carvi
A. flowering and fruiting branch, B. ripe seed, enlarged

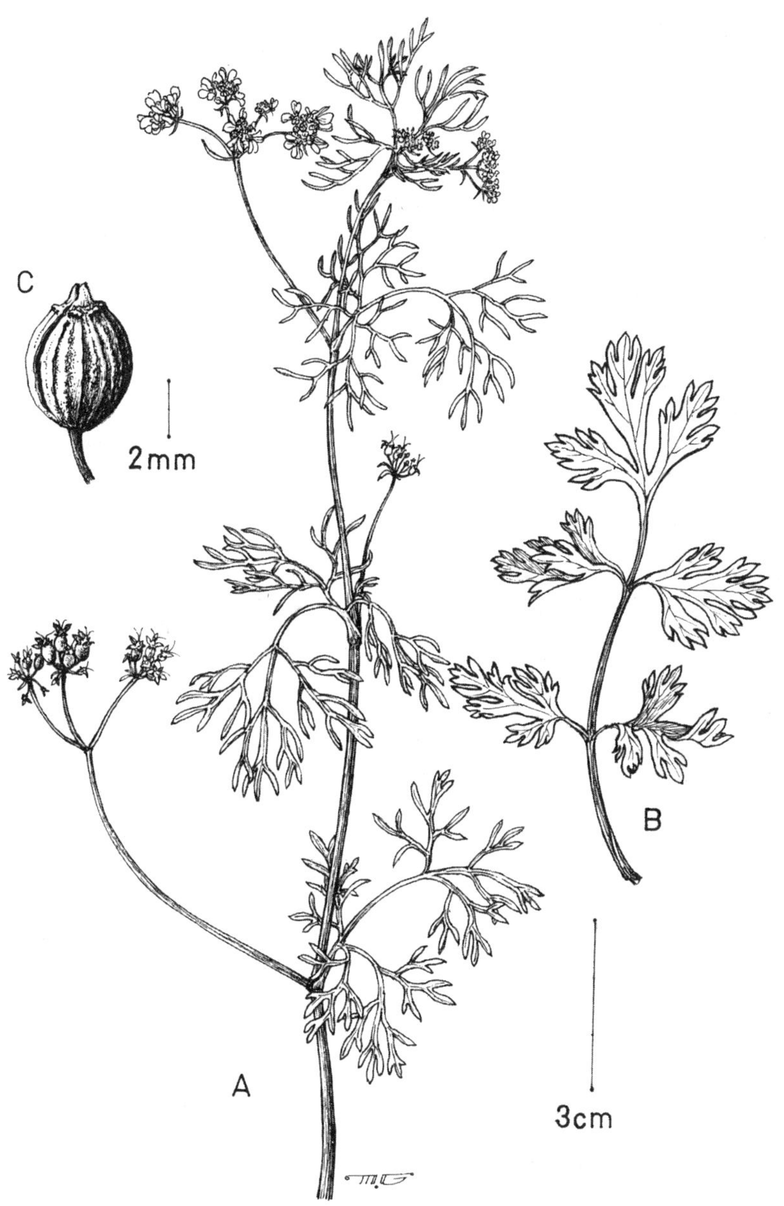

Coriandrum sativum
A. flowering branch, B. basal leaf
C. ripe seed, enlarged

Names: Arabic: Karafs (4, 58, 62); Kerefs el-maa (23, 62). Berber: Kerafess, Krafsa (23, 62). English: Celery, Marsh parsley, Smallage (4); Wild celery (24). French: Céleri (4, 62); Céleri cultivé (62); Ache des marais (23, 24, 45, 62).
Uses: Root, leaves and fruit diuretic. Fruits stimulant, affect the kidneys and bladder, stimulate urine contractions and even, in animals abortion. Tincture prepared from ripe seeds used to treat urine retention and other renal disorders, a traditional remedy for rheumatism and arthritis. Seeds stomachic, resolvent, antiscorbutic, carminative, chologogue, febrifuge, emmenagogue. *Ref:* 23, 24, 25, 45, 56

Carum carvi L. *Area:* Frequently cultivated in North Africa.
Names: Arabic: Karawiya (4, 5, 42, 62). English: Caraway (24); Common caraway (4). French: Carvi (4, 5, 42, 62); Cumin des prés, Kummel (4); Carvi officinal (24).
Uses: Ripe fruits carminative, diuretic, nerve calmative, stomachic, galactogogue, emmenagogue, appetizer, condiment, antiscorbutic, calmative of thirst, aphrodisiac, stimulant, digestive, vermifuge, antispasmodic, diaphoretic, anthelmintic, for scabies. Essence from ripe seeds antispasmodic, carminative, stomachic, promotes milk production; used externally as rubefacient; infusion of seeds for rheumatism and pleurisy. *Ref:* 5, 24, 25, 42, 56

Conium maculatum L. *Area:* Libya to Morocco.
Names: Arabic: Sikran, Djerir (23, 62); Ziata (23, 62, Rabat drug market); Bikhe shoukaran (42); Shawkaran (4); fruit: Harmal el-djezair (23, 62); root: Barbousha (62). Berber: Sellata (23, 62); Guebaba (62). English: Poison-hemlock (4, 25); Hemlock (4, 24, 25). French: Grande ciguë (4, 23, 24, 42, 45); Ciguë tachée (4, 23); Ciguë officinale (23); Ciguë (4).
Uses: Dangerous poisonous plant containing five alkaloids, the main one "coniine", isolated in 1831 and the first plant alkaloid to be synthesized in 1886. Small dose can kill by causing paralysis of the respiratory system; pure coniine used in soothing cancer pains; tincture is prescribed in cases of arteriosclerosis and disorders of the prostate gland; neuromuscular sedative, antispasmodic, used against cancer. Diluted infusion, in small doses, for painful rheumatism; plant analgesic in weak doses. Parts of the body affected by mosquito or other insects; bites are subjected to root fumigant (Rabat drug market). *Ref:* 23, 25, 42, 45, 56

Coriandrum sativum L. *Area:* Frequently cultivated in North Africa. Subspontaneous in some regions.
Names: Arabic: Kusbara (4, 17, 23, 42, 62); Kesbour (5, 23, 42); Debsha (62); fruits: Tabel (23, 62). Berber: Gouzbir (23, 62). English: Coriander (4, 25). French: Coriandre (4, 5, 23, 42, 45).
Uses: Juice of fresh leaves enters in the preparation of eye lotions. Ripe fruits stomachic, carminative, digestive, antihysteric, stimulant. Fruits mixed with honey or raisins are used to heal spreading sores, diseased testes, burns, carbuncles and sore ears, and if woman's milk is added, fluxes of the eyes. Fruits internally used as a general anti-inflammatory, antirheumatic, antiscorbutic, recommended for asthenia of children and aged people, aphrodisiac in large doses, taken in drink with rue for cholera; decoction of fruits used against vomiting, diuretic, anthelmintic, sedative, antipoison for bites of poisonous animals, used for nervous disorders. Intestinal parasites are expelled by coriander seeds. *Ref:* 5, 15, 17, 23, 25, 34, 42, 45

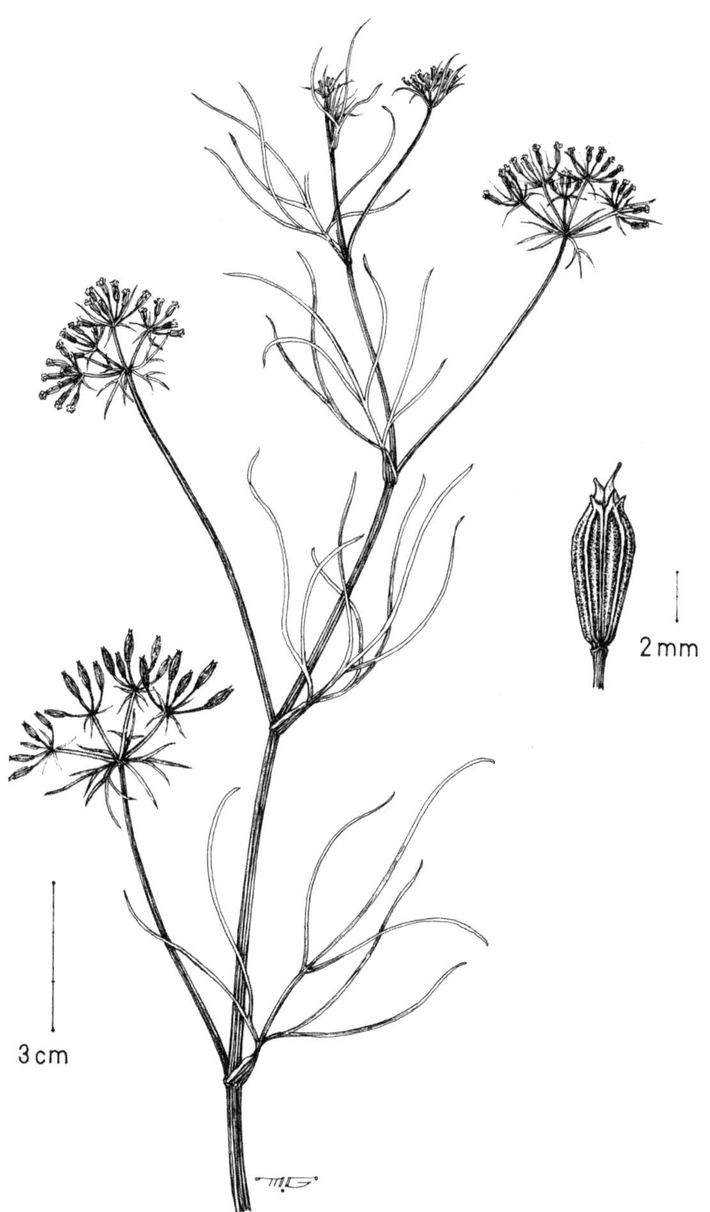

Cuminum cyminum
A. flowering and fruiting branch, B. seed, enlarged

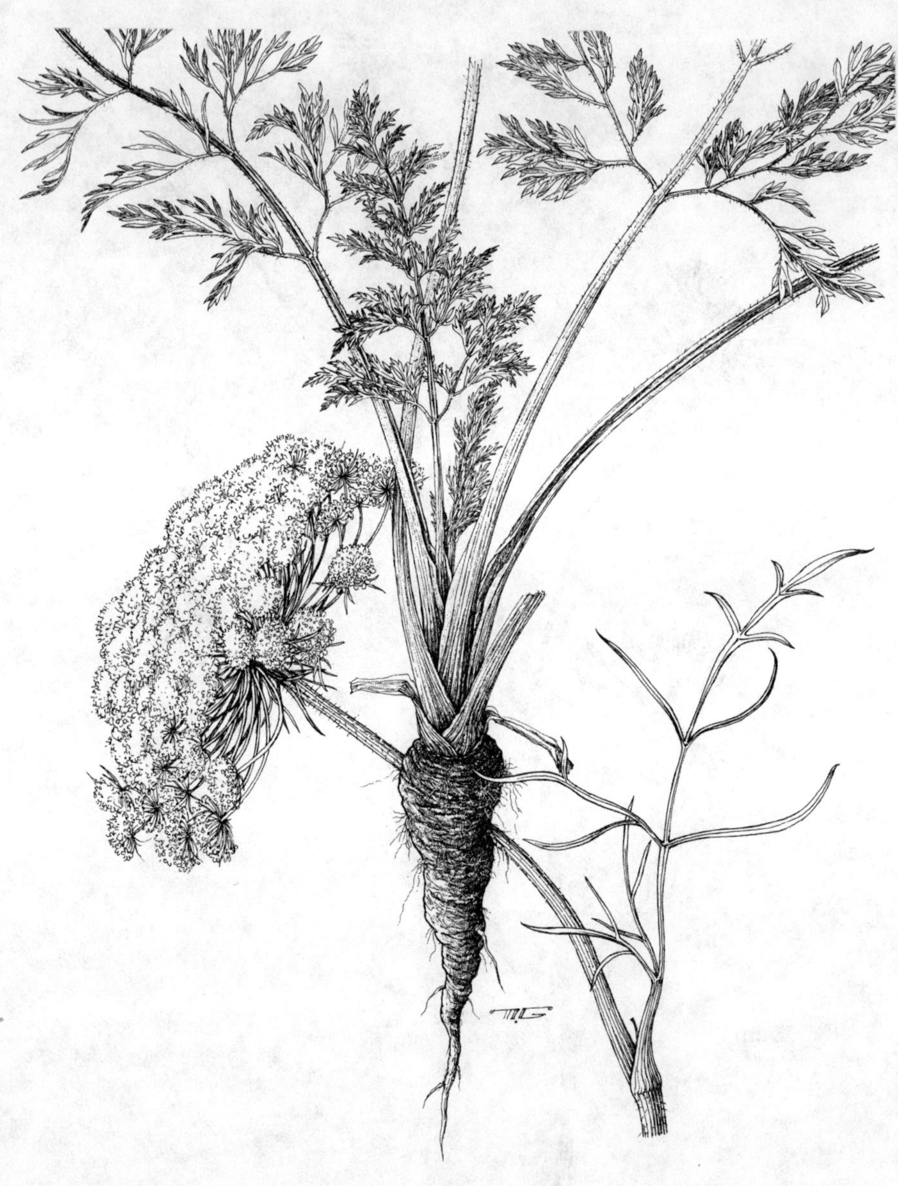

Daucus carota var. *boissieri*

Crithmum maritimum L. *Area:* Egypt to Morocco.
Names: Arabic: Shamar bahariya (4, 23, 62); Selattet el-bahr (23, 62). English: Samphire (4, 25); Rock samphire (25); Sea fennel, Peter's cress (4). French: Perce Pierre (4, 23, 62); Criste marine (23, 24); Fenouil marin, Passe-Pierre, Crithme, Bacille (4).
Uses: Leaves aromatic, depurative, diuretic, and possibly anthelmintic. Fruits and root stimulant, depurative, appetizer, antiscorbutic, diuretic. Essential oil from seeds and juice from leaves an excellent vermifuge. *Ref:* 23, 24, 25

Cuminum cyminum L. *Area:* Frequently cultivated in North Africa.
Names: Arabic: Kemmoun (4, 5, 17, 23, 42, 51, 62). Berber: Acham, Ichammen (23, 62); Ichoumane, Azcar (62). English: Cumin (4, 25). French: Cumin (4, 5, 23, 42, 45, 62).
Uses: Fruits efficient in the treatment of severe colic; infusion of fruits assure easy digestion, stimulant, for colds and fall in body temperature, antispasmodic, anthihysteric, astringent, diuretic, used in veterinary medicine. Seeds carminative, sudorific, galactogogue, emmenagogue, stomachic, used as a cataplasm on the nape of the neck for the treatment of mumps. *Ref:* 5, 17, 23, 24, 25, 42, 45, 51

Daucus carota L. var. **boissieri** Wittm. *Area:* Egypt. Mainly cultivated, often subspontaneous.
Names: Arabic: Gazar baladi (30); Gazar barri (4). English: Parsnip, Wild carrot (4). French: Carotte sauvage, Panias, Pastende (4).
Uses: Fruits possess powerful diuretic, antispasmodic, emmenagogue effects, recommended as anti-inflammatory in urinary tract and uterine infections, to disintegrate urinary calculi and to facilitate pregnancy. *Ref:* 30

Eryngium campestre L. *Area:* Egypt to Morocco.
Names: Arabic: Shouk el-abiod, Qalb el-djadj, Fougga' el-djemel (23, 62); Shaqaqil (4, 62); Garsa'na (42, 62); Shwwiket Ibrahim, Shwika yahoudiya, Bou 'Adjel, Doumiat shouka (62). Berber: Asnan, Azeroual (23, 62); Aiazidh, Taoulouaza (62). English: Common eryngo, Field eryngo (4). French: Panicant (4, 62); Chardon roland (4, 23, 24); Barbe de chèvre, Erynge (4).
Uses: Plant diuretic, appetizer, laxative. Root diaphoretic, expectorant, emetic, for urinary and uterine ailments. Decoction of the root and flowering plant used to treat kidney stones, to remove excess chlorine from the blood, and for some skin diseases.

Eryngium ilicifolium Lam. *Area:* Tunisia to Morocco.
Names: Arabic: Kef ed-dib (62); Zreiga, Shawka zarga, Shawka yahoudiya, Qersa'na (5). French: Panicaut (42).
Uses: Decoction of the root diuretic, spermatogenic, depurative, emmenagogue. *Ref:* 5

Ferula communis L. *Area:* Libya to Morocco.
Names: Arabic: Kelkh (4, 5, 13, 42); Kelkha (5, 13, 62); Keshbur, Besbas harami; gum-resin: 'Ilk el-kelkh (13, 62); Fasoukh (5, 42, 62); inflorescence: Bubal (5). Berber: Aboubal, Toufalt (42, 62); Taggult, Auli (5). English: Giant fennel (4). French: Férule (4, 5, 13, 42, 62); Nard (4).
Uses: Whole plant possesses antispasmodic properties. Gum-resin from the rhizome orally used as diuretic, vermifuge, powerful antialgetic, prescribed for articular pains, skin diseases, feminine sterility, emetic, for rheumatism. Roasted flower buds

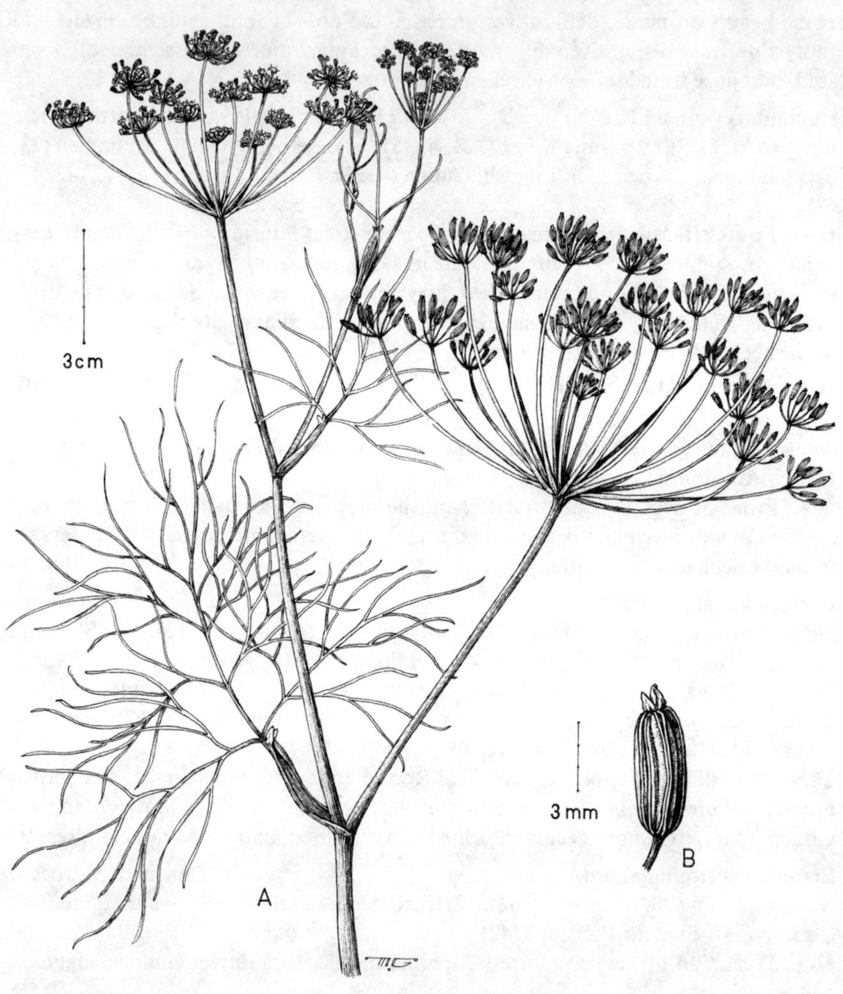

Foeniculum vulgare
A. flowering and fruiting branch, B. ripe seed, enlarged

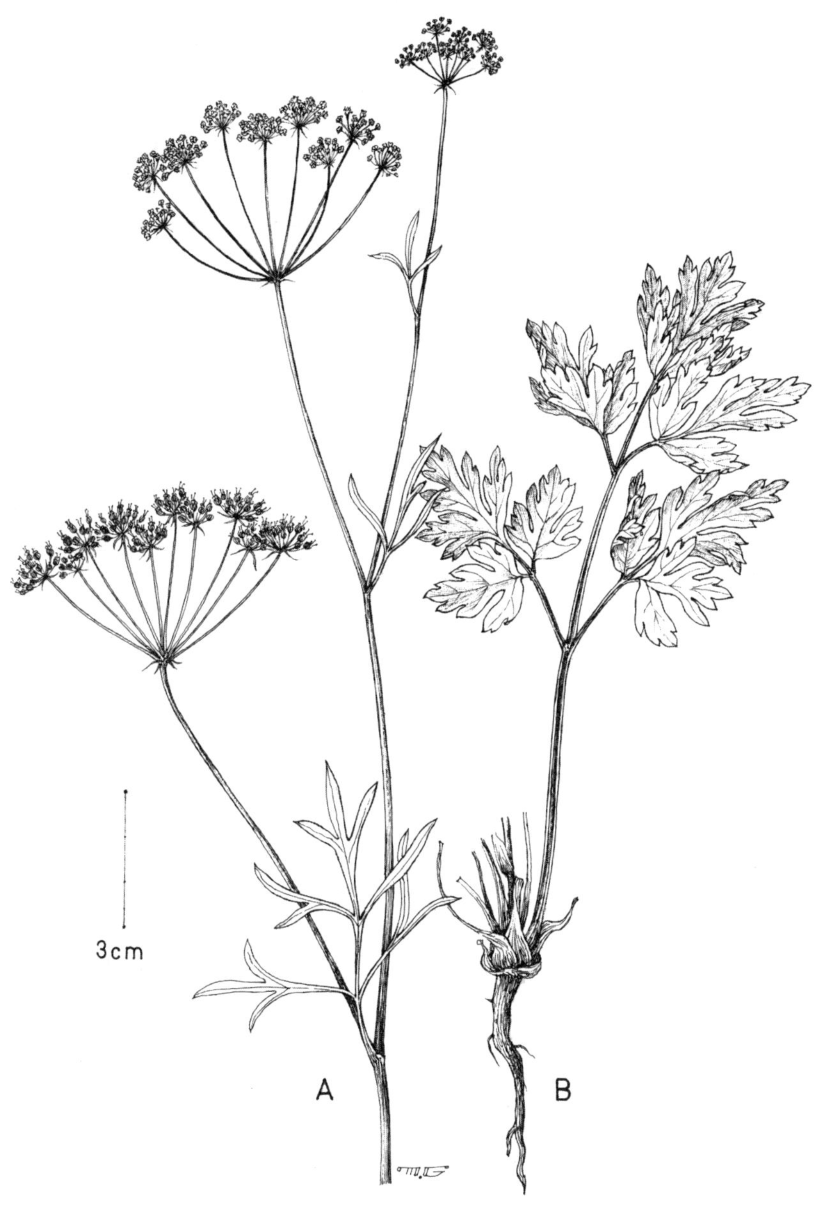

Petroselinum crispum
A. flowering and fruiting branch, B. root and basal leaf

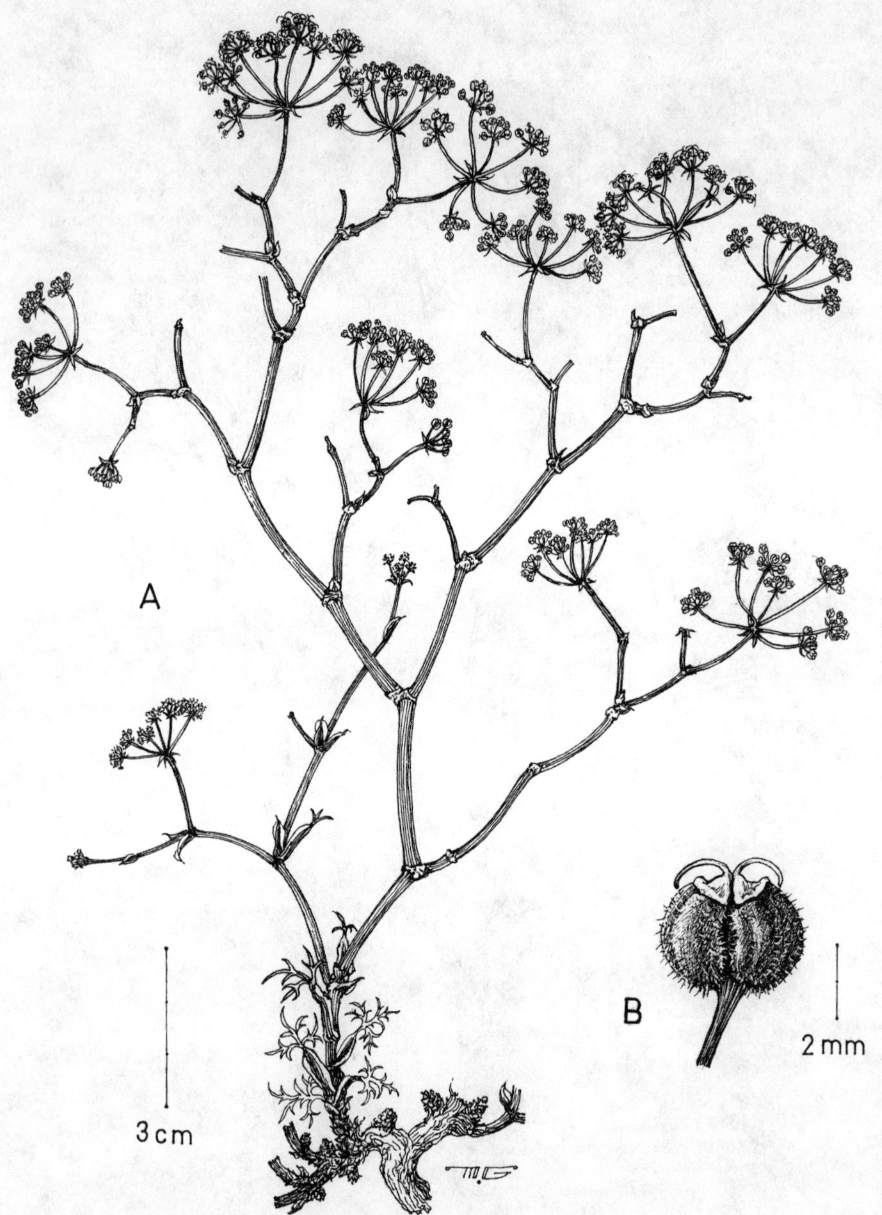

Pituranthos tortuosus
A. flowering and fruiting plant, B. fruit, enlarged

are absorbed as vermifuge, antihysteric, for desentery. *Ref:* 5, 24, 42

Foeniculum vulgare Miller *Area:* Egypt to Morocco. Also cultivated.
Names: Arabic: Besbas (5, 13, 23, 42, 62); Besbasa (23, 47, 62); Shamar (4); fruit: Nafa (5, 23, 42, 62). Berber: Tamessaout, Lemsous (23, 62); Amsa (42). English: Common fennel (4); Fennel (25). French: Fenouil (4, 13, 23, 24, 42, 62); Fenouil doux (5); Aneth doux (4).
Uses: Infusion of entire plant for lumbago and abdominal pains; juice of fresh plant largely used in preparation of eye lotions for cataract. Green plant edible; plant cooked with food or infusion of plant used for liver ailments (Rabat drug market); fresh plant or infusion of dried plant vermifuge (Algiers drug market). Root diuretic. Fruit stimulant, carminative, stomachic, galactogogue, expectorant, antispasmodic, digestive, aphrodisiac, appetizer, tonic, calmative, emmenagogue.
Ref: 23, 24, 25, 34, 42, 56

***Petroselinum crispum** (Miller) A. W. Hill *Area:* Commonly cultivated in North Africa.
Names: Arabic: Bagdouness (23, 62); Ma'adnous (23, 42, 62); Maqdunis rumi (4); Bersil (42). Berber: Imzi (23, 62). English: Common garden parsley (4); Parsley (25). French: Persil (4, 23, 42, 45, 62); Persil cultivé (4).
Uses: Whole plant used as an appetizer, stimulant, sudorific, depurative. Roots diuretic. Seeds carminative, emmenagogue, diuretic, stimulant, stomachic; decoction of seeds taken first thing in the morning as anthelmintic. *Ref:* 17, 23, 24, 25, 42

Pimpinella anisum L. *Area:* Frequently cultivated in North Africa.
Names: Arabic: Yansun (4, 17, 62); Habba helwa (5, 17, 42, 62); Anisun (4, 17); Kemmoun abiad (62); Kammoun helw (4). Berber: Habb talaout (62). English: Anise (4, 25); Sweet cumin, Aniseed plant (4). French: Anis (4, 5, 24); Anis vert (4, 24, 42, 62).
Uses: Essence of anise is diuretic, stomachic, expectorant, spasmolytic, carminative. Infusion of seeds is one of the best carminatives, also used as appetizer, chologogue, digestive, galactogogue, diuretic, stomachic, diaphoretic, aphrodisiac, and very much used against stomach pains and to facilitate digestion after meals. Seeds carminative, stimulant, emmenagogue, for pulmonary conditions, galactogogue if absorbed in small doses mixed with honey before the meals. Decoction of seeds taken orally against bites of poisonous animals. *Ref:* 5, 17, 25, 42, 56

Pituranthos tortuosus (Desf.) Benth. & Hook. fil. *Area:* Egypt to Tunisia.
Names: Arabic: Shabat el-gabal, Qozzah, Qazzah, Kerdwy, Zakouk (58).
Uses: Mannitol, to which its diuretic action may be attributed, is isolated from the plant in appreciable quantities. Plant also used as flavouring agent; tender parts are eaten fresh to bring good appetite (Bedouins, Egypt). *Ref:* 63

Thapsia garganica L. *Area:* Libya to Morocco.
Names: Arabic: Derias (4, 5, 8, 12, 13, 23, 42, 62, Rabat drug market); root: Bou neffa' (5, 12, 13, 23, 42, 62). Berber: Hadriegs, Toufalt (12, 13, 23, 62); Aderias (13, 42). English: Drias plant, Smooth thapsia (4). French: Thapsia (5, 13, 23, 62); Thapsie, Faux fenouil, Faux turbith (4); Sylphium (5); Père de la santé (4).
Uses: Plant dangerous in large doses and should be used with care. Pounded roots are slowly heated in oil or butter for several hours and the resulting liquid is used as a

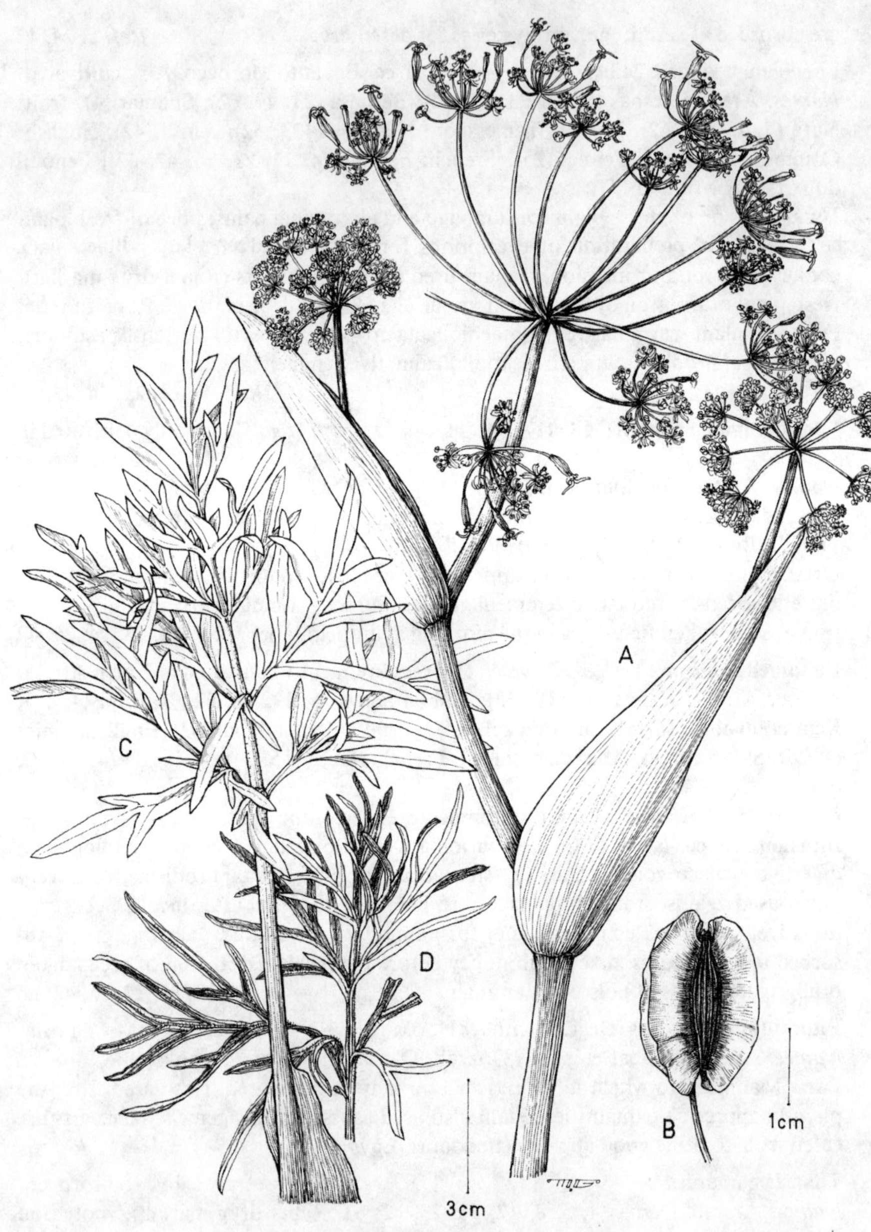

Thapsia garganica

A. flowering branch, B. fruit, enlarged
C. median stem leaf, D. part of basal leaf

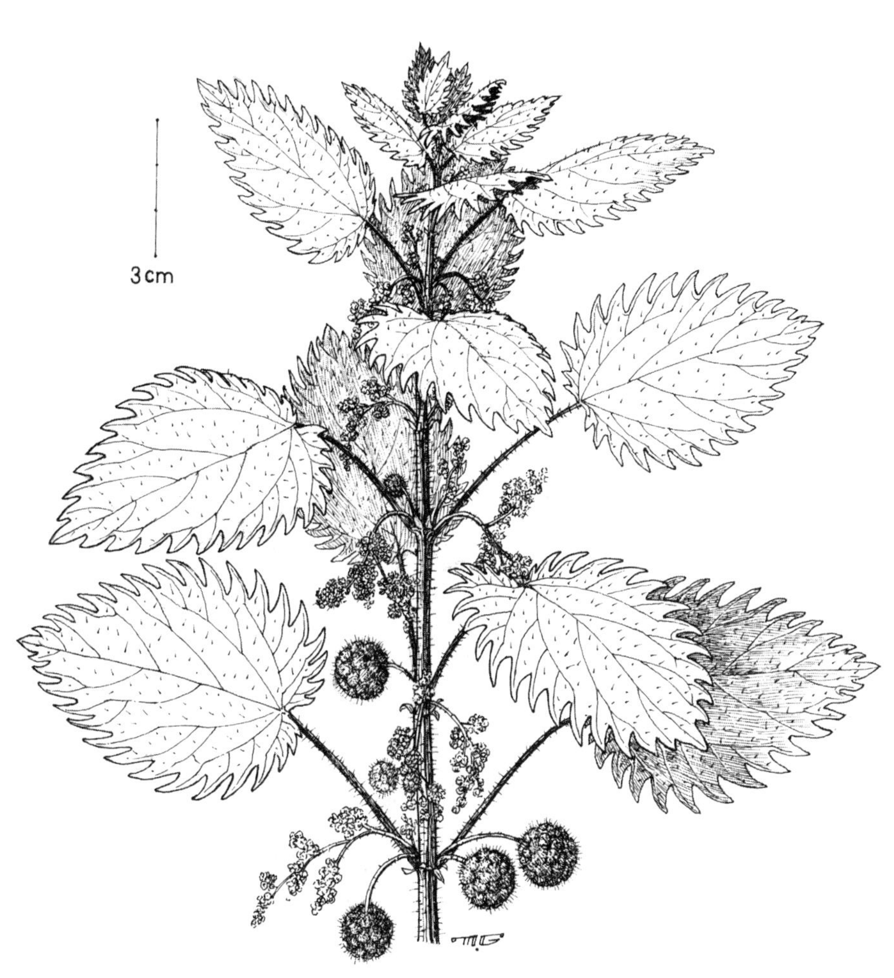

Urtica pilulifera

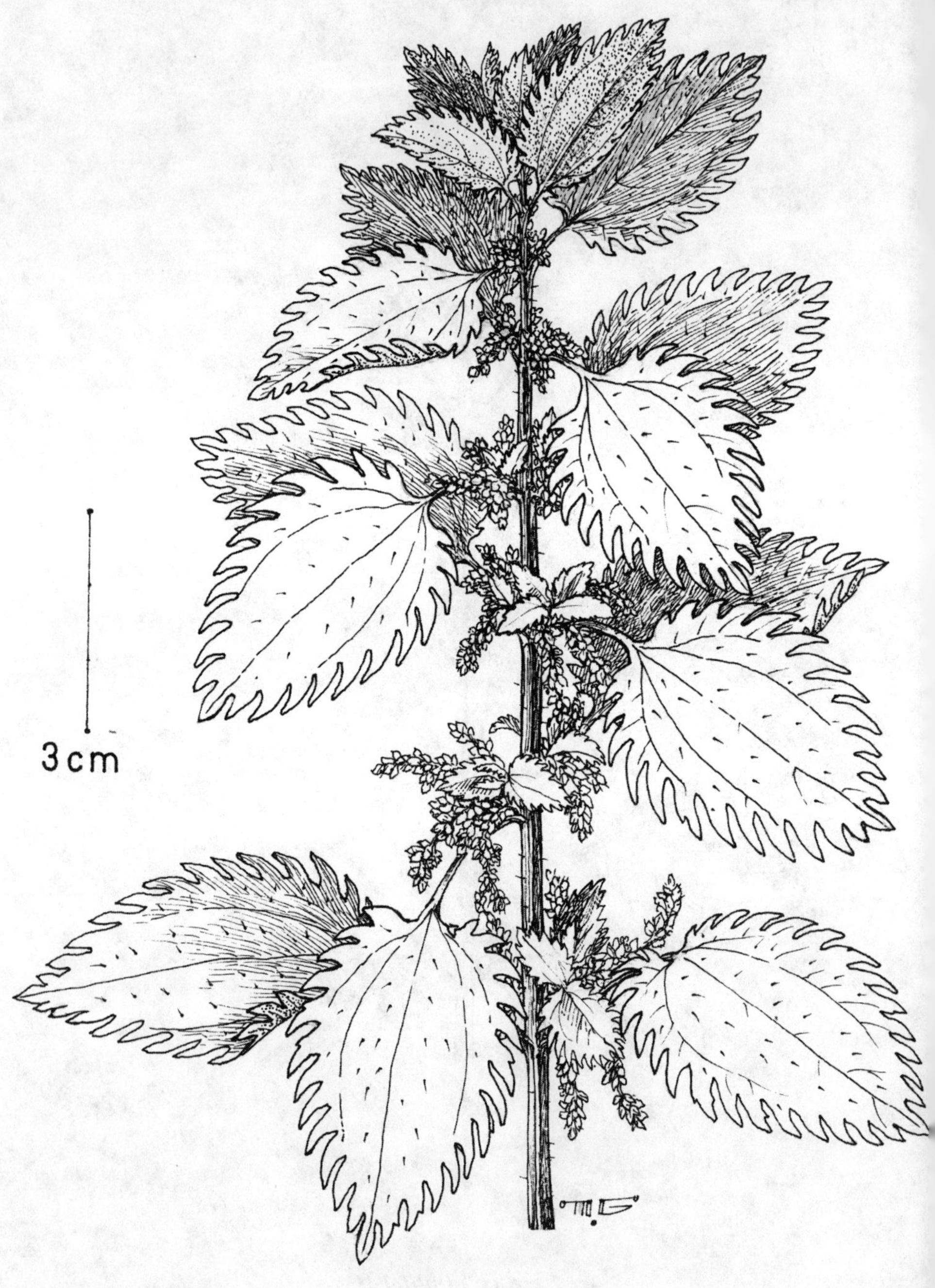

Urtica urens

revulsive, for rheumatism. Root used for rabies, cough, bronchitis, rubefacient, feminine sterility (Rabat drug market), epispastic, for thinness, chest ailments, sterility, gout. Whole plant especially the root bark, contains a gum-resin which is a powerful revulsive and purgative, rubbed on skin as a revulsive in all cases of fall in body temperature and to help in the maturation of abscesses. *Ref:* 5, 23, 25, 42

Urticaceae

Urtica pilulifera L. *Area:* Egypt to Morocco.
Names: Arabic: Qorreis (4, 8, 23, 58, 62); Horreiq (4, 8, 26, 42, 58, 62); Andjira (62); Bent en-nar, Nebat en-nar (42). Berber: Imereksin (23, 62); Imezri, Timezrit (42); Mezri, Tezzount (62). English: Roman nettle (4, 8). French: Ortie romaine (4, 23); Ortie (26, 42, 62); Ortie rude (42); Ozomaine (23).
Uses: Prescribed to cure sore joints by taking a mixture of the plant juice with oil. Contents of stinging hairs provide a cure for rheumatism, hemorrhage. Decoction of summits of the plants diuretic, depurative. Seeds for renal stones and inflammation of the bladder, diuretic, aphrodisiac. *Ref:* 8, 26, 42, 62

Urtica urens L. *Area:* Egypt to Morocco.
Names: Arabic: Horreiq (13, 23, 42, 58, 62); Bent en-nar, Bou khsas, Bou zeqdouf (13, 62); Qorreis (58); Sha'ar el-'agouz (4, 58). Berber: Timezrit (13, 23, 62); Harrous, Iherriqet (13, 62); Timzi, Azekdon (13). English: Small nettle, Dwarf stinger (4). French: Petite ortie, Ortie brûlante (4, 23); Ortie grieche (13).
Uses: Fresh plants used as an effective but painful rub to treat rheumatism, antidiarrhoeic, aphrodisiac, used for hemorrhage, kidney ailments, revulsive. Infusion of entire plant antihemorrhagic, galactogogue. Infusion and decoction of leaves diuretic; extract of fresh leaves used in homeopathy for eczema, dysmenorrhoea, metrorrhagia, nose-bleeding and in lotions to promote hair growth; used externally, it soothes wounds and ulcers. *Ref:* 13, 23, 37, 56

Verbenaceae

***Aloysia triphylla** (L'Hérit.) Britt. *Area:* Cultivated mainly in Algeria and Morocco.
Names: Arabic: Lwiza (4, 23, 62, Rabat and Algiers drug markets). Berber: Ouheireche (23, 62). English: Lemon verbena, Herb Louisa (4). French: Verveine citronelle (23, 24, 62); Verveine odorante (23, 24); Citronelle (4, 23, 24).
Uses: Leaves and flowering summits antispasmodic, stomachic, carminative, febrifuge, for colds (Rabat drug market). *Ref:* 23, 24

Verbena officinalis L. *Area:* Egypt to Morocco.
Names: Arabic: Ben nout (23, 62); Baymut (42, Rabat drug market); Barbina (42); Rigl el-hamam (4). English: Vervain (4, 24); Pigeon's grass, Holy herb (4). French: Verveine (23, 42, 62); Verveine officinale, Herbe sacrée (23, 62).
Uses: Ash of plant used to cure burns and boils (Rabat drug market). Leaves antispasmodic, febrifuge, emmenagogue, diuretic, galactogogue, stimulant, antidiarrhoeic; infusion or decoction for insomnia, stomachic; cataplasm vulnerary.
Ref: 23, 24, 34, 37, 45, 56.

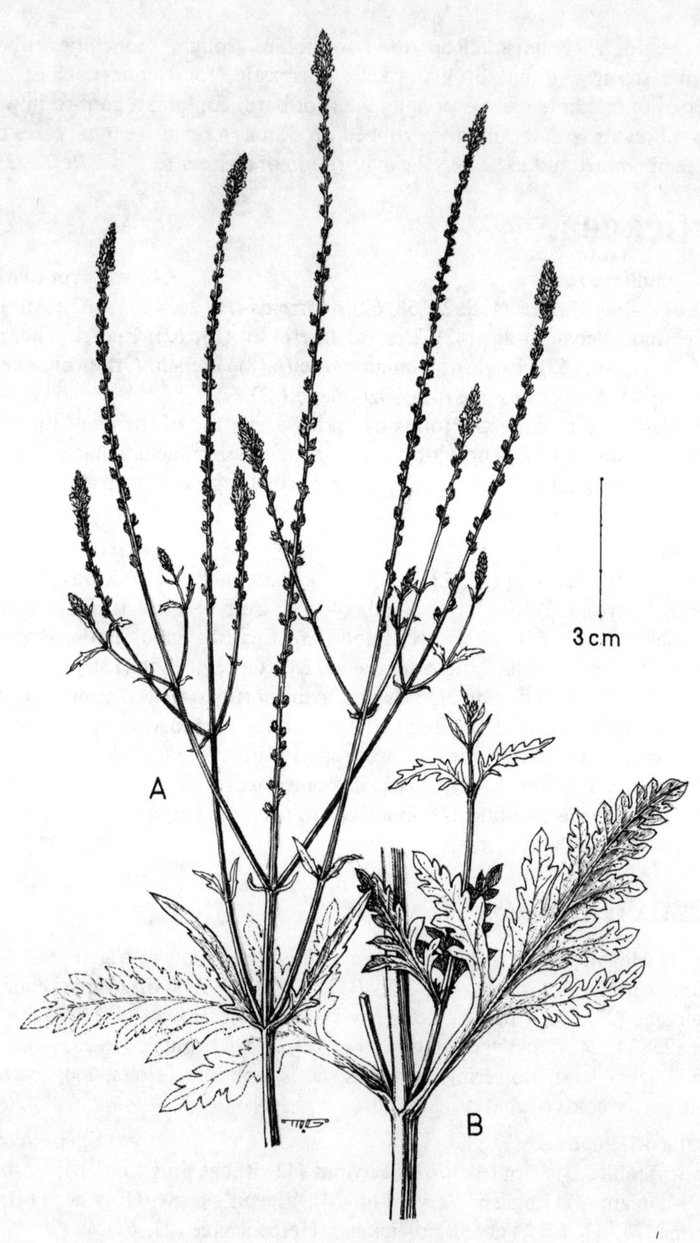

Verbena officinalis
A. flowering branch, B. basal leaves

Vitex agnus-castus L. *Area:* Cultivated in North Africa.
Names: Arabic: Kaf Maryam (4, 23, 62); Ghar (23, 62); Kherwa' (5, 42); Bou metin (62); Bou mentem (23); fruit: Hab el-kheraf (62). Berber: Angarf (6, 23, 42, 62). English: Chaste tree, Agnus castus, Hemp tree, Abraham's balm, Monk's tree (4). French: Gattilier (4, 5, 23, 24, 42, 45, 62); Agneau chaste, Arbre au poivre, Petit poivre (4).
Uses: Fruit anaphrodisiac (Rabat drug market), sedative, soporific, stimulant, appetizer, diuretic, carminative, taken by women to add weight, vermifuge, antispasmodic. *Ref:* 5, 23, 24, 37, 42, 45

Violaceae

Viola odorata L. *Area:* Frequently cultivated in North Africa. Often subspontaneous.
Names: Arabic: Banafsag (4, 23, 42, 62). English: Violet, Sweet violet (4). French: Violette (4, 23, 24, 62); Violette odorante (4, 24, 45).
Uses: Infusions and decoctions of whole plant very effective expectorants for treating respiratory disorders, purgative; tincture used to treat earache, eye infections and whooping cough. Plant sudorific, bechic. Rhizome emetic. Infusion of flowering branches emollient, for fevers, cough and constipation. *Ref:* 23, 24, 42, 56

Viola tricolor L. *Area:* Tunisia to Morocco. Also cultivated in gardens as an ornamental.
Names: Arabic: Belesfendj (47, 62); Pansayh (4). English: Pansy, Heart's ease, Herb trinity (4). French: Pensée (4, 62); Herbe de la trinité (4).
Uses: Infusion of whole plant depurative, mild diuretic, laxative, tonic, emetocathartic in high doses, for skin eruptions in children, diarrhoea, urinary infections. Flowers bechic, expectorant. *Ref:* 24, 56

Zingiberaceae

Alpinia officinarum Hance *Area:* Drug imported from East Asia.
Names: Arabic: Khulingan (4, 5, 42, 62); Hodengal (5, 42). English: Lesser galangal (4). French: Galanga (23, 42, 62); Galanga mineur (4).
Uses: Rhizome aphrodisiac, stomachic, used for kidney conditions, carminative, for aerophagia, bad digestion; rhizome mixed with liquorice root used for cough. *Ref:* 5, 17, 42

***Curcuma zedoaria** (Christm.) Roscoe *Area:* Drug imported from East Asia.
Names: Arabic: Gadwar (4, 5, 42); Kurkum, Khurkum (5); Zingar (42). English: Zedoary, Setwall (4). French: Zédoaire (4, 5, 42); Curcuma zédoaire, Gingembre bâtard (4).
Uses: Rhizome carminative, stimulant; powdered rhizome taken after meals is effective against flatulence; chologogue, anthelmintic, antihemorrhoidal, taken first thing in the morning mixed with honey against conditions of the stomach and intestine, vermifuge, reduces pains caused by hemorrhoids. *Ref:* 5, 12, 42

Zingiber officinale Roscoe *Area:* Drug imported from Southeast Asia.
Names: Arabic: Zenjabil (4, 5, 62); Skengbir (42, 62). English: Common ginger, East

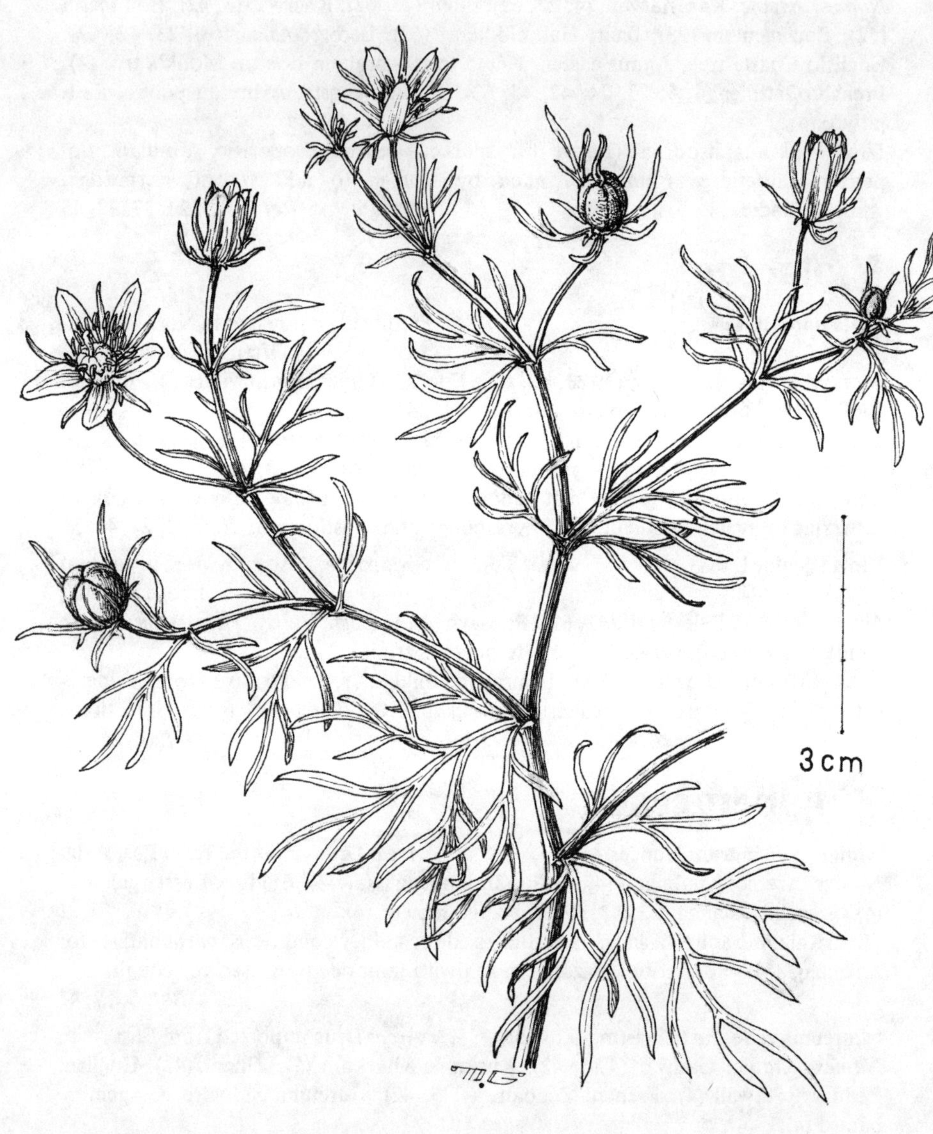

Peganum harmala

Indian ginger (4). French: Gingembre (4, 5, 42, 62); Amome des Indes (4).
Uses: Rhizome stimulant, stomachic, aphrodisiac, for amnesia, weak stomach; olive oil in which powdered rhizome was soaked for several days is used for rubbing the body, after a hot bath, for rheumatism, vertebral pains, stiffness, lumbago. Rhizome mixed with honey taken for conditions of the respiratory system; powdered rhizome mixed with honey is taken daily in small doses as aphrodisiac; decoction of rhizome mixed with an equal amount of black pepper, then added into boiling honey, is taken in the form of pellets twice a day, in the morning and at night, against pectoral diseases. Rhizome is mixed with cloves, honey and oil as a tonic; one teaspoonful of this mixture is taken first thing in the morning with hot water to oppose the action of bites of poisonous animals. *Ref: 5, 42*

Zygophyllaceae

Peganum harmala L. *Area:* Egypt to Morocco.
Names: Arabic: Harmel (5, 13, 23, 42, 58, 62, Rabat and Algiers drug markets); Harmal (4, 8, 58); Mejennena (5, 13, 42); seeds: Harmel sahari (23, 62). English: Harmel, Syrian rue (4). French: Harmel (4, 23, 42, 62); Rue sauvage (4, 23).
Uses: Plant emetic, diuretic. Fresh plants digested in sheep's fat used against rheumatism by rubbing; vapors of burnt plant for headache and neurotic pains; dried powdered plant for the treatment of purulent conjunctivitis; its decoction in oil taken first thing in the morning is effective against hemorrhoids and depurative. Fresh branches revulsive. Seeds anthelmintic; powdered seeds mixed with honey and ginger rubbed on skin for articular pains and rheumatism, cataplasm analgesic; powdered seeds boiled in olive oil used to ameliorate the quality of hair by making it thicker and stronger, for alopecia by massage. Seeds stimulant of the central nervous system, cause paralysis and are poisonous in strong doses. Oil extracted from seeds used for some infectious eye diseases, rheumatic pains and some skin diseases. Seeds eaten in small doses for asthma (Algiers drug market); seeds sudorific, emmenagogue; powdered roasted seeds are taken after meals against bad digestion and diabetes (Rabat drug market). Infusion of seeds is useful for cardiac diseases and its prolonged use helps in cases of sciatica. Pounded roots and seeds mixed with tobacco are smoked in pipes for toothache. *Ref:* 2, 5, 8, 13, 23, 42, 57

Tribulus terrestris L. *Area:* Egypt to Morocco.
Names: Arabic: Hasak (4, 5, 17, 62); Hasaka (5, 62); Adras el-kelb, Hommos el-hamir, Dik 'aroum, Sa'adan (62); Tadrisa (5); Dars el-'agouz (4, 17). Berber: Timgelest (5, 62); Tadjnouft, Tamezlagelt (62); Amagelost, Tagruft (5). English: Caltrops, Land caltrops (4). French: Tribule terrestre, Croix de Malte (4).
Uses: Extract of plant antispasmodic. Fruit used as tonic in spermatorrhea, neurasthenia, vertigo, astringent for oral inflammations, detersive, diuretic, for dysentery and pains of the bladder. *Ref:* 2, 17, 34

Zygophyllum coccineum L. *Area:* Egypt.
Names: Arabic: Rotrayt, Balbal, Bawwal (58); fruit: Kammun karmani (29, 58).
Uses: Fruits used in treatment of rheumatism, gout, asthma, hypertension, diuretic, anthelmintic, antidiabetic. *Ref:* 29

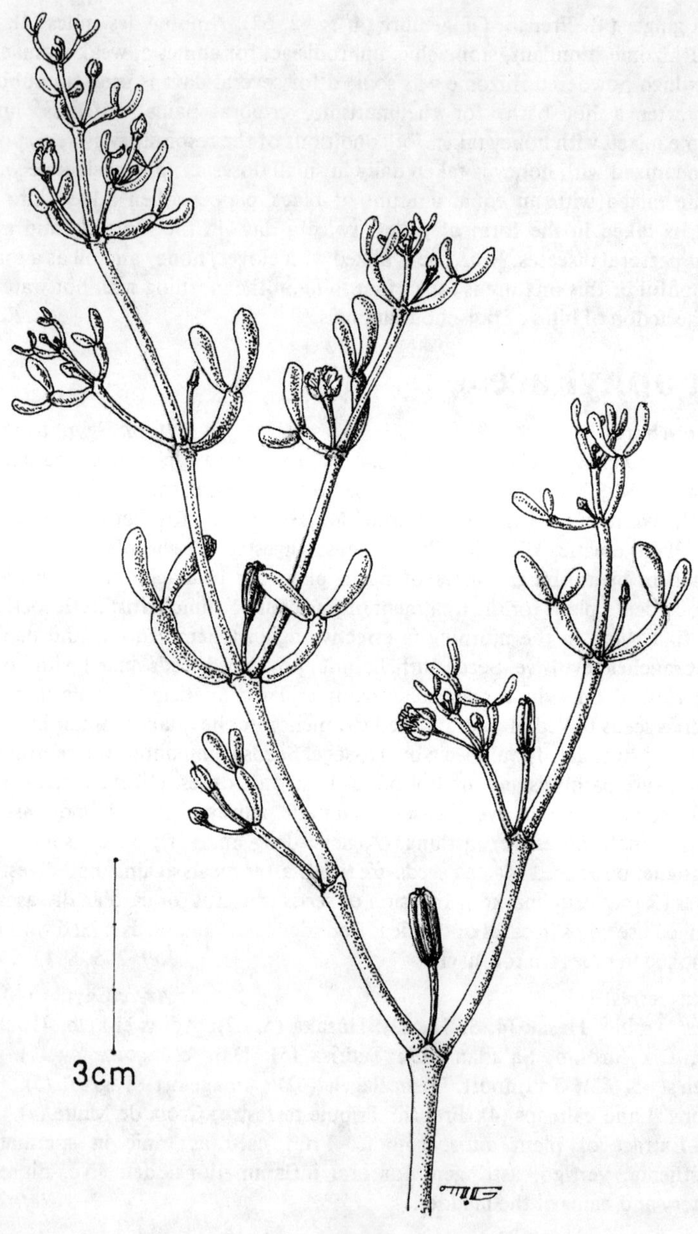

Zygophyllum coccineum

ZYGOPHYLLACEAE

Zygophyllum gaetulum Emberger & Maire *Area:* Endemic to Morocco.
Names: Arabic: Berraya (5). Berber: Aggaya (5).
Uses: Dried powdered leaves hemostatic, used as a plaster on mature boils and abscesses, enter in the treatment of eczema; infusion of leaves used as antiseptic lotion for the hygiene of babies. *Ref:* 5

Notes and Explanations

Synonyms and the names of other taxa included within a species marked by an asterisk (*) in the text, are listed below.

ACANTHACEAE—*Blepharis ciliaris* includes *B. edulis* (Forssk.) Pers.
ADIANTACEAE—The ferns in this volume are located under four families: Adiantaceae, Aspidiaceae, Aspleniaceae, and Polypodiaceae.
ALLIACEAE—*Allium* is sometimes included in Liliaceae.
ASCLEPIADACEAE—*Pergularia tomentosa* includes *Daemia cordata* (Forssk.) R. Br. ex Schult.
Solenostemma argel (Del.) Hayne includes *S. oleifolium* (Nectoux) Bullock & Bruce
ASPLENIACEAE—*Phyllitis scolopendrium* includes *Asplenium scolopendrium* L., *Scolopendrium officinale* Sm., and *Scolopendrium vulgare* Sm.
BORAGINACEAE—*Anchusa azurea* includes *A. italica* Retz.
Echium plantagineum includes *E. maritimum* Willd.
Heliotropium bacciferum includes *H. undulatum* Vahl
Moltkiopsis ciliata includes *Moltkia callosa* (Vahl) Wettst., *Moltkia ciliata* (Forssk.) Maire, and *Lithospermum callosum* Vahl
CAPPARACEAE—*Capparis decidua* includes *C. sodada* R. Br. and *Sodada decidua* Forssk.
Capparis spinosa includes var. *aegyptia,* var. *rupestris,* etc.
CARYOPHYLLACEAE—*Spergularia media* includes *S. marginata* Kettel
Spergularia rubra includes *S. campestris* (L.) Aschers.
Vaccaria pyramidata includes *V. vulgaris* Host, *V. segetalis* Garcke, and *Saponaria vaccaria* L.
CLEOMACEAE—*Cleome* is sometimes included in Capparaceae.
COMPOSITAE—*Artemisia herba-alba* includes *A. inculta* Del.
Chamaemelum nobile includes *Anthemis nobilis* L.
Chamomilla recutita includes *Matricaria recutita* L. and *M. chamomilla* L., partly.
Conyza bonariensis includes *C. ambigua* DC. and *Erigeron crispus* Pourr.
Cotula cinerea includes *Brocchia cinerea* (Del.) Vis.
Eclipta prostrata includes *E. alba* (L.) Hassk.
Inula viscosa includes *Dittrichia viscosa* (L.) W. Greuter
Lactuca serriola includes *L. scariola* L.
Otanthus maritimus includes *Diotis maritima* (L.) Desf. ex Cass. and *D. candidissima* Desf.
Pulicaria crispa includes *Francoeuria crispa* (Forssk.) Cass.
Pulicaria incisa includes *P. desertorum* DC. and *P. undulata* sensu Boiss., non (L.) Kostel.
Senecio anteuphorbium includes *Kleinia pteroneura* DC.
CRUCIFERAE—*Alliaria petiolata* includes *A. officinalis* Andrz. ex Bieb. and *Sisymbrium alliaria* (L.) Scop.

Brassica nigra includes *Sinapis nigra* L.
Lobularia maritima includes *Koniga maritima* (L.) R. Br. and *Alyssum maritimum* (L.) Lam.
Sisymbrium officinale includes *Erysimum officinale* L.
Zilla spinosa includes *Z. macroptera* Coss.

CUCURBITACEAE—*Citrullus colocynthis* includes *Colocynthis vulgaris* Schrader
Lagenaria siceraria includes *L. vulgaris* Ser.
Luffa cylindrica includes *L. aegyptiaca* Miller

CUPRESSACEAE—*Tetraclinis articulata* includes *Callitris articulata* (Vahl) Aschers. & Graebn. and *C. quadrivalvis* Vent.

GENTIANACEAE—*Centaurium erythraea* includes *C. umbellatum* Gilib. and *Erythraea centaurium* Borkh.
Centaurium spicatum includes *Erythraea spicata* (L.) Pers.

GRAMINEAE—*Cymbopogon proximus* includes *C. schoenanthus* (L.) Spreng. subsp. *proximus* (Hochst. ex A. Rich.) Maire & Weiller
Cymbopogon schoenanthus includes *Andropogon schoenanthus* L. and *A. laniger* Desf.
Elymus repens includes *Elytrigia repens* (L.) Desv. ex Nevski, *Agropyron repens* (L.) Beauv., and *Triticum repens* L.
Phragmites australis includes *P. communis* Trin.
Stipagrostis pungens includes *Aristida pungens* Desf.

LABIATAE—*Lavandula angustifolia* includes *L. officinalis* Chaix and *L. vera* DC.
Mentha longifolia subsp. *typhoides* includes *M. sylvestris* L. subsp. *typhoides* Briq.
Mentha spicata includes *M. viridis* (L.) L., *M. crispa* L., and *M. crispata* Schrader
Mentha suaveolens includes *M. rotundifolia* L.
Mentha x *villosa* includes *M. spicata* x *M. suaveolens*
Origanum vulgare subsp. *glandulosum* includes *O. glandulosum* Desf.
Salvia fruticosa includes *S. triloba* L. fil. and *S. libanotica* Boiss. & Gaill.
Stachys officinalis includes *Betonica officinalis* L.
Thymus algeriensis includes *T. zattarellus* Pomel

LEGUMINOSAE—*Acacia nilotica* includes *A. arabica* (Lam.) Willd. var. *nilotica* (L.) Benth.
Acacia raddiana includes *A. tortilis* (Forssk.) Hayne subsp. *raddiana* (Savi) Brenan
Alhagi graecorum includes *A. mannifera* Desv., *nom. nud.* and *A. maurorum* DC., non Medic.
Cassia italica includes *C. obovata* Collad. and *C. aschrek* Forssk.
Cassia senna includes *C. acutifolia* Del. and *C. angustifolia* Vahl
Lupinus albus includes *L. termis* Forssk.
Ononis spinosa includes *O. pungens* Pomel and *O. antiquorum* L.

LILIACEAE—*Androcymbium gramineum* includes *A. punctatum* (Cav.) Baker and *Erythrostictus punctatus* (Cav.) Schlecht.
Asparagus stipularis includes *A. horridus* L. fil.
Asphodelus aestivus includes *A. microcarpus* Salzm. & Viv.
Urginea maritima includes *U. scilla* Steinh. and *Scilla maritima* L.

LYTHRACEAE—*Lawsonia inermis* includes *L. alba* Lam.

MYRISTICACEAE—*Myristica fragrans* includes *M. moschata* Thunb.

MYRTACEAE—*Syzygium aromaticum* includes *Eugenia aromatica* Baill., *E. caryophyllata* Thunb., and *Caryophyllus aromaticus* L.

NYCTAGINACEAE—*Boerhavia repens* is a multiform species including several varieties.

OLEACEAE—*Fraxinus angustifolia* includes *F. oxycarpa* Bieb. ex Willd.

OROBANCHACEAE—*Cistanche phelypaea* includes *C. tinctoria* (Forssk.) G. Beck, *Phelypaea lutea* Desf., and *P. tinctoria* (Forssk.) Brot.

PAEONIACEAE—*Paeonia coriacea* includes *P. corralina* Retz. var. *coriacea* (Boiss.) Maire

PEDALIACEAE—*Sesamum indicum* includes *S. orientale* L.

PISTACIACEAE—*Pistacia* is sometimes included in Anacardiaceae.

PLANTAGINACEAE—*Plantago afra* includes *P. psyllium* L.

POLYGONACEAE—*Rumex vesicarius* includes *R. roseus* Desf., non L.

RANUNCULACEAE—*Adonis annua* includes *A. autumnalis* L.
Ranunculus macrophyllus includes *R. lanuginosus* Poir.

RHAMNACEAE—*Ziziphus zizyphus* includes *Z. jujuba* Miller, *Z. sativa* Gaertn., *Z. vulgaris* Lam. and *Rhamnus zizyphus* L.

ROSACEAE—*Crataegus monogyna* includes *C. oxyacantha* L.

RUBIACEAE—*Galium odoratum* includes *Asperula odorata* L.

RUTACEAE—*Citrus aurantium* includes *C. bigaradia* Duh.

SOLANACEAE—*Hyoscyamus faleslez* includes *H. muticus* L. subsp. *faleslez* (Coss.) Maire

TAMARICACEAE—*Tamarix aphylla* includes *T. articulata* Vahl

TYPHACEAE—*Typha domingensis* includes *T. australis* Schum., *T. angustata* Bory & Chaub., and *T. angustifolia* L.

UMBELLIFERAE—*Ammoides pusilla* includes *A. verticillata* (Duby) Briq., *Ptychotis ammoides* Koch, and *Carum ammoides* (L.) Ball
Petroselinum crispum includes *P. sativum* Hoffm.

VERBENACEAE—*Aloysia triphylla* includes *A. citriodora* (Cav.) Ort., *Verbena citriodora* Cav., *V. triphylla* L'Hérit., and *Lippia citriodora* H.B.K.

ZINGIBERACEAE—*Curcuma zedoaria* includes *C. pallida* Lour.

GLOSSARY

ABORTION—interruption of pregnancy, usually during the first three months when the contents of the womb are emptied.

ABORTIVE—effecting an abortion.

ABSCESS—localized collection of pus or liquid derived from blood in any part of the body.

ACNE—skin eruption due to inflammation of sebaceous glands, common in adolescence, and characterized by red pimples, especially on the face.

AEROPHAGY (AEROPHAGIA)— spasmodic swallowing of air, followed by eructations.

ALBUGO—a white corneal opacity.

ALBUMINURIA—presence of albumin in the urine, sometimes indicating kidney disease.

ALOPECIA—baldness, with the scalp wholly or partly hairless; a natural or abnormal condition.

AMENORRHEA—abnormal suppression or absence of menstruation.

AMNESIA—loss of memory.

ANEMIA (ANAEMIA)—deficiency of red blood corpuscles or their haemoglobin, often causing paleness.

ANALEPTIC—a drug with restorative effect.

ANALGESIC—a drug producing analgesia, that relieves or reduces the pain.

ANAPHRODISIAC—a drug or agent that reduces the sexual desire.

ANESTHETIC—a drug used to produce anesthesia, a partial or total loss of the sense of pain, touch, temperature, etc.

ANGINA PECTORIS—a disease of the heart signaled by acute constricting pains in the chest.

ANTHELMINTIC (= VERMIFUGE)—a drug which kills or causes the destruction and expulsion of intestinal worms.

ANTIALGETIC—a drug acting against or reducing pain.

ANTIBIOTIC—a substance that inhibits the growth of micro-organisms.

ANTICOLIC—See Colic.

ANTIDIABETIC—a drug that checks diabetes, which is a metabolic disorder characterized by excessive discharge of glucose-containing urine, with persistent thirst.

ANTIDIARRHOEIC—a drug or substance that acts against diarrhoea.

ANTIDOTE—a drug or substance that counteracts a poison.

ANTIFEBRILE (= ANTIPYRETIC, FEBRIFUGE).

ANTIHELMINTHOID—a drug acting against worms.

ANTIHEMORRHAGIC—a drug or substance that stops hemorrhage, or bleeding.

ANTIHEMORRHOID—a drug acting against hemorrhoids.

ANTIHYSTERIC—drug or substance that helps to arrest hysteria, which is a functional disturbance of the nervous system, of psychoneurotic origin.

ANTILEPROUS—effective against leprosy, a chronic contagious disease due to infection with lepra bacillus.

ANTIMITOTIC—inhibiting or preventing mitosis, the process of cell division.

ANTINEURALGIC—a drug that arrests the intense intermittent pain, usually of head or face, caused by neuralgia.

ANTIPHLOGISTIC—acting against inflammation and fever.

ANTIPRURIGINOUS—a drug acting against prurigo, which is a chronic inflammatory skin disease producing eruptions and severe itching.

ANTIPYRETIC (=ANTIFEBRILE, FEBRIFUGE)—a drug that reduces or prevents fever.

ANTIRABIC—a drug or substance which prevents or cures rabies.

ANTISCORBUTIC—a drug or substance that corrects or cures scurvy.

ANTISCROFULOUS—See Scrofula.

ANTISPASMODIC—spasmolytic; a drug or agent that prevents or relieves spasm or the involuntary and irregular contractions of the body muscles.

ANTISYPHILITIC—a drug which is effective against, or a remedy for syphilis, a venereal disease caused by *Treponema pallidum.*

ANTITUSSIVE—a drug that reduces or prevents cough.

ANTIVIRAL—a drug or substance that weakens or abolishes the action of virus.

APHRODISIAC—a drug or agent that causes the stimulation of sexual passions.

APHTHA (plural, APHTHAE)—an ulcer of the mucous membrane, usually oral.

ARTERIOSCLEROSIS—hardening of the walls of the arteries.

ARTHRITIS—inflammation of joints.

ASTHENIA—general weakness or loss of strength and energy due to some disorder.

ASTHMA—a disorder characterized by wheezing, difficult breathing, coughing and suffocating feeling.

ASTRINGENT—a drug that contracts the body tissues to check the discharge of secretions or arrests capillary bleeding.

ATONY—insufficient muscular tone.

BACTERIOSTATIC—a drug or substance that inhibits the growth and reproduction of bacteria.

BECHIC—a tonic or other remedy that controls coughing.

BILHARZIASIS (BILHARZIA)—See Schistosoma.

BLENNORRHAGIA—gonorrhea, an inordinate secretion and discharge of mucous.

BLEPHARITIS—inflammation of the eyelids.

BLISTER—thin vesicle on the skin, filled with serum, and caused by rubbing, friction, burn, etc.

BOIL—a localized pyrogenic infection originating in a hair follicle, often painful.

BOURDONNEMENT—a humming or buzzing sound, whether subjective or ausculatory.

BRONCHITIS—an illness caused by the inflammation of bronchial mucous membrane.

BRUISE—contusion, injury by a blow to the body tissue without breaking the skin but causing discoloration.

CALCULUS (plural, CALCULI)—deposit of solid matter composed of mineral substances and salts formed in any portion of the body, such as kidney stone.

CALEFACIENT—a drug or substance that causes a sense of warmth.

CANCER—a malignant new growth or tumor in any part of the body.

CANKER—ulcer-like sore, especially in the mouth, that spreads.

CARDIODYNIA—pain of the heart.
CARMINATIVE—drug or substance which prevents formation of or promotes expulsion of flatus (wind generated in the stomach or bowels).
CATAPLASM—poultice; a paste of plant part or drug applied to sore or inflamed part of the body to supply moisture or to act as a local stimulant.
CATARACT—progressive opacity or clouding of the lens of the eye.
CATARRH—mild inflammation of mucous membranes, especially those of the air passages of the nose and throat.
CATHARTIC—a drug having a purgative action on the bowels.
CEPHALALGIA—headache.
CHANCROID—the hard and soft forms of sores caused by all venereal infections other than syphilis.
CHILL—a shivering or shaking, accompanied by a sense of cold.
CHOLOGOGUE—choleretic; a drug which stimulates the flow of bile by the liver.
CHOLERA—an acute, specific, infectious disease caused by *Vibrio,* resulting in profuse, effortless diarrhoea, vomiting, collapse, muscular cramps, and suppression of urine.
CHOLERETIC—See Cholagogue.
COLIC—pain resulting from excessive or sudden abnormal spasmodic contractions of muscles in the intestine wall, bile ducts or ureter, following the stretching of the walls by gas or solid substances.
CONDIMENT—a spice for seasoning the food.
CONGESTION—abnormal accumulation of blood in an organ.
CONJUNCTIVA—the mucous membrane lining the inner eyelid and front of eyeball.
CONJUNCTIVITIS—inflammation of the conjunctiva.
CONSTIPATION—condition of bowels in which defecation is irregular and difficult.
CONTUSION—See Bruise.
CONVULSION—violent irregular motion of limb or body due to involuntary contraction of muscles.
CORN—horny induration of cuticle with hard center and root, often penetrating deep into subjacent tissue, caused by pressure of shoes or feet.
CORYZA—inflammation of the mucous membrane of the nose and sinuses.
CRAMP—sudden painful involuntary contraction of muscles.
CYSTITIS—inflammation of the urinary bladder.
DANDRUFF—scurf, dead skin in small scales among the hair.
DECOCTION—liquid preparation obtained by boiling the plant in water and extracting the soluble drug by straining.
DECONGESTIVE—a drug that reduces congestion.
DEMULCENT—a drug substance used for its soothing and protective action, allaying irritation of surfaces, especially mucous membranes.
DEPILATORY—a drug or agent for removing or destroying the hair.
DEPURATIVE—a drug or agent that induces the excretion and removal of waste material.
DERMATITIS—inflammation of the skin causing discomforts such as eczema.
DETERSIVE—a detergent or cleansing agent.

DIAPHORETIC—a drug that causes an increase of perspiration as a result of the stimulation of sweat glands.

DIARRHOEA (DIARRHEA)—increased frequency of stool discharge as a result of gastro-intestinal disorder.

DISINFECTANT—a drug or substance that cleanses from infection, destroys harmful germs, bacteria, viruses, etc.

DISTOMATOSIS—infection with distoma, a group of trematode worms.

DIURETIC—a drug that has the ability to stimulate the kidneys to increase the secretion and flow of urine.

DIZZINESS—a condition of feeling giddy or unsteady.

DROPSY (HYDROPSY)—a leakage of the watery part of the blood into any of the tissues or cavities of the body.

DYSENTERY—a disease caused by bacteria or protozoa, bringing inflammation of mucous membrane and glands of large intestine, accompanied by painful diarrhoea and bloody evacuations.

DYSMENORRHEA (DYSMENORRHOEA)—painful spasmodic or continuous pains during the menstruation period.

DYSPEPSIA—indigestion.

ECZEMA—acute or chronic non-contagious inflammation of the skin, often accompanied by itching.

EDEMA (OEDEMA)—a condition in which excessive clear fluid passes from the blood into the tissues.

ELEPHANTIASIS—chronic enlargement of cutaneous and subcutaneous tissues, results from obstruction of lymphatics.

EMETIC—a drug or agent having the power to empty the stomach by vomiting.

EMMENAGOGUE—a drug that stimulates the menstrual flow.

EMOLLIENT—a drug or substance applied externally to soften the surface tissues or internally to soothe inflamed or irritated surface.

ENTERITIS—acute or chronic intestinal inflammation.

ENTERORRHAGIA—gastric bleeding.

EPILEPSY—a nervous disorder involving temporary loss of consciousness with or without convulsions and muscular spasms.

EPISPASTIC—a drug or substance with blistering action.

EPISTAXIS—nose bleeding.

ERUCTATION—the act of belching.

ERYSIPELAS—an acute inflammation of the skin and subcutaneous tissues, characterized by serious toxic symptoms of high fever and great prostration (St. Anthony's Fire).

ESCHAROTIC—a çorrosive or caustic agent or drug.

EXANTHEMA—a disease accompanied by eruptions of the skin, such as measles or scarlet fever.

EXPECTORANT—a drug that promotes or modifies the ejection of mucous or other secretions by coughing from the upper respiratory tract, especially the mouth.

FEBRIFUGE (= ANTIFEBRILE, ANTIPYRETIC).

FELON—See Whitlow.

FLATULENCE—the presence of an excessive amount of gas in the stomach and intestines.

FRECKLES—spotted pigmentation of skin.

FURUNCLE—a boil that usually is the result of an infection of a hair follicle.

GALACTOGOGUE—a drug that induces or increases the secretion of milk.

GANGLION—a group of nerve cells forming a center for reception and transmission of impulses.

GASTRALGIA—gastric pains.

GASTRO-INTESTINAL—pertaining to the stomach and intestines.

GINGIVITIS—inflammation of the gums.

GLOSSITIS—inflammation of the tongue.

GONORRHOEA (GONORRHEA)—a venereal disease due to gonococcus that causes specific infectious inflammations of the mucous membrane of the urethra and adjacent cavities.

GOUT—paroxysmal disease with painful inflammation of smaller joints due to excessive uric acid in the blood and formation of chalk-stones.

HALLUCINOGENIC—a drug or substance that produces hallucinations, imaginary things apparently seen or heard.

HEMOPTYSIS (HAEMOPTYSIS)—spitting of blood from the bronchi, larynx, lungs or trachea.

HEMORRHAGE—bleeding.

HEMORRHOID—enlarged or dilated blood vessels or veins in swollen tissue of the anal canal or the lower portion of the alimentary tract.

HEMOSTATIC—a drug or substance that arrests hemorrhage.

HEPATIC—pertaining to or occurring in the liver.

HERNIA—the abnormal protrusion of an organ through its containing wall; it may occur in any part of the body, but especially associated with the abdominal cavity.

HERPES—acute inflammation of skin or mucous membrane, characterized by the development of groups of vesicles on an inflammatory base.

HICCUP—involuntary spasm of respiratory organs, with sudden closure of glottis and characteristic sound.

HOARSENESS—to have a rough and husky voice.

HOMEOPATHY—a system of treatment for certain diseases by small doses of drugs that in a healthy person and in large doses would produce symptoms like those of the disease.

HYDRAGOGUE—a cathartic which causes watery purgation.

HYDROPSY—See Dropsy.

HYPERTENSIVE—causing high blood pressure.

HYPERTROPHY—an abnormal increase in the size of an organ or tissue.

HYPOGLYCEMIC—low concentration of sugar in the blood.

HYPOTENSIVE—causing low blood pressure.

HYPOTHERMY—fall in the temperature of the body.

HYSTERIA—See Antihysteric.

IMPOTENCE—inability to engage in sexual intercourse.

INCONTINENCE—a condition in which the patient is unable to control the natural discharge of the contents of the bladder and bowel.

INFLUENZA—acute infectious febrile disorder, caused by a virus.

INFUSION—the liquid extract that results from steeping a drug or substance in water and contains its active principles.

INSOLATION—exposure to sun's rays.

INSOMNIA—sleeplessness.

ITCH—to feel an irritating sensation on the skin, with the desire to scratch.

JAUNDICE—yellowness of the skin, mucous membranes and secretions due to bile pigments in the blood.

KERATOLYTIC—pertaining to or producing keratolysis, which is separation or peeling of the horny layer of epidermis.

LARYNGITIS—inflammation of the membrane lining of the larynx.

LAXATIVE—a drug having the action of loosening the bowels, stimulating defecation.

LENITIVE—a drug with soothing effect.

LEPROSY (HANSEN'S DISEASE)—chronic contagious disease due to infection with lepra bacillus.

LETHARGY—prolonged and unnatural drowsiness.

LEUCODERMA (LEUKODERMA)—a skin condition characterized by defective whitish pigmentation, especially a congenital absence of pigments in spots or bands.

LEUCOMA (LEUKOMA)—milky-white opacity of the cornea.

LEUKORRHEA (LEUKORRHOEA)—a white or yellowish mucopurulent discharge from the vagina.

LITHONTRIPTIC (LITHOTRIPTIC)—pertaining to or producing lithotripsy: the crushing of a calculus within the bladder.

LOTION—a liquid preparation used for washing, soothing, healing, etc.

LUMBAGO—muscular rheumatism, a general term for backache in the lumbar region.

LYMPHANGITIS—inflammation of lymphatic vessels.

MALARIA—acute or chronic protozoan disease caused by the genus *Plasmodium* and transmitted by the *Anopheles* mosquito, causing intermittent fever, anemia and debility.

MASTICATORY (SIALOGOGUE)—a drug or substance chewed to increase salivation.

MASTITIS—inflammation of the breast.

MEASLES—an acute infectious disease, which is often epidemic; true measles may produce a high mortality in children.

MELANODERMA—an abnormal deposit of melanin in the skin.

MENORRHALGIA—distress associated with menstruation, including premenstrual tension, pelvic vascular conjection and dysmenorrhea.

METRITIS—inflammation of the uterus.

METRORRHAGIA—an abnormal uterine hemorrhage, especially bleeding from the uterus during the intermenstrual period.

MIGRAINE—a recurring and intensely painful headache, often accompanied by vomiting, giddiness, and disturbance of the vision.

MUMPS—virus infection which causes acute inflammation of parotid gland and consequent swelling of neck and face.

MYDRIATIC—a drug which causes marked dilation of the pupil of the eye.
NARCOTIC—drug or substance that relieves pain, induces drowsiness, sleep, stupor or insensibility.
NAUSEA—a feeling of sickness at the stomach, with an urge to vomit.
NEPHRITIC—pertaining to or occuring in the kidney.
NEURALGIA—sudden severe pains radiating along the course of a nerve, without demonstrable structural changes occurring.
NEURASTHENIA—nervous exhaustion characterized by abnormal fatigability.
NEURITIS—inflammation of nerves.
ODONTALGIC—pertaining to or marked by toothache.
OEDEMA—See Edema.
OPHTHALMIA—severe inflammation of the conjunctiva of the eye or the eyeball.
ORCHITIS—inflammation of the testis.
OTITIS—inflammation of the ear.
PALPITATION—a rapid pulsation or throbbing of the heart.
PARASYMPATHOLYTIC—producing effects resembling those of interruption of the parasympathetic nerve supply to a part.
PECTORAL—pertaining to the breast or chest.
PERITONITIS—inflammation of a part of the peritoneum.
PESSARY—a contraceptive device worn in the vagina.
PILES (= HEMORRHOIDS).
PLAGUE—any epidemic disease of wide prevalence and of excessive mortality, e.g. Bubonic Plague.
PLEURISY—inflammation of the pleura membrane enveloping the lung.
PNEUMONIA—refers to a large number of conditions that include the inflammation or passive congestion of the lungs resulting in portions of the lungs becoming solid.
POULTICE (= CATAPLASM).
PROSTATISM—a morbid state of mind and body due to prostatic disease, especially the condition which results from obstruction to urination due to prostatic hypertrophy.
PRURITUS—itching of skin.
PSORIASIS—a chronic inflammatory skin disease characterized by reddish patches covered with white scales.
PULMONARY—pertaining to the lungs.
PURGATIVE—a drug that when taken internally produces the evacuation of the bowels.
PURGE—See Purgative.
PYORRHEA—a purulent discharge that contains or consists of pus.
RABIES—canine madness, an infectious virus disease passed on to man by the bite of an infected animal causing choking, convulsions, etc.
RACHITIS (RICKETS)—a vitamin D deficiency disease of the young, often marked by the faulty ossification of bone.
RASH (plural, RASHES)—eruptions of the skin in spots or patches.
REFRIGERANT—a cooling remedy, relieving fever and thirst or reducing heat.
RESOLVENT—drug or substance that reduces swellings or inflammation.
RESTORATIVE—a remedy that is efficient in restoring health and strength.

REVULSIVE—producing revulsion; the treatment of a disordered organ by acting upon another.

RHEUMATISM—diseases of muscle, tendon, joint, bone or nerve, resulting in discomfort or disability.

RHINITIS—inflammation of the mucous membrane of the nose.

RICKETS—See Rachitis.

RUBEFACIENT—a drug or agent that reddens the skin by producing active or passive hyperemia.

SCABIES—a contagious parasitic disease of the skin caused by the mite *Sarcoptes scabi.*

SCHISTOSOMA—bilharzia, trematode worms causing genito-urinary or intestinal bilharzia.

SCHISTOSOMAL WORMS—See Schistosoma.

SCIATICA—neuralgic pain along the course of the sciatic nerve caused by inflammation or injury to the nerve.

SCLEROSIS—pathological hardening of soft tissue resulting from an overgrowth of fibrous tissue.

SCROFULA—turberculosis of the lymphatic glands, especially of the neck, in which the glands become enlarged.

SCURVY—a nutritional disorder caused by deficiency of vitamin C, characterized by extreme weakness, spongy gums, a tendency to develop hemorrhages under the skin, from the mucous membranes and under the periosteum.

SCYBALOUS—pertaining to a hardened fecal mass, or scybalum.

SEDATIVE—a drug which quiets nervous activity.

SIALOGOGUE—See Masticatory.

SINUSITIS—inflammation of the sinus.

SMALLPOX—a severe, eruptive contagious disease marked by chills, high fever, headache and backache.

SOPORIFIC—a drug that causes deep sleep.

SPASMOLYTIC—See Antispasmodic.

SPERMATOGENIC—producing semen or spermatozoa.

SPERMATOPOIETIC—subserving or promoting the secretion of semen or spermatoza.

SPERMATORRHEA (SPERMATORRHOEA)—the involuntary discharge of semen without an orgasm.

SPLEEN—the organ that filters blood and prevents infection.

SPRAIN—to wrench or twist a ligament or muscle of a joint, especially the ankle or wrist, without dislocating the bones.

STERNUTATORY—a drug or substance used as a snuff and causing sneezing.

STIMULANT—a drug or agent that causes increased functional activity.

STOMACHIC—a drug or substance which promotes the functional activity of the stomach.

STOMATITIS—inflammation of the mucous membranes of the mouth.

STUPOR—mental or moral dullness or apathy.

SUDORIFIC—a drug or agent producing sweating.

SUPPURATION—formation or secretion of pus.

SYMPATHOMIMETIC—producing effects simulating those caused by stimulation of the sympathetic nervous system.

SYPHILIS—See Antisyphilitic.

TAPEWORM—See Tenia.

TENIA (TAENIA)—tapeworm, a parasitic worm of the class *Cestoidea,* a segmented ribbon-like flatworm that develops in the alimentary canal of vertebrates.

TINCTURE—solution of a drug in alcohol.

TONIC—a drug that invigorates or improves the normal tone of an organ or of the patient generally.

TONSILLITIS—inflammation of the tonsils.

TRANQUILIZER—a drug used in calming persons suffering from nervous tension, anxiety, etc.

TUBERCULOSIS—infectious disease caused by tubercle bacillus, attacking all tissues, especially the lungs.

TYPHOID—infectious disease caused by bacteria and acquired through contaminated food, it causes fever and intestinal disorders.

TYPHUS—an infectious disease caused by the microorganism *Rickettsia,* characterized by high fever and delirium.

ULCER—open sore on external or internal surface of the body, secreting pus, other than a wound.

URTICARIA—hives or nettle rash, a transient skin eruption characterized by the appearance of intensely itching wheals or welts.

VARICES—abnormally dilated or knotted blood vessels.

VARICOCELE—varicose swelling of spermatic veins.

VARICOSE—pertaining to varices.

VARIOLA—virus diseases, including smallpox, cowpox, etc., characterized by pustular eruptions.

VARIX—denoting varices in the singular sense.

VASO-CONSTRICTOR—a drug causing constriction of the blood vessels.

VASO-DILATOR—a drug causing dilation or relaxation of the blood vessels.

VENEREAL—pertaining to or produced by sexual intercourse.

VERMIFUGE—See Anthelmintic.

VESICATORY (VESICANT)—a drug or agent that produces blisters on the skin.

VULNERARY—a drug or agent that heals wounds.

WHITLOW—an old general term for any suppurative inflammation on a finger or toe, synonymous with felon.

Bibliography

1. Ayensu, E.S. 1978. *Medicinal Plants of West Africa.* Reference Publications, Inc.: Algonac, Michigan.

2. Ayensu, E.S. 1979. Plants for Medicinal Uses with Special Reference to Arid Zones, p. 117-178, In: Goodin, J.R. and Northington, D.K. (eds.), *Arid Land Plant Resources.* Lubbock, Texas.

3. Balbaa, S.I., Zaki, A.Y. & El- Zalabani, S.M. 1975. Preliminary Phytochemical Study of *Anthemis pseudocotula* Boiss. *Egypt. J. Pharm. Sci.* 16: 323-338.

4. Bedevian, A. 1936. *Illustrated Polyglottic Dictionary of Plant Names.* Argus & Papazian Presses: Cairo.

5. Bellakhdar, J. 1978. *Médecine traditionelle et toxicologie ouest-saharienne, contribution à l'étude de la pharmacopée marocaine.* Edition techniques nord-africaines: Rabat.

6. Bonnet, E. & Barratte, G. 1896. *Catalogue raisonné des plantes vasculaires de la Tunisie.* Paris.

7. Boulos, L. 1966. Flora of the Nile Region in Egyptian Nubia. *Feddes Repert.* 73: 184-215.

8. Boulos, L. 1970. *Medicinal Herbs in Libya.* Al Hasad 16. Esso Standard Libya Inc. Publ.

9. Boulos, L. 1971. *Wild Trees and Shrubs in Libya.* Al Hasad 20. Esso Standard Libya Inc. Publ.

10. Boulos, L. 1978. Notes on the Flora of Egypt 1. Six Species New to the Flora of Egypt. *Egypt. J. Bot.* 21: 223-226.

11. Boulos, L. 1982. Flora of Gebel Uweinat and Some Neighboring Regions of Southwestern Egypt. *Candollea* 37: 257-276.

12. Bouquet, J. 1921. Matière medicale indigène de l'Afrique du Nord. *Bull. Soc. Pharmacol.* 28: 22-36, 73-84.

13. Charnot, A. 1945. La toxicologie au Maroc. *Mém. Soc. Sci. Nat. Maroc* 47: 1-823.

14. Chopra, I.C., Abrol, B.K. & Handa, K.L. 1960. *Medicinal Plants of the Arid Zones. Part 1.* UNESCO: Paris.

15. Darby, W.J., Ghalioungui, P. & Grivetti, L. 1977. *Food: the Gift of Osiris.* vol. 2. Academic Press: London, New York, San Francisco.

16. Doreau, M. 1961. *Considerations actuelles sur l'alimentation, ainsi que sur la*

pharmacopée et la thérapeutique traditionnelles au Sahara. Thèse, Faculté de Pharmacie, Strasbourg.

17. Ducros, A.H. 1930. Essai sur le droguier populaire arabe de l'inspectorat des pharmacies du Caire. *Mém. Inst. Egypt* 15: i-viii, 1-162, pl. I-IX.

18. Duncan, G.R., Levi, D.D. & Pyttel, R. 1968. Bitter Principles of the Cucurbitaceae: *Bryonia dioica. Planta Medica* 16: 224-230.

19. El-Kiey, M.A., Abd-El-Wahab, S.M., Zaki, A.Y. & Wassel, G.M. 1967. A Pharmacognostical Study of the Corms of *Eminium spiculatum* Blume and *Arisarum vulgare* Schott Growing in Egypt. Part 1. Macro and Micromorphology. *J. Pharm. Sci. U.A.R.* 8: 147-157.

20. El-Menshawi, B., Karawya, M., Wassel, G., Reisch, J. & Kjaer, A. 1980. Glucosinolates in the Genus *Zilla* (Brassicaceae). *J. Nat. Products* 43: 534-536.

21. El-Moghazy Shoaib, A.M. 1967. The Study of the Egyptian *Cyperus rotundus* L. Part I.A Pharmacognostical Study of the Tuber. *J. Pharm. Sci. U.A.R.* 8: 35-48.

22. Fell, K.R. & Peck, Janet M. 1968. The Anatomy of the Leaf and Flower of *Borago officinalis* L. *Planta Medica* 16: 29-42.

23. Fourment, P. & Roques, H. 1941. *Répertoire des plantes médicinales et aromatiques d'Algérie.* Documents et renseignements agricoles, Bull. 61. Alger.

24. Fournier, P. 1947-1948. *Le livre des plantes médicinales et vénéneuses de France.* 3 vols. Lechevalier: Paris.

25. French, D.H. 1971. p. 385-412, In: Heywood, V.H. (ed), The Biology and Chemistry of the Umbelliferae. Linnean Soc. London. Academic Press: London, Beccles and Colchester.

26. Gattefossé, J. 1921. Les plantes dans la thérapeutique indigène au Maroc. In: *Sur les productions végétales du Maroc.* Rapport de la mission Perrot-Gentil, chap. 4: 73-123. Notice 10. Off. Nat. Matières Premières Végétales. Paris, Larose.

27. Gattefossé, J. 1952. L'*Ammi visnaga* et la Khelline. *Mém. Inst. Bot. Appl. et Agric. Trop.*, mars-avril No. 353-354: 116-123.

28. Haddad, D.Y., Khafagy, S.M. & El-Fatatry, L. 1960. A Contribution to the Study of *Achillea santolina* L. Isolation of Two Crystalline Principles Santolin and Santolinol. *J. Pharm. Sci. U.A.R.* 1: 75-81.

29. Hifny Saber, A. & El-Moghazy Shoaib, A.M. 1966. The Study of the Root of *Zygophyllum coccineum* L. Part I. The Chemistry. *J. Pharm. Sci. U.A.R.* 7: 117-123.

30. Hilal, S.H., El-Shamy, A.M. & Haggag,M. Y. 1975. A Study of the Volatile and Fixed Oils of the Fruits of *Daucus carota* L. var. *boissieri. Egypt. J. Pharm. Sci.* 16: 509-520.

31. Holdsworth, D.K. 1977. *Medicinal Plants of Papua New Guinea.* Technical Paper No. 175. Noumea, New Caledonia.

32. Humphries, C.J. 1979. A Revision of the genus *Anacyclus* L. (Compositae: Anthemideae). *Bull. British Museum (Natural History)* 7(3): 83-142.

33. Karawya, M.S., Hilal, S.H. & El-Hawary, S.S. 1974. Macro and Micromorphology of *Centaurea calcitrapa* L. Part I. Root and Stem. *Egypt. J. Pharm. Sci.* 15: 303-310.

34. Keys, J.D. 1976. *Chinese Herbs, their Botany, Chemistry and Pharmacodynamics.* Charles E. Tuttle Company: Rutland, Vermont, and Tokyo.

35. Khafagy, S.M. & Mnajed, H.K. 1967. The Chemical Study of the Glycosidal Substance Isolated from *Centaurium spicatum* Growing in Egypt. *J. Pharm. Sci. U.A.R.* 8: 187-199.

36. Khafagy, S.M. & Sabri, N.N. 1969. Pharmacognostical Study of *Withania somifera* Dunal, Morphology and Histology of the Flowers, Fruits, Leaves and Roots. *Abstracts Confr. Pharmaceutical Sci. Cairo* 1969:57.

37. Lemordant, D., Boukef, K. & Bensalem, M. 1977. Plantes utiles et toxiques de Tunisie. *Fitoterapia* 48: 191-214.

38. Louis, A. 1979. *Nomades d'hier et d'aujourd'hui dans le Sud tunisien.* Edisud Mondes méditerranéens: Aix en Provence, France. Imprimé à Gap, France.

39. Mahfouz, M. & El-Dakhakhny, M. 1960. The Isolation of a Crystalline Active Principle from *Nigella sativa* L. Seeds. *J. Pharm. Sci. U.A.R.* 1: 9-19.

40. Mahran, G.H., Hifny Saber, A. & Khairy, N.H. 1968. A Phytochemical Investigation of *Pergularia tomentosa* Linné Growing Wild in Egypt. *J. Pharm. Sci. U.A.R.* 8: 101-125.

41. Mahran, G.H., Hilal, S.H. & El-Alfy, T.S. 1972. Phytochemical Investigation of *Hedera helix* L. Growing in Egypt. *Abstracts XII Confr. Pharmaceutical Sci. Cairo* 1971:97.

42. Nauroy, J. 1954. *Contribution à étude de la pharmacopée marocaine traditionnelle (drogues végétales).* Thèse, Univ. Paris. Jouve, éditeur, Paris.

43. Nazir, W. 1970. *Plant Wealth in Ancient Egypt* (in Arabic). Egyptian Organization for Publishing: Cairo.

44. Osborn, D.J. 1968. Notes on Medicinal and Other Uses of Plants in Egypt. *Economic Botany* 22: 165-177.

45. Perrot, E. & Paris, R. 1971. *Les plantes médicinales,* 2 vols. Presses Universitarires de France: Vendome.

46. Purseglove, J.W. 1972. *Tropical Crops, Monocotyledons.* 2 vols. Longmans: London and Harlow.

47. Quézel, P. & Santa, S. 1962-1963. *Nouvelle flore de l'Algérie.* 2 vols. C.N.R.S. Paris.

48. Reynolds, G.W. 1966. *The Aloes of Tropical Africa and Madagascar.* Trustees of the Aloes Book Fund, Mbabane, Swaziland: Cape Town.

49. Rizkallah, M.M., Mahran, G.H. & Hifny Saber, A. 1967. *Calotropis procera* (Ait.) R.Br. Part III. The Root, its Macro and Micromorphology. *J. Pharm. Sci. U.A.R.* 8: 71-80.

50. Sabbah-Salomon, C. 1948. *Contribution à l'étude du droguier marocain.* Thèse, Faculté de Pharmacie, Strasbourg.

51. Saleh, M.R.I. & Gabr, O. 1963. Isolation of a Crystalline Principle "Cuminin" from the fruits of *Cuminum cyminum* L. *J. Pharm. Sci. U.A.R.* 4: 35-40.

52. Saleh, M.R.I. & Gabr, O. 1965. *Fumaria judaica* Boiss. Part I. Isolation of Three Crystalline Alkaloids from the Leaves, Stems and Roots. *J. Pharm. Sci. U.A.R.* 6: 61-70.

53. Saleh, M.R.I. & Gharbo, S. 1963. Isolation of a Crystalline Principle. "Alexandrin" from the Leaves of *Centaurea alexandrina* Del. *J. Pharm. Sci. U.A.R.* 4: 17-24.

54. Saleh, M.R.I., Nazmi, N. & Haddad, D.Y. 1965. Macro and Microscopical Characters of the Stems and Leaves of *Salvia triloba* L. *J. Pharm. Sci. U.A.R.* 6: 1-10.

55. Saleh, M.R.I. & Sarg, T.M. 1965. Macro and Micromorphology of the Stems and Leaves of *Thymelaea hirsuta* L. *J. Pharm. Sci. U.A.R.* 6: 147-162.

56. Schauenberg, P. & Paris, P.S.F. 1977. *Guide to Medicinal Plants.* Lutterworth Press: Guildford and London.

57. Täckholm, V. 1939. The Drug Plants of the Sinai Peninsula. *Horticultural Review Cairo* 28 (101): 22-23.

58. Täckholm, V. 1974. *Students' Flora of Egypt.* Second Edition. Publisher: Cairo University. Cooperative Printing Co.: Beirut.

59. Täckholm, V. & Drar, M. 1950. *Flora of Egypt,* vol. 2. Bull. Fac. Sci. Fouad I Univ. 28.

60. Täckholm, V. & Drar, M. 1954. *Flora of Egypt,* vol. 3. Bull. Fac. Sci. Cairo Univ. 30.

61. Täckholm, V., Täckholm G. & Drar, M. 1941. *Flora of Egypt,* vol. 1. Bull. Fac. Sci. Fouad I Univ. 17.

62. Trabut, L. 1935. *Répertoire des noms indigènes des plantes spontanées, cultivées et utilisées dans le Nord de l'Afrique.* Collection du Centenaire de l'Algérie, Alger.

63. Wassel, G.M. 1971. Macro and Micromorphology of *Pithyranthus tortuosus* (Desf.) Benth. and Hook. Growing in Egypt. Stem and Fruit. *J. Pharm. Sci. U.A.R.* 12: 381-392.

64. Willis, J.C. 1973. *A Dictionary of the Flowering Plants and Ferns.* ed. 8. Cambridge University Press: London.

65. Zohary, M. 1966. *Flora Palaestina* 1. Israel Acad. Sci. and Humanities: Jerusalem.

66. Zohary, M. 1972. *Flora Palaestina* 2. Israel Acad. Sci. and Humanities: Jerusalem.

INDEXES

MEDICINAL INDEX

Abdominal ailments
Mentha pulegium 104

Abdominal pains
Cleome amblyocarpa 52
Foeniculum vulgare 187
Glycyrrhiza glabra 123
Juniperus phoenicea 79
Ricinus communis 86

Abdominal problems
Glycyrrhiza glabra 123

Abortion
Apium graveolens 175

Abortive
Atractylis gummifera 57
Citrullus colocynthis 73
Daphne gnidium 172
Echinops spinosus 64
Euphorbia echinus 83
Juniperus communis 79
Juniperus thurifera 80
Nerium oleander 25
Nigella sativa 150
Paeonia coriacea 138
Pergularia tomentosa 32
Retama raetam 126
Rosmarinus officinalis 110
Rubia peregrina 154
Rubia tinctorum 155
Ruta montana 158
Sesamum indicum 142
Tetraclinis articulata 80
Urginea maritima 130

Abscesses
Artemisia herba-alba 57
Asphodelus aestivus 130
Atractylis gummifera 57
Heliotropium bacciferum 37
Myrtus communis 135
Olea europaea 137
Plantago coronopus 146
Portulaca oleracea 149
Ricinus communis 86
Rosmarinus officinalis 110
Thapsia garganica 187
Vaccaria pyramidata 45
Ziziphus spina-christi 153
Zygophyllum gaetulum 197

Abscesses of the breast
Asphodelus aestivus 130

Absorbent
Populus nigra 158

Aches, *See* pains

Aching of decayed teeth
Asphodelus aestivus 130

Acne
Piper nigrum 142

Acute arthritis
Phragmites australis 96

Aerophagy
Citrus aurantium 155
Viola tricolor 193

Ailments
Zilla spinosa 73

Air infection
Punica granatum 149

Albugo
Lycium intricatum 167

Albuminurea
Cynara scolymus 64

Allergic
Ricinus communis 86

Alopecia
Euphorbia resenifera 83
Juniperus communis 79
Peganum harmala 195

Amenorrhea
Aloe perryi 128
Cyperus rotundus 82

Amnesia
Zingiber officinale 193

Analeptic
Cyperus rotundus 82
Iris pseudacorus 97
Trigonella foenum-graecum 128

Analgesic
Cannabis sativa 40
Capparis decidua 40
Conium maculatum 180
Cyperus rotundus 82
Luffa cylindrica 79
Papaver somniferum 140
Penganum harmala 195
Pistacia lentiscus 145
Plantago coronopus 146
Solanum nigrum 168

Anaphrodisiac
Portulaca oleracea 149
Vitex agnus-castus 193

Anemia
Centaurium erythraea 89
Cynara scolymus 64
Haplophyllum tuberculatum 155
Inula viscosa 64
Marrubium vulgare 101
Rubia tinctorum 155
Trigonella foenum-graecum 128

Anesthetic
Cannabis sativa 40
Datura stramonium 164
Hyoscyamus albus 164
Hyoscyamus faleslez 167
Withania somnifera 168

Angina pectoris
Ammi majus 175
Ammi visnaga 175

Anthelmintic
Achillea fragrantissima 52
Achillea santolina 52
Agrimonia eupatoria 153
Allium sativum 23
Artemisia absinthium 54
Artemisia arborescens 54
Balanites aegyptiaca 35
Capparis decidua 40
Carum carvi 180
Chenopodium ambrosioides 46
Chenopodium vulvaria 46
Citrullus colocynthis 73
Coriandrum sativum 180
Cotula coronopifolia 61
Crithmum maritimum 183
Cucurbita pepo 75
Curcuma zedoaria 193
Cyperus rotundus 82
Lagenaria siceraria 75
Peganum harmala 195
Pergularia tomentosa 32
Petroselinum crispum 187
Polygonum aviculare 146
Santolina chamaecyparissus 67
Thymelaea hirsuta 172
Urginea maritima 130
Ziziphus spina-christi 153
Ziziphus zizyphus 153
Zygophyllum coccineum 195

Antihysteric
Cuminum cyminum 183

Anti-epileptic
Withania somnifera 168

Anti-inflammatory
Blepharis ciliaris 23
Coriandrum sativum 180
Daucus carota 183

Anti-leprosy
Coriandrum sativum 180

Anti-scabies
Ruta montana 158

Antialgetic
Heliotropium bacciferum 37

Antiallergic
Ferula cummunis 183

Antiamoebic
Chamomilla recutita 60

Antiasthmatic
Alliaria petiolata 70
Chenopodium ambrosioides 46
Datura stramonium 164
Ephedra alata 82
Allium sativum 23
Centaurea alexandrina 60
Olea europaea 137

Antibiotic
Centaurea alexandrina 60

Anticatarrhal
Hypericum perforatum 96
Laurus nobilis 116
Mentha pulegium 104
Nasturtium officinale 71
Salvia sclarea 110
Stachys officinalis 112
Ziziphus zizyphus 153

Anticathartic
Laurus nobilis 116

Anticolic
Opuntia ficus-indica 40
Solenostemma arghel 32

Antidiabetic
Allium cepa 23
Anthemis pseudocotula 54
Artemisia arborescens 54
Centaurea alexandrina 60
Geranium robertianum 92
Juglans regia 98
Marrubium vulgare 101
Nasturtium officinale 71
Olea europaea 137
Portulaca oleracea 149
Zygophyllum coccineum 195

Antidiarrhoeic
Acacia nilotica 116
Acacia raddiana 116
Ajuga iva 98
Artemisia herba-alba 57
Capparis spinosa 40
Citrus aurantium 155
Cupressus sempervirens 79

Erodium cicutarium 92
Fragaria vesca 153
Geranium robertianum 92
Juniperus phoenicea 79
Linum usitatissimum 131
Lycium intricatum 167
Lythrum salicaria 131
Myrtus communis 135
Opuntia ficus-indica 40
Origanum compactum 109
Polygonum aviculare 146
Polygonum maritimum 146
Potentilla reptans 154
Punica granatum 49
Ricinus communis 86
Rosa canina 154
Rubia peregrina 154
Rubia tinctorum 155
Urtica urens 191
Verbena officinalis 191
Ziziphus spina-chtisti 153
Ziziphus zizyphus 153

Antidote
Allium sativum 23
Balanites aegyptiaca 35
Iris germanica 97
Nigella sativa 150
Olea europaea 137

Antiemetic
Anethum graveolens 175
Calendula officinalis 60
Phragmites australis 96

Antiepileptic
Citrullus colocynthis 73

Antifebrile
Centaurea calcitrapa 60

Antifungal
Calendula officinalis 60

Antihelminthoid
Cucurbita pepo 75

Antihelmintic
Ajuga iva 98
Dryopteris filix-mas 32
Punica granatum 149

Antihemorrhagic
Convolvulus arvensis 68
Cupressus sempervirens 79
Geranium robertianum 92
Lycopus europaeus 101
Opuntia ficus-indica 40
Urtica urens 191

Antihemorrhoidal
Blepharis ciliaris 23
Capsicum annuum 164
Capsicum frutescens 164
Cupressus sempervirens 79
Curcuma zedoaria 193

Antihysteric
Chenopodium vulvaria 46
Coriandrum sativum 180
Ferula communis 183

Antileprous
Coriandrum sativum 180

Antimitotic, *See* Preventing cell division

Antineuralgic
Androcymbium gramineum 128

Antiophthalmic
Centaurea calcitrapa 60

Antiparasitic
Juniperus oxycedrus 79

Antiphlogistic
Portulaca oleracea 149
Raphanus sativus 73

Antipoison
Anethum graveolens 175
Coriandrum sativum 180
Ficus carica 134
Haplophyllum tuberculatum 155
Iris pseudacorus 97
Juglans regia 98
Lactuca serriola 67
Nerium oleander 25
Nigella sativa 150
Olea europaea 137
Ranunculus macrophyllus 151
Ruta montana 158
Verbascum sinuatum 162

Antipruriginous
Fumaria parviflora 89

Antipyretic
Ageratum conyzoides 52
Berberis hispanica 35
Imperata cylindrica 94
Morus alba 135
Phragmites australis 96

Antirabic
Lycium intricatum 167
Cynara scolymus 64

Antirheumatic
Asphodelus aestivus 130
Chenopodium vulvaria 46
Conyza bonariensis 61
Coriandrum sativum 180
Cymbopogon schoenanthus 94
Cynara scolymus 64
Fraxinus angustifolia 137
Lavandula stoechas 101
Marrubium vulgare 101
Sambucus ebulus 42
Sambucus nigra 42
Solanum dulcamara 168
Withania somnifera 168

Antirheumatic liniments
Lawsonia inermis 131

Antiscorbutic
Alisma plantago-aquatica 23
Alliaria petiolata 70
Allium cepa 23
Apium graveolens 175
Berberis hispanica 35
Brassica nigra 70
Capparis spinosa 40
Carum carvi 180
Coriandrum sativum 180
Crithmum maritimum 183
Eruca sativa 71
Lepidium sativum 71
Nasturtium officinale 71
Portulaca oleracea 149
Potentilla reptans 154
Raphanus sativus 73
Rosa canina 154
Sisymbrium officinale 73

Antiscrofulous
Fumaria officinalis 89
Juglans regia 98

Antiseptic
Aloe perryi 128
Artemisia absinthium 54
Artemisia herba-alba 57
Atropa bella-donna 162
Eucalyptus globulus 135
Hypericum perforatum 96
Juniperus communis 79
Juniperus oxycedrus 79
Lavandula angustifolia 101
Lawsonia inermis 131
Mentha pulegium 104
Myrtus communis 135
Nicotiana rustica 167
Ononis spinosa 126
Origanum compactum 109
Pinus halepensis 142
Rosmarinus officinalis 110
Salix alba 158
Salvia officinalis 110
Salvia sclarea 110
Spergularia rubra 45
Thymus broussonettii 112
Zygophyllum gaetulum 197

Antispasmodic
Acacia nilotica 116
Aloysia triphylla 191
Ammi visnaga 175
Anethum graveolens 175
Ballota nigra 101
Calendula officinalis 60
Cannabis sativa 40
Carum carvi 180
Chamaemelum nobile 60
Chamomilla recutita 60
Chenopodium ambrosioides 46
Chenopodium vulvaria 46
Citrus aurantium 155
Conium maculatum 180
Crataegus monogyna 153
Cuminum cyminum 183
Datura stramonium 164
Daucus carota 183
Eucalyptus globulus 135
Ferula communis 183
Foeniculum vulgare 187
Glycyrrhiza glabra 123
Hedera helix 27
Herniaria hirsuta 45
Iris foetidissima 97
Luctuca serriola 67
Laurus nobilis 116
Lavandula angustifolia 101
Lavandula stoechas 101
Meliotus indica 126
Melissa officinalis 104
Mentha pulegium 104
Nigella sativa 150
Paeonia coriacea 138
Papaver somniferum 140
Rosmarinus officinalis 110
Ruta montana 158
Salix alba 158
Salvia sclarea 110
Santolina chamaecyparissus 67
Thymus algeriensis 112
Tribulus terrestris 195
Verbena officinalis 191
Vicia faba 128
Vitex agnus-castus 193

Antisyphilitic
Boerhavia repens 137
Nerium oleander 25
Salvadora persica 158
Smilax aspera 162
Solanum dulcamara 168
Solenostemma arghel 32

Antitumor
Anthemis pseudocotula 54
Solanum dulcamara 168

Antitumor activity
Solanum dulcamara 168

Antitussive
Cucumis melo 75
Morus alba 135
Pistacia lentiscus 145

Antiviral
Morus alba 135

Anxiety
Rosa damascena 154

Aphrodisiac
Aceras anthropophorum 138
Anacyclus pyrethrum 52
Argania spinosa 162
Asparagus stipularis 130

Atropa bella-donna 162
Cannabis sativa 40
Capparis spinosa 40
Capsicum annuum 164
Capsicum frutescens 164
Carum carvi 180
Cicer arietinum 123
Coriandrum sativum 180
Corrigiola telephiifolia 42
Crocus sativus 97
Cynara cardunculus 61
Cynomorium coccineum 80
Cyperus esculentus 80
Cyperus rotundus 82
Daphne gnidium 172
Datura stramonium 164
Delphinium staphisagria 150
Eruca sativa 71
Foeniculum vulgare 187
Fraxinus angustifolia 137
Globularia alypum 92
Haplophyllum tuberculatum 155
Hyoscyamus faleslez 167
Juglans regia 98
Lactuca sativa 67
Lepidium sativum 71
Melissa officinalis 104
Mentha spicata 104
Myristica fragrans 135
Nasturtium officinale 71
Origanum compactum 109
Origanum majorana 109
Paronychia arabica 45
Paronychia argentea 45
Phoenix dactylifera 140
Pimpinella anisum 187
Piper cubeba 142
Piper nigrum 142
Rubia peregrina 154
Rubia tinctorum 155
Ruta montana 158
Solanum dulcamara 168
Solanum nigrum 168
Thymus algeriensis 112
Trigonella foenum-graecum 128
Urginea maritima 130
Urtica pilulifera 191
Urtica urens 191
Viola tricolor 193
Zingiber officinale 193

Aphtha
Olea europaea 137
Tamarindus indica 126

Appetite stimulant
Olea europaea 137
Tamarindus indica 126

Appetizer
Ammi visnaga 175
Artemisia absinthium 54
Artemisia arborescens 54
Asparagus stipularis 130
Capparis spinosa 40
Capsicum frutescens 164
Carum carvi 180
Centaurea calcitrapa 60
Cichorium intybus 61
Crithmum maritimum 183
Eryngium campestre 183
Eupatorium cannabinum 64
Foeniculum vulgare 187
Fragaria vesca 153
Iris foetidissima 97
Mentha spicata 104
Nasturtium officinale 71
Paronychia argentea 45
Petroselinum crispum 187
Pimpinella anisum 187
Pituranthos tortuosus 187
Ranunculus sceleratus 151
Raphanus sativus 73
Rubia tinctorum 155
Ruscus aculeatus 155
Ruta montana 158
Silybum marianum 68
Stachys officinalis 112
Thymus broussonettii 112
Vitex agnus-castus 193

Aromatic
Aceras anthropophorum 138
Ammodaucus leucotrichus 175
Anethum graveolens 175
Cotula cinerea 61
Crithmum maritimum 183
Hypericum perforatum 96
Myristica fragrans 135
Myrtus communis 135

Aromatic baths
Rosmarinus officinalis 110

Aromatic condiment
Syzygium aromaticum 137

Aromatic spice
Ammodaucus leucotrichus 175

Aromatic stomachic
Cyperus rotundus 82

Aromatic tonic
Chamaemelum nobile 60

Arresting cell division at metaphase, *See* Preventing cell division

Arrow poison
Balanites aegyptiaca 35

Arteriosclerosis
Capparis spinosa 40
Conium maculatum 180
Cynara scolymus 64

Arthritis
Apium graveolens 175
Avena sativa 92
Colchicum autumnale 130

Globularia alypum 92
Lolium temulentum 96
Ranunculus sceleratus 151

Articular pains
Ferula communis 183
Peganum harmala 195
Thymus broussonettii 112

Asthenia
Peganum harmala 195

Asthenia of children
Olea europaea 137

Asthma
Adiantum capillus-veneris 23
Ambrosia maritima 52
Ammi majus 175
Ammi visnaga 175
Anacyclus pyrethrum 52
Calotropis procera 27
Capparis decidua 40
Cistus ladanifer 46
Cistus monspeliensis 52
Colchicum autumnale 130
Convolvlus althaeoides 68
Crocus sativus 97
Datura stramonium 164
Eucalyptus globulus 135
Euphorbia peplis 83
Hyoscyamus muticus 167
Morus alba 135
Myrtus communis 135
Nigella sativa 150
Peganum harmala 195
Plantago major 146
Ranunculus scelaratus 151
Viscum cruciatum 131
Zygophyllum coccineum 195

Asthma of aged people
Coriandrum sativum 180

Astringent
Agrimonia eupatoria 153
Alisma plantago-aquatica 23
Alkanna tinctoria 35
Ambrosia maritima 52
Anthyllis vulneraria 119
Arbutus pavari 82
Asplenium adiantum-nigrum 32
Asplenium trichomanes 32
Capparis decidua 40
Capparis spinosa 40
Capsella bursa-pastoris 71
Centaurea acaulis 60
Ceratonia siliqua 119
Ceterach officinarum 32
Cistus ladanifer 46
Citrullus colocynthis 73
Cuminum cyminum 183
Cupressus sempervirens 79
Cymbopogon schoenanthus 94
Cynoglossum officinale 37
Cynomorium coccineum 80
Cyperus rotundus 82
Eclipta prostrata 64
Ephedra alata 82
Erodium cicutarium 92
Eucalyptus globulus 135
Fragaria vesca 153
Fumaria parviflora 89
Geranium robertianum 92
Geum urbanum 153
Herniaria hirsuta 45
Hypericum perforatum 96
Hyphaene thebaica 138
Inula viscosa 64
Juglans regia 98
Lawsonia inermis 131
Lycopus europaeus 101
Lythrum salicaria 131
Malva parviflora 134
Malva sylvestris 134
Myrtus communis 135
Olea europaea 137
Opuntia ficus-indica 40
Phyllitis scolopendrium 35
Pinus halepensis 142
Pistacia lentiscus 145
Plantago coronopus 146
Plantago major 146
Polygonum aviculare 146
Polygonum maritimum 146
Polypodium vulgare 149
Potentilla reptans 154
Punica granatum 149
Quercus coccifera 86
Rhamnus alaternus 151
Rosa canina 154
Rubia peregrina 154
Rubus ulmifolius 154
Salix alba 158
Salvia officinalis 110
Stellaria media 45
Tamarix aphylla 172
Teucrium polium 112
Tribulus terrestris 195
Ulmus campestris 172
Viscum cruciatum 131
Ziziphus spina-christi 153

Atony
Cichorium intybus 61

Auricular affections
Rosa damascena 154

Babies agitations
Citrus aurantium 155

Babies cough
Lactuca virosa 67

Babies sleeping agent
Citrus aurantium 155

Bactericide
Portulaca oleracea 149

Bacteriostatic
Allium cepa 23
Anthemis pseudocotula 54

Bathing
Malva sylvestris 134

Bechic
Alliaria petiolata 70
Ceratonia siliqua 119
Ceterach officinarum 32
Malva parviflora 134
Mentha pulegium 104
Punica granatum 149
Sisymbrium officinale 73
Viola odorata 193
Viola tricolor 193
Ziziphus zizyphus 153

Bilary disorders
Marrubium vulgare 101

Bilary obstruction
Cynomorium coccineum 80

Bilary stones
Ceratonia siliqua 119

Bile
Centaurium erythraea 89

Bile secretion
Cichorium intybus 61

Bilharziasis
Alhagi graecorum 119
Ambrosia maritima 52
Hyphaene thebaica 138

Bites
Plantago coronopus 146

Bites of poisonous animals
Coriandrum sativum 180
Euphorbia echinus 83
Hyphaene thebaica 138
Pimpinella anisum 187
Salvadora persica 158
Zingiber officinale 193

Bitter tonic
Aloe perryi 128
Artemisia absinthium 54
Berberis hispanica 35
Centaurium erythraea 89
Chamaemelum nobile 60
Cupressus sempervirens 79
Teucrium chamaedrys 112

Bitter astringent
Centaurea calcitrapa 60

Blacken the hair
Myrtus communis 135

Bladder
Urtica pilulifera 191

Bladder diseases
Ceterach officinarum 32

Bladder irritation
Hyoscyamus muticus 167

Bladder pains
Tribulus terrestris 195

Bladder troubles
Ricinus communis 86

Blennorrhagia *See* Gonorrhoea
Althaea officinalis 134
Lavandula stoechas 101
Piper cubeba 142

Blennorrhagial affections
Rosa damascena 154

Blepharitis
Phoenix dactylifera 140
Plantago major 146

Blood circulation
Myrtus communis 135
Thymus algeriensis 112

Blood depurative
Thymus algeriensis 112

Blood diseases
Rubia tinctorum 155

Blood pressure
Cymbopogon proximus 92

Boils
Atractylis gummifera 57
Balanites aegyptiaca 35
Capparis decidua 40
Globularia alypum 92
Hedera helix 27
Heliotropium bacciferum 37
Linum usitatissimum 131
Luffa cylindrica 79
Myrtus communis 135
Olea europaea 137
Pistacia lentiscus 145
Ricinus communis 86
Salvadora persica 158
Verbena officinalis 191
Zygophyllum gaetulum 197

Bone fractures
Viscum cruciatum 131

Bourdonnement of the ears
Ruta montana 158

Brain clearing
Balanites aegyptiaca 35

Breast milk secretion
Ricinus communis 86

Bronchia
Mentha pulegium 104

Bronchial asthma
Nigella sativa 150

Bronchial catarrhs
Anacyclus pyrethrum 52
Plantago major 146

Bronchital calmative
Cupressus sempervirens 79

Bronchitis
Adiantum capillus-veneris 23
Artemisia herba-alba 57
Chamomilla recutita 60
Inula viscosa 64
Iris germanica 97
Lepidium sativum 71
Mandragora autumnalis 167
Morus alba 135
Nasturtium officinale 71
Origanum compactum 109
Plantago major 146
Polygonum aviculare 146
Silybum marianum 68
Thapsia garganica 187

Broncho-Pulmonary affections
Trigonella foenum-graecum 128

Broncho-pulmonary conditions
Cotula cinerea 61

Bronchodilator
Ephedra alata 82

Bruises
Borago officinalis 37
Helianthus annuus 64
Inula viscosa 64
Rosmarinus officinalis 110

Buccal inflammations
Ricinus communis 86

Burns
Ageratum conyzoides 52
Coriandrum sativum 180
Cynoglossum officinale 37
Hedera helix 27
Lawsonia inermis 131
Narcissus tazetta 25
Plantago coronopus 146
Polygonum maritimum 146
Senecio anteuphorbium 68
Solanum nigrum 168
Verbena officinalis 191

Burnt parts
Solanum nigrum 168

Calculus
Rumex vesicarius 149

Calefacient
Artemisia absinthium 54
Euphorbia echinus 83
Myristica fragrans 135

Calefacient properties to bread
Mentha suaveolens 109

Calmative
Avena sativa 92
Citrus aurantium 155
Cynoglossum officinale 37
Dryopteris filix-mas 32
Foeniculum vulgare 187
Fragaria vesca 153
Fumaria officinalis 89
Hyoscyamus albus 164
Lactuca sativa 67
Lactuca serriola 67
Lactuca virosa 67
Mandragora autumnalis 167
Papaver rhoeas 140
Papaver somniferum 140
Physalis alkekengi 168
Pistacia lentiscus 145
Plantago major 146
Populus nigra 158
Portulaca oleracea 149
Rosa damascena 154
Salix alba 158
Senecio anteuphorbium 68
Solanum nigrum 168
Spergularia rubra 45
Withania somnifera 168
Zea mays 96
Ziziphus zizyphus 153

Calmative for stomach
Citrus aurantium 155

Calmative of stomach pains
Artemisia herba-alba 57

Calmative of thirst
Carum carvi 180

Camel skin diseases
Citrullus colocynthis 73

Cancer
Clematis flammula 150
Colchicum autumnale 130
Conium maculatum 180
Cucurbita pepo 75
Ricinus communis 86

Cancer pains
Conium maculatum 180

Cancer growths
Hedera helix 27

Carbuncles
Coriandrum sativum 180
Pistacia lentiscus 145
Ricinus communis 86

Cardiac affections
Pistacia lentiscus 145

Cardiac diseases
Peganum harmala 195

Cardiac troubles
Marrubium vulgare 101
Papaver rhoeas 140

Cardiodynia
Pistacia lentiscus 145

Cardiotonic
Adonis aestivalis 150
Calotropis procera 27
Corronilla scorpioides 123
Nerium oleander 25

Cardiotoxic
Viscum cruciatum 131

Carminative
Aloysia triphylla 191
Ammi majus 175
Ammi visnaga 175
Ammodaucus leucotrichus 175
Anethum graveolens 175
Apium graveolens 175
Capparis spinosa 40
Carum carvi 180
Chamomilla recutita 60
Chenopodium ambrosioides 46
Citrus aurantium 155
Coriandrum sativum 180
Cuminum cyminum 183
Curcuma zedoaria 193
Cymbopogon schoenanthus 94
Cyperus rotundus 82
Foeniculum vulgare 187
Juniperus communis 79
Laurus nobilis 116
Lavandula angustifolia 101
Lepidium sativum 71
Melissa officinalis 104
Mentha longifolia subsp. *typhoides* 104
Mentha pulegium 104
Mentha spicata 104
Mentha x *villosa* 109
Nigella sativa 150
Ocimum basilicum 109
Petroselinum crispum 187
Piper nigrum 142
Rosmarinus officinalis 110
Salvadora persica 158
Salvia officinalis 110
Syzygium aromaticum 137
Viola tricolor 193
Vitex agnus-castus 193

Carminative
Pimpinella anisum 187

Catalepsy
Cannabis sativa 40

Cataract
Blepharis ciliaris 23
Foeniculum vulgare 187
Verbascum sinuatum 162

Catarrh
Cistus ladanifer 46
Mentha pulegium 104
Spergularia rubra 45
Urginea maritima 130

Catarrh of head and nostrils
Mentha pulegium 104

Catarrh of the bladder
Piper cubeba 142

Cathartic
Aloe perryi 128
Bryonia dioica 73
Convolvulus arvensis 68
Euphorbia resenifera 83
Ricinus cummunis 86
Thymelaea hirsuta 172
Urginea maritima 130

Cephalalgia
Ajuga iva 98
Artemisia herba-alba 57
Centaurea calcitrapa 60
Ephedra alata 82
Maerua crassifolia 42
Origanum compactum 109

Cephalics
Origanum majorana 109
Rosa damascena 154

Chancroid
Polygonum aviculare 146

Chest ailments
Papaver somniferum 140
Thapsia garganica 187

Chest diseases
Adiantum capillus-veneris 23
Atractylis gummifera 57
Capparis spinosa 40
Euphorbia peplis 83

Childbirth
Acacia seyal 116
Anastatica hierochuntica 70
Atractylis gummifera 57
Echinops spinosus 64
Erodium cicutarium 92
Haplophyllum tuberculatum 155
Juniperus phoenicea 79

Juniperus thurifera 80
Paeonia coriacea 138
Pistacia lentiscus 145
Trigonella foenum-graecum 128

Cholera
Coriandrum sativum 180

Choleretic
Cynara scolymus 64

Chologogue
Allium sativum 23
Aloe perryi 128
Apium graveolens 175
Artemisia absinthium 54
Calendula officinalis 60
Cichorium intybus 61
Convolvulus arvensis 68
Curcuma zedoaria 193
Cuscuta epithymum 70
Cuscuta planiflora 70
Cynara scolymus 64
Eupatorium cannabinum 64
Fumaria officinalis 89
Hypericum perforatum 96
Lavandula angustifolia 101
Marrubium vulgare 101
Mentha pulegium 104
Olea europaea 137
Pimpinella anisum 187
Polypodium vulgare 149
Rosmarinus officinalis 110
Rubia peregrina 154
Salvia officinalis 110
Vicia faba 128

Chronic enlargements
Ricinus communis 86

Circumcision
Myristica fragrans 135
Rosmarinus officinalis 110

Circumcision wound
Rosmarinus officinalis 110

Colds
Adiantum capillus-veneris 23
Ajuga iva 98
Allium sativum 23
Aloysia triphylla 191
Anastatica hierochuntica 70
Artemisia judaica 57
Balanites aegyptiaca 35
Corrigiola telephiifolia 42
Cuminum cyminum 183
Euphorbia falcata 83
Iris germanica 97
Juncus acutus 98
Lepidium sativum 71
Marrubium vulgare 101
Mentha pulegium 104
Mentha x *villosa* 109
Origanum compactum 109
Origanum majorana 109
Ruta chalepensis 158
Salvia officinalis 110
Solenostemma arghel 32
Teucrium polium 112
Thymus broussonettii 112
Withania somnifera 168

Colds of the back
Capparis spinosa 40

Colic
Ageratum conyzoides 52
Cuminum cyminum 183
Cymbopogon proximus 92
Cyperus rotundus 82
Ricinus communis 86

Combat bad breath
Juglans regia 98

Condiment
Anethum graveolens 175
Capsicum annuum 164
Capsicum frutescens 164
Carum carvi 180
Cistus ladanifer 46
Crocus sativus 97
Cynomorium coccineum 80
Cyperus rotundus 82
Fraxinus angustifolia 137
Iris pseudacorus 97
Juniperus communis 79
Laurus nobilis 116
Lepidium sativum 71
Origanum majorana 109
Piper cubeba 142
Piper nigrum 142
Syzygium aromaticum 137
Thymus algeriensis 112

Congestion of prostate gland
Capsicum annuum 164

Congestions
Bryonia dioica 73

Conjunctiva
Ficus carica 134

Conjunctivitis
Peganum harmala 195
Plantago major 146

Constipation
Haplophyllum tuberculatum 155
Helianthus annuus 64
Ocimum basilicum 109
Olea europaea 137
Plantago afra 145
Ricinus communis 86
Rumex vesicarius 149
Sesamum indicum 142
Sinapis alba 73
Viola odorata 193

Contractions of the uterus
Erodium cicutarium 92
Paeonia coriacea 138

Contusions
Anthyllis vulneraria 119
Cistanche phelypaea 138
Heliotropium bacciferum 37
Rubia tinctorum 155
Salvadora persica 158
Tamus communis 82
Viscum cruciatum 131

Convalescence
Marrubium vulgare 101
Sesamum indicum 142
Ziziphus lotus 151

Convulsions
Ziziphus lotus 151

Convulsions of infants
Paeonia coriacea 138

Cooling agent
Plantago afra 145

Cornea
Atractylis gummifera 57

Corns
Hedera helix 27

Coryza
Corrigiola telephiifolia 42
Juglans regia 98
Thymus broussonettii 112

Cosmetic powders
Corrigiola telephiifolia 42
Iris germanica 97

Cough,
Allium sativum 23
Althaea officinalis 134
Artemisia herba-alba 57
Asplenium adiantum-nigrum 32
Asplenium trichomanes 32
Capparis decidua 40
Convolvuus althaeoides 68
Corrigiola telephiifolia 42
Cupressus sempervirens 79
Cynodon dactylon 94
Datura stramonium 164
Dryopteris filix-mas 32
Fraxinus angustifolia 137
Glycyrrhiza glabra 123
Hyoscyamus albus 164
Hyoscyamus muticus 167
Lactuca virosa 67
Lavandula multifida 101
Lepidium sativum 71
Malva sylvestris 134
Mandragora autumnalis 167
Morus alba 135
Nigella sativa 150
Ocimum basilicum 109
Olea europaea 137
Paeonia coriacea 138
Papaver somniferum 140
Phoenix dactylifera 140
Piper nigrum 142
Pistacia lentiscus 145
Rosmarinus officinalis 110
Salvia fruticosa 110
Silybum marianum 68
Solenostemma arghel 32
Tamarindus indica 126
Thapsia garganica 187
Thymus capitatus 112
Viola odorata 193
Viola tricolor 193

Cough drops
Ziziphus lotus 151

Cough mixtures
Urginea maritima 130

Cramps
Dryopteris filix-mas 32

Criminal purposes
Hyoscyamus faleslez 167

Cutaneous affections
Daphne gnidium 172
Plumbago europaea 146

Cystitis
Capsella bursa-pastoris 71
Zea mays 96

Dandruff
Daphne gnidium 172
Thymelaea hirsuta 172

Dangerous in large doses
Thymelaea hirsuta 172

Decongestive eye lotion
Thapsia garganica 187

Degenerative neuritis
Sesamum indicum 142

Delayed menses
Nigella sativa 150

Delirium
Euphorbia resenifera 83

Demulcent
Borago officinalis 37
Ocimum basilicum 109

Dental pains
Ocimum basilicum 109

Depilatory
Pergulaira tomentosa 32
Pistacia lentiscus 145

Depurative
Ajuga iva 98
Alisma plantago-aquatica 23
Allium sativum 23
Anthyllis vulneraria 119
Berberis hispanica 35
Buxus sempervirens 37
Calendula officinalis 60
Centaurium erythraea 89
Cichorium intybus 61
Crithmum maritimum 183
Cuscuta epithymum 70
Cynodon dactylon 94
Echinops spinosus 64
Elymus repens 94
Ephedra alata 82
Eryngium ilicifolium 183
Euphorbia peplis 83
Fumaria officinalis 89
Fumaria parviflora 89
Globularia alypum 92
Glycyrrhiza glabra 123
Herniaria hirsuta 45
Nasturtium officinale 71
Ononis spinosa 126
Peganum harmala 195
Petroselinum crispum 187
Plantago major 146
Potentilla reptans 154
Rosmarinus officinalis 110
Smilax aspera 162
Solanum dulcamara 168
Teucrium polium 112
Urtica pilulifera 191
Viola tricolor 193

Dermal affections
Solanum nigrum 168

Dermal diseases
Daphne gnidium 172
Tetraclinis articulata 80

Dermal infections
Vaccaria pyramidata 45

Dermal inflammations
Tetraclinis articulata 80

Dermatitis
Cedrus atlantica 142
Fumaria judaica 89
Fumaria officinalis 89

Desentery
Fumaria judaica 89

Desiccative
Ferula communis 183

Detersive
Aloe perryi 128
Tribulus terrestris 195

Diabetes
Acacia nilotica 116
Ajuga iva 98
Ambrosia maritima 52
Centaurium erythraea 89
Centaurium spicatum 89
Citrullus colocynthis 73
Cymbopogon proximus 92
Lupinus albus 123
Marrubium vulgare 101
Peganum harmala 195

Dialator for urinary tract
Juniperus phoenicea 79

Diaphoretic
Aceras anthropophorum 138
Asparagus stipularis 130
Borago officinalis 37
Caltropis procera 27
Capparis decidua 40
Carum carvi 180
Citrus aurantium 155
Clematis flammula 150
Cyperus rotundus 82
Echinops spinosus 64
Eryngium campestre 183
Eucalyptus globulus 135
Hyphaene thebaica 138
Lavandula stoechas 101
Phragmites australis 96
Pimpinella anisum 187
Smilax aspera 162
Solanum dulcamara 168
Thymus algeriensis 112

Diarrhoea
Acacia nilotica 116
Ageratum conyzoides 52
Agrimonia eupatoria 153
Ceratonia siliqua 119
Cistanche phelypaea 138
Crataegus monogyna 153
Cyperus rotundus 82
Juniperus phoenicea 79
Lolium perenne 94
Malva sylvestris 134
Ocimum basilicum 109
Olea europaea 137
Origanum compactum 109
Papaver somniferum 140
Phoenix dactylifera 140
Plantago afra 145
Polygonum aviculare 146
Portulaca oleracea 149
Reseda luteola 151
Retama raetam 126
Ricinus communis 86
Viola tricolor 193

Digestant
Raphanus sativus 73

Digestion
Ageratum conyzoides 52
Aloe perryi 128

Cuminum cyminum 183
Myristica fragrans 135
Peganum harmala 195
Polypodium vulgare 149
Rumex vesicarius 149
Viola tricolor 193

Digestion after meals
Pimpinella anisum 187

Digestive
Allium sativum 23
Ammi majus 175
Ammodaucus leucotrichus 175
Ammoides pusilla 157
Anethum graveolens 175
Artemisia absinthium 54
Carum carvi 180
Chenopodium ambrosioides 46
Cistus albidus 46
Citrus aurantium 155
Coriandrum sativum 180
Cucumis melo 75
Foeniculum vulgare 187
Hypericum perforatum 96
Melissa officinalis 104
Mentha x *villosa* 109
Origanum compactum 109
Pimpinella anisum 187
Piper nigrum 142
Salvia officinalis 110
Teucrium chamaedrys 112
Thymus broussonettii 112

Digestive disorders
Malva sylvestris 134

Digestive tract
Ajuga iva 98
Punica granatum 149

Digestive tract inflammations
Punica granatum 149

Digestive troubles
Chamaemelum nobile 60
Cichorium intybus 61
Thymus broussonettii 112

Digestive troubles due to fear
Cichorium intybus 61

Disinfectant
Acacia raddiana 116
Capparis decidua 40
Capparis spinosa 40
Cynodon dactylon 94
Juniperus communis 79
Mentha pulegium 104
Origanum compactum 109
Piper cubeba 142

Distomatosis of sheep
Dryopteris filix-mas 32

Diuretic
Adonis aestivalis 150
Adonis annua 150
Agrimonia eupatoria 153
Alisma plantago-aquatica 23
Alliaria petiolata 70
Allium cepa 23
Ambrosia maritima 52
Ammi majus 175
Ammi visnaga 175
Anchusa azurea 35
Anethum graveolens 175
Apium graveolens 175
Artemisia absinthium 54
Artemisia arborescens 54
Artemisia herba-alba 57
Asparagus stipularis 130
Asphodelus aestivus 130
Avena sativa 92
Borago officinalis 37
Brassica nigra 70
Bryonia dioica 73
Capparis spinosa 40
Capsicum annuum 164
Carum carvi 180
Centaurea calcitrapa 60
Ceratonia siliqua 119
Ceterach officinarum 32
Chenopodium ambrosioides 46
Cichorium intybus 61
Cistanche phelypaea 138
Citrullus colocynthis 73
Clematis flammula 150
Colchicum autumnale 130
Conyza bonariensis 61
Coriandrum sativum 180
Corrigiola telephiifolia 42
Crithmum maritimum 183
Cuminum cyminum 183
Cupressus sempervirens 79
Cuscuta epithymum 70
Cuscuta planiflora 70
Cymbopogon proximus 92
Cymbopogon schoenanthus 94
Cynara cardunculus 61
Cynara scolymus 64
Cynodon dactylon 94
Cyperus rotundus 82
Daucus carota 183
Ecballium elaterium 75
Echinops spinosus 64
Echium plantagineum 37
Elymus repens 94
Eryngium campestre 183
Eryngium ilicifolium 183
Eupatorium cannabinum 64
Euphorbia peplis 83
Ferula communis 183
Ficus carica 134
Foeniculum vulgare 187
Fragaria vesca 153
Fraxinus angustifolia 137
Fumaria officinalis 89
Fumaria parviflora 89

Galium odoratum 154
Geranium robertianum 92
Globularia alypum 92
Glycyrrhiza glabra 123
Herniaria hirsuta 45
Hypericum perforatum 96
Hyphaene thebaica 138
Imperata cylindrica 94
Iris foetidissima 97
Iris germanica 97
Iris pseudacorus 97
Juniperus communis 79
Juniperus oxycedrus 79
Lactuca serriola 67
Lactuca virosa 67
Lagenaria siceraria 75
Laurus nobilis 116
Lavandula angustifolia 101
Lavandula stoechas 101
Leptadenia pyrotechnica 27
Marrubium vulgare 101
Mercurialis annua 86
Morus alba 135
Nasturtium officinale 71
Nigella sativa 150
Ocimum basilicum 109
Olea europaea 137
Ononis spinosa 126
Paronychia argentea 45
Peganum harmala 195
Petroselium crispum 187
Phragmites australis 96
Phyllitis scolopendrium 35
Physalis alkekengi 168
Pimpinella anisum 142
Piper nigrum 142
Pistacia lentiscus 145
Pituranthos tortuosus 187
Plantago major 146
Polygonum aviculare 146
Portulaca oleracea 149
Punica granatum 149
Raphanus sativus 73
Rosa canina 154
Rosmarinus officinalis 110
Rubia peregrina 154
Rubia tinctorum 155
Ruta montana 158
Ruscus aculeatus 155
Salvadora persica 158
Salvia officinalis 110
Sambucus ebulus 42
Sambucus nigra 42
Sisymbrium officinale 73
Smilax aspera 162
Solanum dulcamara 168
Spartium junceum 126
Spergularia rubra 45
Stellaria media 45
Syzygium aromaticum 137
Tamus communis 82
Thymus broussonettii 112
Tribulus terrestris 195
Ulmus campestris 172
Urginea maritima 130
Urtica pilulifera 191
Urtica urens 191
Verbena officinalis 191
Vicia faba 128
Viola tricolor 193
Vitex agnus-castus 193
Withania somnifera 168
Zea mays 96
Ziziphus zizyphus 153
Zygophyllum coccineum 195
Ruta montana 158

Dizziness
Ricinus communis 86
Rosa damascena 154

Dog bites
Rosa damascena 154

Dorsal pains
Iris germanica 97

Dropsy
Borago officinalis 37
Bryonia dioica 73
Capparis spinosa 40
Colchicum autumnale 130

Dryness of mouth and throat
Bryonia dioica 73

Dyeing the hair black
Daphne gnidium 172

Dysentery
Calotropis procera 27
Cistus ladanifer 46
Citrus aurantium 155
Luffa cylindrica 79
Lythrum salicaria 131
Ocimum basilicum 109
Plantago afra 145
Polygonum aviculare 146
Portulaca oleracea 149
Tamarindus indica 126
Tribulus terrestris 195

Dysentry of babies
Lythrum salicaria 131

Dysmenorrhoea (dysmenorrhea)
Capparis spinosa 40
Capsella bursa-pastoris 71
Cyperus rotundus 82
Echinops spinosus 64
Hedera helix 27
Urtica urens 191

Dyspepsia
Aloe perryi 128
Cynara scolymus 64
Cyperus rotundus 82

Ear ailments
Origanum majorana 109

Ear drops
Origanum majorana 109
Ruta chalepensis 158
Solanum nigrum 168

Ear troubles
Ruta chalepensis 158

Earache
Asphodelus aestivus 130
Viola odorata 193

Ears
Ruta chalepensis 158

Ears discharging liquids
Coriandrum sativum 180

Eczema
Euphorbia echinus 83
Fumaria officinalis 89
Marrubium vulgare 101
Ononis spinosa 126
Ranunculus scelaratus 151
Rosmarinus officinalis 110
Urtica urens 191
Zygophyllum gaetulum 197

Edible
Lycium intricatum 167
Pituranthos tortuosus 187
Salvadora persica 158

Elephantiasis
Pituranthos tortuosus 187

Emetic
Ageratum conyzoides 52
Ammi visnaga 175
Anagyris foetida 119
Atractylis gummifera 57
Atriplex halimus 45
Balanites aegyptiaca 35
Brassica nigra 70
Buxus sempervirens 37
Calotropis procera 27
Cucumis melo 75
Delphinium staphisagria 150
Ecballium elaterium 75
Eryngium campestre 183
Eupatorium cannabinum 64
Euphorbia peplis 83
Euphorbia resenifera 83
Ferula communis 183
Marrubium vulgare 101
Mentha spicata 104
Peganum harmala 195
Ranunculus macrophyllus 151
Retama raetam 126
Ricinus communis 86
Stachys officinalis 112
Tamus communis 82
Urginea maritima 130
Viola odorata 193
Viscum cruciatum 131
Withania somnifera 168

Emetic-cathartic
Arisarum vulgare 25
Arum italicum 27
Spergularia media 45

Emetocathartic
Hedera helix 27
Iris germanica 97
Rhamnus alaternus 151
Viola tricolor 193

Emmenagogue
Adiantum capillus-veneris 23
Adonis aestivalis 150
Agrimonia eupatoria 153
Aloe perryi 128
Ammi visnaga 175
Anagyris foetida 119
Anastatica hierochuntica 70
Apium graveolens 175
Artemisia absinthium 54
Artemisia atlantica 57
Artemisia herba-alba 57
Ballota nigra 101
Calendula officinalis 60
Carum carvi 180
Chamaemelum nobile 60
Chenopodium ambrosioides 46
Chenopodium vulvaria 46
Crocus sativus 97
Cuminum cymium 183
Cymbopogon schoenanthus 94
Cynodon dactylon 94
Cyperus rotundus 82
Daucus carota 183
Eryngium ilicifolium 183
Foeniculum vulgare 187
Glycyrrhiza glabra 123
Hedera helix 27
Hypericum perforatum 96
Juniperus phoenicea 79
Juniperus thurifera 80
Laurus nobilis 116
Lavandula angustifolia 101
Marrubium vulgare 101
Nigella sativa 150
Origanum majorana 109
Otanthus maritimus 67
Papaver somniferum 140
Peganum harmala 195
Petroselinum crispum 187
Pimpinella anisum 187
Piper nigrum 142
Pistacia lentiscus 145
Ricinus communis 86
Rosmarinus officinalis 110
Rubia peregrina 154
Rubia tinctorum 155
Ruta chalepensis 158
Ruta montana 158
Salvia officinalis 110
Salvia sclarea 110
Santolina chamaecyparissus 67
Senecio vulgaris 68
Sesamum indicum 142
Thymus broussonettii 112

Urginea maritima 130
Vaccaria pyramidata 45
Verbena officinalis 191

Emollient
Acanthus mollis 23
Adiantum capillus-veneris 23
Althaea officinalis 134
Ambrosia maritima 52
Anethum graveolens 175
Asplenium adiantum-nigrum 32
Asplenium trichomanes 32
Blepharis ciliaris 23
Borago officinalis 37
Ceterach officinarum 32
Cynodon dactylon 94
Cynoglossum officinale 37
Cyperus esculentus 80
Elymus repens 94
Ficus carica 134
Glycyrrhiza glabra 123
Lactuca sativa 67
Lactuca serriola 67
Linum usitatissimum 131
Lupinus albus 123
Malva parviflora 134
Malva sylvestris 134
Melilotus indica 126
Opuntia ficus-indica 40
Physalis alkekengi 168
Plantago afra 145
Plantago major 146
Polygonum aviculare 146
Portulaca oleracea 149
Ricinus communis 86
Sambucus nigra 42
Senecio vulgaris 68
Solanum nigrum 168
Stellaira media 45
Trigonella foenum-graecum 128
Ulmus campestris 172
Verbascum sinuatum 162
Viola odorata 193
Ziziphus lotus 151
Ziziphus spina-christi 153
Ziziphys zizyphus 153

Emotions calmative
Artemisia herba-alba 57

Enhance fertility
Phoenix dactylifera 140

Enigmatic
Phoenix dactylifera 140

Enteritis
Ajuga iva 98
Polygonum aviculare 146
Senecio anteuphorbium 68
Tamarix aphylla 172

Enterorrhagia
Luffa cylindrica 79
Portulaca oleracea 149

Epilepsy
Alisma plantago-aquatica 23
Anacyclus pyrethrum 52
Anastatica hierochuntica 70
Atractylis gummifera 57
Lavandula stoechas 101
Ricinus communis 86
Ruta montana 158
Viscum cruciatum 131

Epilepsy attacks
Paeonia coriacea 138

Epileptic crises
Bryonia dioica 73

Epispastic
Thapsia graganica 187

Epistaxis
Imperata cylindrica 94

Erysipelas
Ranunculus sceleratus 151

Escharotic
Ruta montana 158

Exanthema
Fumaria officinalis 89

Expectorant
Adiantum capillus-veneris 23
Allium sativum 23
Arum italicum 27
Asplenium adiantum-nigrum 32
Asplenium trichomanes 32
Calotropis procera 27
Capparis spinosa 40
Cucumis melo 75
Cupressus sempervirens 79
Eryngium campestre 183
Eucalyptus globulus 135
Euphorbia peplis 83
Foeniculum vulgare 187
Glycyrrhiza glabra 123
Herniaria hirsuta 45
Iris germanica 97
Lepidium sativum 71
Marrubium vulgare 101
Mentha pulegium 104
Morus alba 135
Phyllitis scolopendrium 35
Pimpinella anisum 187
Pistacia lentiscus 145
Plantago major 146
Polypodium vulgare 149
Raphanus sativus 73
Rubia tinctorum 155
Sisymbrium officinale 73
Solanum dulcamara 168
Spergularia media 45
Thymelaea hirsuta 172
Urginea maritima 130
Viola odorata 193
Viola tricolor 193

Eye diseases
Centaurea calcitrapa 60
Verbascum sinuatum 162

Eye drops
Verbascum sinuatum 162

Eye hygiene
Verbascum sinuatum 162

Eye infections
Viola odorata 193

Eye inflammations
Ruta montana 158

Eye lotion
Ageratum conyzoides 52
Coriandrum sativum 180
Euphorbia echinus 83
Foeniculum vulgare 187
Lawsonia inermis 131
Lycium intricatum 167
Myrtus communis 135
Phoenix dactylifera 140
Ricinus communis 86
Rosa damascena 154
Solanum nigrum 168

Eye pains
Berberis hispanica 35
Nicotiana rustica 167

Eye powder
Nicotiana rustica 167

Eye troubles
Haplophyllum tuberculatum 155
Retama raetam 126

Eye wash
Retama raetam 126

Eyes
Ficus carica 134
Hyoscyamus albus 164
Rosa damascena 154

Facilitate the period
Hyoscyamus albus 164

Fall in body temperature
Clematis flammula 150
Cuminum cyminum 183
Iris pseudacorus 97
Thapsia garganica 187

Fall of hair
Juglans regia 98
Lycium intricatum 167
Nerium oleander 25

Fattener, *See* Weight adding

Febrifuge
Adonis aestivalis 150
Aloysia triphylla 191
Apium graveolens 175
Artemisia absinthium 54
Artemisia herba-alba 57
Balanites aegyptiaca 35
Brassica nigra 70
Buxus sempervirens 37
Capparis spinosa 40
Centaurea calcitrapa 60
Centaurium erythraea 89
Chamaemelum nobile 60
Chamomilla recutita 60
Chenopodium ambrosioides 46
Cichorium intybus 61
Convolvulus arvensis 68
Cupressus sempervirens 79
Cymbopogon schoenanthus 94
Cynara scolymus 64
Eucalyptus globulus 135
Eupatorium cannabinum 64
Fraxinus angustifolia 137
Geum urbanum 153
Glycyrrhiza glabra 123
Haplophyllum tuberculatum 155
Hedera helix 27
Lobularia maritima 71
Lycopus europaeus 101
Maerua crassifolia 42
Marrubium vulgare 101
Morus alba 135
Nasturtium officinale 71
Nerium oleander 25
Otanthus maritimus 67
Paronychia argentea 45
Potentilla reptans 154
Retama raetam 126
Ruscus aculeatus 155
Salix alba 158
Salvadora persica 158
Salvia officinalis 110
Silybum marianum 68
Teucrium chamaedrys 112
Trigonella foenum-graecum 128
Verbena officinalis 191
Withania somnifera 168
Ziziphus lotus 151
Ziziphus spina-christi 153

Feeble sight
Blepharis ciliaris 23

Feminine sterility
Ajuga iva 98
Capparis spinosa 40
Ferula communis 183
Teucrium polium 112
Thapsia garganica 187

Fertility
Lactuca sativa 67

Fertility to women
Capparis spinosa 40
Cymbopogon proximus 92
Ocimum basilicum 109
Ricinus communis 86

Fever of children and babies
Ruta chalepensis 158

Fevers
Acacia nilotica 116
Acacia seyal 116
Ageratum conyzoides 52
Capparis decidua 40
Centaurium erythraea 89
Marrubium vulgare 101
Plantago coronopus 146
Rosa damascena 154
Ruta chalepensis 158
Tamarindus indica 126
Teucrium polium 112
Viola odorata 193

Flatulence
Curcuma zedoaria 193
Nigella sativa 150

Flavouring agent
Pituranthos tortuosus 187

Flesh-forming
Phoenix dactylifera 140

Food poisoning
Phragmites australis 96

Fortifier
Nigella sativa 150

Fortify the sight
Ruta montana 158

Freckles
Ficus carica 134
Piper nigrum 142

Fumigant
Piper nigrum 142

Fungus infections
Origanum compactum 109

Furuncles
Vaccaria pyramidata 45
Ziziphus lotus 151
Ziziphus spina-christi 153

Galactogenic
Ziziphus lotus 151

Galactogogue
Alisma plantago-aquatica 23
Anethum graveolens 175
Carum carvi 180
Chenopodium ambrosioides 46
Cuminum cyminum 183
Cyperus esculentus 80
Foeniculum vulgare 187
Lepidium sativum 71
Nigella sativa 150
Pimpinella anisum 187
Piper nigrum 142
Thymus broussonettii 112
Trigonella foenum-graecum 128
Urtica urens 191
Vaccaria pyramidata 45
Verbena officinalis 191

Gall stones
Silybum marianum 68

Ganglions
Capparis spinosa 40

Gastralgia
Centaurium erythraea 89
Cyperus rotundus 82
Pistacia lentiscus 145
Tamarix aphylla 172

Gastric Acidity
Cyperus rotundus 82

Gastric ailments
Rhus tripartita 25

Gastric antispasmodic
Ocimum basilicum 109

Gastric disorders
Mercurialis annua 86

Gastric pains
Haplophyllum tuberculatum 155

Gastric secretion
Capsicum frutescens 164

Gastric stimulant
Laurus nobilis 116

Gastric troubles
Ammodaucus leucotrichus 175
Centaurium erythraea 89

Gastric ulcers
Acacia seyal 116
Ammi visnaga 175
Glycyrrhiza glabra 123
Psoralea plicata 126

Gastritis
Glycyrrhiza glabra 123

Gastro-duodenal ulcers
Plantago afra 145

Gastro-intestinal ailments
Malva parviflora 134

Gastro-intestinal cramps
Artemisia judaica 57
Solenostemma arghel 32

Gastro-intestinal disorders
Solenostemma arghel 32

Gastro-intestinal hemorrhages
Ricinus cummunis 86

Gastro-intestinal troubles
Trigonella foenum-graecum 128

General antiseptic
Marrubium vulgare 101

General preventive for all diseases
Allium sativum 23

Genital ailments of women
Papaver somniferum 140

Genital diseases
Mandragora autumnalis 167

Genital organs
Mandragora autumnalis 167
Melilotus indica 126

Genital sedative
Salix alba 158

Gingivitis
Melilotus indica 126

Glossitis
Iris germanica 97

Gonorrhoea *see* Blennorrhagia
Citrullus colocynthis 73
Euphorbia echinus 83
Ocimum basilicum 109
Opuntia ficus-indica 40
Ranunculus sceleratus 151
Salvadora persica 158
Withania somnifera 168

Good appetite
Salvadora persica 158

Gout
Adonis annua 150
Anacyclus pyrethrum 52
Capparis spinosa 40
Colchicum autumnale 130
Euphorbia peplis 83
Ocimum basilicum 109
Physalis alkekengi 168
Ruta montana 158
Similax aspera 162
Thapsia garganica 187
Urginea maritima 130
Zygophyllum coccineum 195

Gum disease
Salvadora persica 158

Gum strengthener
Nerium oleander 2
Punica granatum 149

Gums
Malva parviflora 134
Plumbago europaea 146

Gums reddening
Plumbago europaea 146

Hair
Juglans regia 98

Hair coloring
Lycium intricatum 167

Hair growth
Daphne gnidium 172
Eclipta prostrata 64
Urtica urens 191

Hair lotions
Urtica urens 191

Hair strengthening
Peganum harmala 195

Hair thicker and stronger
Peganum harmala 195

Hair tonic
Eucalyptus globulus 135
Myrtus communis 135
Olea europaea 137
Rosa damascena 154

Hallucinogenic
Cannabis sativa 40
Hyoscyamus faleslez 167

Headache
Ageratum conyzoides 52
Asparagus stipularis 130
Centaurium erythraea 89
Datura stramonium 164
Lavandula stoechas 101
Marrubium vulgare 101
Nigella sativa 150
Peganum harmala 195
Ricinuis communis 86
Ruta montana 158

Healing
Nicotiana rustica 167

Healing burns
Marrubium vulgare 101

Healing of small pox
Cicer arietinum 123

Healing of sores
Maeura crassifolia 42

Healing of wounds
Artemisia herba-alba 57

Maerua crassifolia 42

Heart diseases
Adonis aestivalis 150
Pulicaria incisa 67
Urginea maritima 130

Heart sedative
Pulicaria incisa 67

Hemoptysis
Imperata cylindrica 94

Hemorrhage
Atractylis gummifera 57
Lolium perenne 94
Lolium temulentum 96
Urtica pilulifera 191
Urtica urens 191

Hemorrhagic wounds
Lolium perenne 94

Hemorrhoids
Allium sativum 23
Asparagus stipularis 130
Curcuma zedoaria 193
Juniperus communis 79
Juniperus thurifera 80
Luffa cylindrica 79
Nigella sativa 150
Ocimum basilicum 109
Peganum harmala 195
Plantago afra 145
Plantago coronopus 146
Polygonum aviculare 146
Populus nigra 158
Portulaca oleracea 149
Ruscus aculeatus 155

Hemostatic
Capparis decidua 40
Capsella bursa-pastoris 71
Cistus ladanifer 46
Echinops spinosus 64
Eclipta prostrata 64
Erodium cicutarium 92
Imperata cylindrica 94
Luffa cylindrica 79
Lythrum salicaria 131
Moltkiopsis ciliata 37
Plantago coronopus 146
Polygonum aviculare 146
Punica granatum 149
Rosa damascena 154
Senecio anteuphorbium 68
Senecio vulgaris 68
Typha domingensis 172
Zygophyllum gaetulum 197

Hepatic affections
Cynara scolymus 64

Hepatic ailments
Iris pseudacorus 97

Olea europaea 137
Rumex vesicarius 149
Vicia faba 128

Hepatic fever
Marrubium vulgare 101

Hernia
Fumaria judaica 89

Herpes
Balanites aegyptiaca 35
Ranunculus sceleratus 151

Hiccup
Ranunculus sceleratus 151

Hoarseness of voice
Glycyrrhiza glabra 123

Homeopathy
Allium cepa 23
Calendula officinalis 60
Capsella bursa-pastoris 71
Colchicum autumnale 130
Lactuca sativa 67
Lolium temulentum 96
Urtica urens 191

Hydragogue
Arum italicum 27
Thymelaea hirsuta 172

Hydropsy
Adonis annua 150
Convolvulus althaeoides 68
Euphorbia peplis 83
Iris foetidissima 97
Smilax aspera 162

Hygiene of babies
Zygophyllum gaetulum 197

Hypertension
Centaurium spicatum 89
Echinops spinosus 64
Eminium spiculatum 27
Ephedra alata 82
Morus alba 135
Rubia tinctorum 155
Zygophyllum coccineum 195

Hypertrophy of the prostate gland
Echinops spinosus 64

Hypoglycemic
Allium cepa 23
Olea europaea 137

Hypotensive
Acacia nilotica 116
Allium sativum 23
Arbutus pavari 82
Crataegus monogyna 153
Olea europaea 137

Hypothermy
Ricinus communis 86

Hypotonic
Lactuca virosa 67
Withania somnifera 168

Hysteria
Atractylis gummifera 57
Citrus aurantium 155
Crocus sativus 97
Hyoscyamus albus 164
Hyoscyamus muticus 167
Viscum cruciatum 131

Hysteric affections
Santolina chamaecyparissus 67

Ill health
Narcissus tazetta 25

Impotence
Lactuca sativa 67

Incontinence of urine
Althaea officinalis 134
Lolium temulentum 96

Increase the girth of women
Iris pseudacorus 97

Indurations of mammary gland
Ricinus communis 86

Infected hairy skins
Maerua crassifolia 42

Infections of the throat
Mentha pulegium 104

Infectious eye diseases
Peganum harmala 195

Inflamed breasts of suckling mothers
Cyperus rotundus 82

Inflammations
Acadia seyal 116
Capparis decidua 40
Cynoglossum officinale 37
Linum usitatissimum 131
Plantago coronopus 146
Tribulus terrestris 195
Urtica pilulifera 191
Verbascum sinuatum 162
Ziziphus spina-christi 153

Inflammations of eyes
Berberis hispanica 35
Borago officinalis 37

Inflammations of the skin
Malva sylvestris 134

Inflammatory affections
Ricinus communis 86

Smilax aspera 162

Influenza
Corrigiola telephiifolia 42
Cymbopogon proximus 92
Juglans regia 98
Nigella sativa 150
Salvia fruticosa 110

Insect bites
Cymbopogon proximus 92

Insecticide
Aloe perryi 128
Artemisia herba-alba 57
Atractylis gummifera 57
Citrullus colocynthis 73
Eucalyptus globulus 135
Lawsonia inermis 131
Mentha pulegium 104
Nerium oleander 25
Rosmarinus officinalis 110

Insolation
Tetraclinis articulata 80

Insomnia
Crataegus monogyna 153
Juncus maritimus 98
Morus alba 135
Verbena officinalis 191

Intelligence
Juncus maritimus 98

Intermittent fevers
Centaurea calcitrapa 60
Globularia alypum 92

Internal bleeding
Centaurium erythraea 89

Intestinal ailments
Psoralea plicata 126
Rhus tripartita 25

Intestinal antiseptic
Rhus tripartita 25

Intestinal astringent
Populus nigra 158

Intestinal cramps
Lolium temulentum 96

Intestinal diseases
Maerua crassifolia 42

Intestinal disinfectant
Allium cepa 23
Juniperus phoenicea 79

Intestinal disorders
Papaver somniferum 140

Intestinal hemorrhage
Phoenix dactylifera 140

Intestinal pains
Ajuga iva 98
Cyperus rotundus 82

Intestinal parasites
Coriandrum sativum 180
Nigella sativa 150

Intestinal stimulant
Nigella sativa 150

Intestinal troubles
Artemisia arborescens 54
Cuscuta epithymum 70
Origanum compactum 109
Ruta chalepensis 158
Teucrium polium 112

Intestinal worms
Allium sativum 23
Haplophyllum tuberculatum 155

Intestine
Thymus broussonettii 112

Intestine conditions
Haplophyllum tubereulatum 155

Intoxicant
Curcuma zedoaria 193

Irritability
Lavandula stoechas 101
Rosa damascena 154

Irritable cough
Hyoscyamus muticus 167

Irritation to the skin
Urginea maritima 130

Itch
Bryonia dioica 73
Chrysanthemum coronarium 61
Cicer arietinum 123
Citrullus colocynthis 73
Clematis flammula 150
Daphne gnidium 172
Delphinium staphisagria 150
Lupinus albus 123
Nerium oleander 25
Ricinus communis 86
Teucrium polium 112
Trigonella foenum-graecum 128

Itching cracks of the skin
Sesamum indicum 142

Jaundice
Acacia raddiana 116
Aloe perryi 128
Asparagus stipularis 130
Asphodelus aestivus 130
Atractylis gummifera 57
Borago officinalis 37
Chamaemelum nobile 60
Cornulaca monacantha 46
Cressa cretica 68
Cuscuta epithymum 70
Cuscuta planiflora 70
Cynara scolymus 64
Ecballium elaterium 75
Fumaria judaica 89
Marrubium vulgare 101
Ononis tournefortii 126
Phoenix dactylifera 140
Phragmites australis 96
Ricinus communis 86
Rumex vesicarius 149
Silybum marianum 68
Thymus broussonettii 112

Joints
Urtica pilulifera 191

Keratolyic
Blepharis ciliaris 23

Kidney affections
Aloe perryi 128

Kidney ailments
Urtica urens 191

Kidney conditions
Viola tricolor 193

Kidney diseases
Ceterach officinarum 32

Kidney inflammations
Juniperus communis 79

Kidney or ureter stones
Lavandula dentata 101

Kidney stones
Centaurium spicatum 89
Eryngium campestre 183
Ononis spinosa 126
Zilla spinosa 73

Kidney stones expeller
Eryngium campestre 183

Kidney troubles
Ricinus communis 86

Lacteral tumors
Ricinus communis 86

Laryngitis
Datura stramonium 164

Lathyrism
Cicer arietinum 123

Laxative
Alhagi graecorum 119
Avena sativa 92
Balanites aegyptiaca 35
Brassica nigra 70
Capparis decidua 40
Capparis spinosa 40
Cassia senna 119
Ceratonia siliqua 119
Cichorium intybus 61
Colutea arborescens 123
Cuscuta epithymum 70
Cuscuta planiflora 70
Eryngium campestre 183
Euphorbia helioscopia 83
Ficus carica 134
Fragaria vesca 153
Fraxinus angustifolia 137
Fumaria officinalis 89
Fumaria parviflora 89
Globularia alypum 92
Juniperus phoenicea 79
Lactuca virosa 67
Linum usitatissimum 131
Malva sylvestris 134
Mercurialis annua 86
Pergularia tomentosa 32
Physalis alkekengi 168
Polypodium vulgare 49
Rhamnus alaternus 151
Rubia peregrina 154
Sambucus nigra 42
Senecio vulgaris 68
Sinapis alba 73
Solanum dulcamara 168
Tamarinuds indica 126
Trigonella foenum-graecum 128
Viola tricolor 193
Withania somnifera 168
Ziziphus spina-christi 153

Lenitive
Sesamum indicum 142

Leprosy
Acacia albida 116
Bryonia dioica 73
Cicer arietinum 123
Ficus carica 134
Lawsonia inermis 131
Nigella sativa 150
Piper nigrum 142
Ricinus communis 86

Lethargy
Anacyclus pyrethrum 52

Leucoderma (Leukoderma)
Balanites aegyptiaca 35
Citrullus colocynthis 73

Leucoma
Asphodelus aestivus 130

Leukorrhea
Punica granatum 149

Lice
Hysocyamus faleslez 167
Tamarix aphylla 172

Liniment
Salvadora persica 158

Lithontriptic
Ammi visnaga 175

Liver affections
Agrimonia eupatoria 153
Cedrus atlantica 142
Ricinus communis 86

Liver ailments
Asparagus stipularis 130
Foeniculum vulgare 187

Liver diseases
Agrimonia eupatoria 153
Echinops spinosus 64
Thymus broussonettii 112

Liver disorders
Euphorbia peplis 83
Silybum marianum 68

Liver infections
Avena sativa 92
Marrubium vulgare 101

Liver inflation
Marrubium vulgare 101

Liver problems
Cynara humilis 64

Liver sclerosis
Ocimum basilicum 109

Liver swelling
Iris germanica 97

Liver troubles
Cuscuta epithymum 70
Cuscuta planiflora 70

Local analgesic
Periploca laevigata 32

Local sedative
Populus nigra 158

Loose teeth
Cuscuta planiflora 70

Loosen teeth
Calotropis procera 27

Loss of consciousness
Anacyclus pyrethrum 52

Lumbago
Dryopteris filix-mas 32

Foeniculum vulgare 187
Ricinus communis 86
Zingiber officinale 193

Lungs
Mentha pulegium 104

Lymphangitis
Vaccaria pyramidata 45

Malaria
Balanites aegyptiaca 35
Haplophyllum tuberculatum 155
Inula viscosa 64
Marrubium vulgare 101
Plantago coronopus 146

Malignant ulcers
Haplophyllum tuberculatum 155

Malignant wounds
Cyperus papyrus 82

Masticatory
Balanites aegyptiaca 35

Mastitis
Pistacia lentiscus 145
Vaccaria pyramidata 45

Measles
Papaver dubium 140
Vicia sativa 128
Ziziphus lotus 151
Ziziphus spina-christi 153

Melanoderma
Vicia sativa 128

Memory
Piper nigrum 42
Tribulus terrestris 195

Menorrhagia
Capsella bursa-oastoris 71

Menstrual flow
Ricinus communis 86

Metritis
Cyperus rotundus 82

Metrorrhagia
Echinops spinosus 64
Luffa cylindrica 79
Urtica urens 191

Migraine
Anagyris foetida 119
Chamaemelum nobile 60
Nigella sativa 150
Rosa damascena 154
Ruta montana 158
Tetraclinis articulata 80

Milk production
Chamaemelum nobile 60

Milk secretion for mothers
Sesamum indicum 142

Mint tea
Mentha suaveolens 109
Mentha x *villosa* 109

Miscarriage
Mentha x *villosa* 109

Mosquito bites
Ephedra alata 82

Mosquitos
Ricinus communis 86

Mothers after childbirth
Sesamum indicum 142

Mouth ailments
Olea europaea 137

Mouth care
Plumbago europaea 146

Mucous membrane inflammations
Malva sylvestris 134

Mumps
Cunimum cyminum 183

Muscle pains
Hyoscyamus muticus 167

Mydriatic
Conium maculatum 180

Mydriatic eye lotion
Solanum nigrum 168

Narcotic
Cannabis sativa 40
Crocus sativus 97
Cynoglossum officinale 37
Lactuca virosa 67
Mandragora autumnalis 167
Papaver somniferum 140
Solanum dulcamara 168
Solanum nigrum 168
Withania somnifera 168

Nasal affections
Rosa damascena 154

Nasal diseases
Ruta chalepensis 158

Nasal douche
Ocimum basilicum 109

Nausea
Cotula cinerea 61
Haplophyllum tuberculatum 155
Lolium temulentum 96
Rosa damascena 54

Neck pains
Tetraclinis articulata 80

Nephritic colics
Physalis alkekengi 168

Nephritic pains
Vicia faba 128

Nerve calmative
Haplophyllum tuberculatum 155

Nerve sedative
Citrus aurantium 155
Crataegus monogyna 153

Nerves
Urginea maritima 130

Nervous disorders
Coriandrum sativum 180
Ricinus communis 86

Nervous gastralgia
Ricinus communis 86

Nervous irritation
Hyoscyamus albus 164

Nervous troubles
Cyperus rotundus 82

Nervousness
Ruta chalepensis 158

Neuralgia
Anacyclus pyrethrum 52
Delphininum staphisagria 150
Lolium temulentum 96

Neurasthenia
Morus alba 135
Tribulus terrestris 195

Neuromuscular sedative
Tribulus terrestris 195

Neuroparalysis
Sesamum indicum 142

Neurotic diseases
Cymbopogon proximus 92

Neurotic pains
Peganum harmala 195

Nocturnal incontinence of urine
Cupressus sempervirens 79

Non-striated muscles
Hyoscyamus muticus 167

Nose drops
Ecballium elaterium 75
Nerium oleander 25
Ruta chalepensis 158

Nose-bleeding
Crocus sativus 97
Lolium temulentum 96
Urtica urens 191

Nourishing
Cyperus esculentus 80
Juglans regia 98
Lepidium sativum 71
Sesamum indicum 142

Nourishing for livestock
Lepidum sativum 71

Obstructions
Asparagus stipularis 130

Obstructions of spleen
Adiantum capillus-veneris 23

Obstructions of liver
Adiantum capillus-veneris 23

Occular affections
Acacia seyal 116

Occular ailments
Malva sylvestris 134

Odontalgic
Mentha spicata 104
Piper nigrum 142
Plumbago europaea 146
Syzygium aromaticum 137

Oedema
Anagyris foetida 119
Heliptropium bacciferum 37
Ruta montana 158
Urginea maritima 130

Oedema of spleen
Tamarix aphylla 172

Oestrogenic
Eucalyptus globulus 135
Punica granatum 149

Oestrogenic hormones
Punica granatum 149

On diet
Malva parviflora 134

Ophthalmia
Ricinus communis 86

Ophthalmic diseases
Artemisia herba-alba 57
Cassia italica 119
Euphorbia echinus 83
Lycium intricatum 167

Orchitis
Luffa cylindrica 79

Otitis
Allium sativum 23
Marrubium vulgare 101
Rosa damascena 154
Ruta montana 158

Pain of aching parts of the body
Maerua crassifolia 42

Pain of bone fractures
Maerua crassifolia 42

Painful articular conditions
Linum usitatissimum 131

Painful organs
Myrtus communis 135

Pains
Althaea officinalis 134
Anastatica hierochuntica 70
Balanites aegyptiaca 35
Curcuma zedoaria 193
Haplophyllum tuberculatum 155
Hyoscyamus albus 164
Hyoscyamus muticus 167
Linum usitatissimum 131
Mandragora autumnalis 167
Myristica fragrans 135
Myrtus communis 135
Narcissus tazetta 25
Papaver somniferum 140
Peganum harmala 195
Polypodium vulgare 149
Ricinus communis 86
Senecio anteuphorbium 68
Thymus broussonettii 112
Tribulus terrestris 195
Zingiber officinale 193

Pains of the eyes
Berberis hispanica 35

Palpitation
Crataegus monogyna 153

Palsy
Anastatica hierochuntica 70

Paralyse respiratory system
Conium maculatum 180

Paralysis
Asphodelus aestivus 130
Atractylis gummifera 57
Avena sativa 92
Nigella sativa 150
Peganum harmala 195
Ruta montana 158

Paralysis of arms and legs
Ricinus communis 86

Paralysis of lips
Atractylis gummifera 57

Paralysis of muscles
Vaccaria pyramidata 45

Paralysis of the tongue
Anacyclus pyrethrum 52

Parasiticide
Delphinium staphisagria 150
Laurus nobilis 116
Lupinus albus 123
Nicotiana rustica 167

Parasiticide in veterinary medicine
Laurus nobilis 116

Parasympatholytic
Capsicum annuum 164

Pectoral
Anchusa azurea 35
Borago officinalis 37
Ceterach officinarum 32
Cyperus esculentus 80
Echium plantagineum 37
Lavandula stoechas 101
Malva sylvestris 134
Marrubium vulgare 101
Origanum majorana 109
Papaver rhoeas 140

Pectoral ailments
Ziziphus zizyphus 153

Pectoral pastes
Glycyrrhiza foetida 123

Pectoral troubles
Punica granatum 149
Zingiber officinale 193

Peptic ulcer
Pistacia lentiscus 145

Perfumery
Iris germanica 97

Peritonitis
Silybum marianum 68

Pharyngeal inflammations
Ricinus communis 86

Piles
Ecballium elaterium 75
Ocimum basilicum 109

Plague
Allium sativum 23
Punica granatum 49

Pleasant excitement producer
Punica granatum 149

Pleurisy
Carum carvi 180

Pneumonia
Urginea maritima 130

Pneumonia in children
Cannabis sativa 40

Poisoning
Narcissus tazetta 25

Poisonous
Arisarum vulgare 25
Atriplex halimus 45
Colutea arborescens 123
Conium maculatum 180
Delphinium staphisagria 150
Eminium spiculatum 27
Euphorbia balsamifera 83
Hyoscyamus faleslez 167
Nerium oleander 25
Nigella sativa 150
Peganum harmala 195
Tamus communis 82

Poisonous bites
Euphorbia granulata 83
Nigella sativa 150

Poisonous to sheep and goats
Nigella sativa 150

Poultice
Pergularia tomentosa 32

Pregnancy
Daucus carota 183

Preventing cell division
Crotalaria aegyptiaca 123
Cucurbita pepo 75

Probe wounds
Stipagrostis pungens 96

Prostate gland
Conium maculatum 180

Prostate gland congestion
Colchicum autumnale 130

Prostatism
Echinops spinosus 64

Pruritus
Polygonum aviculare 146
Ranunculus sceleratus 151

Psoriasis
Stellaria media 45

Pulmonary
Ranunculus sceleratus 151

Pulmonary abscesses
Phragmites australis 96

Pulmonary affections
Sesamum indicum 142

Pulmonary conditions
Pimpinella anisum 187

Pulmonary diseases
Acacia raddiana 116
Imperata cylindrica 94
Lepidium sativum 71

Pulmonary stimulant
Lepidium sativum 71

Pulmonary troubles
Atractylis gummifera 57
Marrubium vulgare 101

Pulmonary tuberculosis
Plantago major 146

Purgative
Ageratum conyzoides 52
Alhagi graecorum 119
Aloe perryi 128
Ammi visnaga 175
Anagyris foetida 119
Anthyllis vulneraria 119
Arum italicum 27
Atractylis gummifera 57
Balanites aegyptiaca 35
Boerhavia repens 137
Bryonia dioica 73
Buxus sempervirens 37
Cassia italica 119
Cassia senna 119
Citrullus colocynthis 73
Clematis flammula 150
Colchicum autumnale 130
Colutea arborescens 123
Convolvlus althaeoides 68
Convolvulus arvensis 68
Convolvulus hystrix 68
Coronilla scorpioides 123
Cuscuta epithymum 70
Cynara cardunculus 61
Daphne gnidium 172
Ecballium elaterium 75
Eupatorium cannabinum 64
Euphorbia echinus 83
Euphorbia helioscopia 83
Euphorbia lathyrus 83
Euphorbia resenifera 83
Fraxinus angustifolia 137
Globularia alypum 92
Iris foetidissima 97
Iris germanica 97
Iris pseudacorus 97
Marrubium vulgare 101
Mercurialis annua 86
Olea europaea 137
Plantago afra 145
Ranunculus macrophyllus 151
Retama raetam 126
Rhammus alaternus 151
Ricinus communis 86
Sambucus ebulus 42
Sambucus nigra 42
Sinapis alba 73
Spartium junceum 126

Stachys officinalis 112
Tamus communis 82
Thapsia garganica 187
Urginea maritima 130
Viola odorata 193

Purge
Cressa cretica 68
Phoenix dactylifera 140

Purifying the blood
Phoenix dactylifera 140

Purify the breath
Pistacia lentiscus 145

Pyorrhea
Juglans regia 98
Malva parviflora 134

Rabies
Alisma plantago-aquatica 23
Thapsia garganica 187

Rachitis
Thapsia garganica 187

Rash
Ricinus communis 86
Withania somnifera 168

Rat poison
Urginea maritima 130

Reconstituent
Lepidium sativum 71

Redden the lips
Juglans regia 98

Reduce pain
Hyoscyamus albus 164

Refreshing agent
Capparis spinosa 40
Cynodon dactylon 94
Elymus repens 94
Fragaria vesca 153
Mentha spicata 104
Portulaca oleracea 149

Refreshing beverage
Cyperus esculentus 80

Refrigerant
Borago officinalis 37
Cucumis melo 75

Reinvigorative
Cicer arietinum 123
Cucumis melo 75

Remove excess chlorine from blood
Eryngium campestre 183

Renal affections
Anagyris foetida 119
Cynara scolymus 64
Plantago afra 145

Renal calculi
Cyperus rotundus 82

Renal disorders
Apium graveolens 175
Colchicum autumnale 130

Renal inflammations
Plantago afra 145

Renal pains
Colchicum autumnale 130

Renal stones
Ammi visnaga 175
Asparagus stipularis 130
Centaurea calcitrapa 60
Urtica pilulifera 191

Renal stones expeller
Paronychia argentea 45

Renal troubles
Ambrosia maritima 52
Cynodon dactylon 94

Resolvent
Anagyris foetida 119
Anethum graveolens 175
Apium graveolens 175
Arum italicum 27
Citrullus colocynthis 73
Eupatorium cannabinum 64
Lavandula stoechas 101
Lupinus albus 123
Morus alba 135
Nigella sativa 150
Origanum majorana 109
Pupulus nigra 158
Salvia officinalis 110
Sambucus ebulus 42
Sambucus nigra 42
Senecio vulgaris 68
Silybum marianum 68
Tamus communis 82
Ulmus campestris 172
Vicia sativa 128

Respiratory affections
Nigella sativa 150

Respiratory ailments
Glycyrrhiza glabra 123
Myrtus communis 135
Psoralea plicata 126

Respiratory disorders
Marrubium vulgare 101
Viola odorata 193

Respiratory oppression
Viola odorata 193

Respiratory organs
Nigella sativa 150

Respiratory system
Acacia seyal 116
Eucalyptus globulus 135
Myrtus communis 135
Ruta montana 158
Zingiber officinale 193

Respiratory tracts
Eucalyptus globulus 135

Restorative
Trigonella foenum-graecum 128

Revulsive
Brassica nigra 70
Bryonia dioica 73
Capsicum annuum 164
Capsicum frutescens 164
Cistus ladanifer 46
Daphne gnidium 172
Euphorbia resenifera 83
Peganum harmala 195
Ruta montana 158
Solanum dulcamara 168
Thapsia garganica 187
Urtica urens 191

Rheumatic conditions
Physalis alkekengi 168
Ranunculus scelaratus 151

Rheumatic pains
Acacia seyal 116
Alhagi graecorum 119
Ambrosia maritima 52
Cleome amblyocarpa 52
Euphorbia falcata 83
Haplophyllum tuberculatum 155
Inula viscosa 64
Iris pseudacorus 97
Polypodium vulgare 149
Ricinus communis 86
Ruta chalepensis 158
Salvia fruticosa 110
Senecio anteuphorbium 68
Stellaria media 45
Stipagrostis pungens 96
Withania somnifera 168

Rheumatism
Acacia seyal 116
Ageratum conyzoides 52
Anacyclus pyrethrum 52
Apium graveolens 175
Artemisia absinthium 54
Artemisia herba-alba 57
Asparagus stipularis 130
Atractylis gummifera 57
Avena sativa 92
Borago officinalis 37
Bryonia dioica 73
Buxus sempervirens 37
Capparis decidua 40
Capparis spinosa 40
Carum carvi 180
Chamaemelum nobile 60
Colchicum autumnale 130
Conium maculatum 180
Cotula cinerea 61
Dryopteris filix-mas 32
Euphorbia resenifera 83
Ferula communis 183
Globularia alypum 92
Glycyrrhiza glabra 123
Haplophyllum tuberculatum 155
Iris germanica 97
Laurus nobilis 116
Lolium perenne 94
Lolium temulentum 96
Mercurialis annua 86
Peganum harmala 195
Periploca laevigata 32
Pistacia lentiscus 145
Ricinus communis 86
Rosmarinus officinalis 110
Rubia peregrina 154
Salix alba 158
Smilax aspera 162
Tamus communis 82
Thapsia garganica 187
Thymus broussonettii 112
Urginea maritima 130
Urtica pilulifera 191
Urtica urens 191
Vicia sativa 128
Zingiber officinale 193
Zygophyllum coccineum 195

Rheumatism of the head
Anacyclus pyrethrum 52

Rheumatism of the tongue
Anacyclus pyrethrum 52

Rhinitis
Ranunculus sceleratus 151

Rubefacient
Alliaria petiolata 70
Anacyclus pyrethrum 52
Capsicum annuum 164
Carum carvi 180
Daphne gnidium 172
Eruca sativa 71
Juniperus communis 79
Ruta montana 158
Tamus communis 82
Thapsia garganica 187
Urginea maritima 130

Scabies
Calotropis procera 27
Carum carvi 180
Clematis flammula 150

Fumaria judaica 89
Vaccaria pyramidata 45

Scabies of camels and goats
Capparis decidua 40
Carum carvi 180

Scalp
Daphne gnidium 172

Scalp hair growth
Eclipta prostrata 64

Schistosomal snails
Calotropis procera 27

Sciatica
Anacyclus pyrethrum 52
Capparis spinosa 40
Centaurium spicatum 89
Dryopteris filix-mas 32
Iris germanica 97
Iris pseudacorus 97
Peganum harmala 195
Ranunculus sceleratus 151
Ricinus communis 86
Rubia peregrina 154
Rubia tinctorum 155

Sclerosis of spleen
Ocimum basilicum 109

Scorpion bites
Artemisia arborescens 54
Cotula cinerea 61
Hyoscyamus albus 164
Lactuca serriola 67

Scorpion repellant
Ruta chalepensis 158

Scorpion stings
Citrullus colocynthis 73
Cyperus rotundus 82
Ricinus communis 86

Scrofula
Anagyris foetida 119
Capparis spinosa 40
Pistacia atlantica 145

Scrofulous ulcers
Lepidium sativum 71
Rosmarinus officinalis 110

Scurf
Lupinus albus 123

Scurvy
Capparis spinosa 40

Sedative
Aceras anthropophorum 138
Anthum graveolens 175
Atropa bella-donna 162
Cannabis sativa 40
Chenopodium vulvaria 46
Citrus aurantium 155
Conium maculatum 180
Coriandrum sativum 180
Cupressus sempervirens 79
Cyperus rotundus 82
Datura stramonium 164
Fumaria officinalis 89
Fumaria parviflora 89
Hyoscyamus faleslez 167
Iris foetidissima 97
Juniperus phoenicea 79
Mandragora autumnalis 167
Papaver somniferum 140
Pistacia lentiscus 145
Populus nigra 158
Salix alba 158
Santolina chamaecyparissus 67
Senecio anteuphorbium 68
Solanum nigrum 168
Vitex agnus-castus 193

Sialogogue
Anethum graveolens 175

Sight ameliorating
Verbascum sinuatum 162

Sight weakness
Verbascum sinuatum . 162

Sinusitis
Ajuga iva 98
Nigella sativa 150
Ocimum basilicum 109

Skin
Pinus halepensis 142
Sesamum indicum 142

Skin conditions
Sesamum indicum 142

Skin diseases
Acacia nilotica 116
Artemisia judaica 57
Avena sativa 92
Corrigiola telephiifolia 42
Delphinium staphisagria 150
Eryngium campestre 183
Ferula communis 183
Hedera helix 27
Juniperus communis 79
Juniperus oxycedrus 79
Mentha longifolia subsp. *typhoides* 104
Nasturtium officinale 71
Ocimum basilicum 109
Peganum harmala 195
Pergularia tomentosa 32
Ricinus communis 86
Smilax aspera 162
Thymus capitatus 112

Skin disorders
Cynara scolymus 64

Skin eruptions in children
Viola tricolor 193

Skin irritant
Artemisia judaica 57

Skin tonic
Borago officinalis 37

Sleeping sickness
Anacyclus pyrethrum 52

Smallpox
Myrtus communis 135
Teucrium polium 112
Vicia sativa 128
Ziziphus lotus 151

Snake bites
Artemisia arborescens 54
Citrullus colocynthis 73
Euphorbia resenifera 83
Haloxylon scoparium 46
Hyoscyamus albus 164
Lactuca serriola 67
Ruta montana 158
Ziziphus spina-christi 153

Sneezing
Citrullus colocynthis 73

Snuff
Nicotiana rustica 167
Ruta chalepensis 158

Soothing
Chamomilla recutita 60
Malva sylvestris 134

Soporific
Hyoscyamus albus 164
Mandragora autumnalis 167
Papaver rhoeas 140
Papaver somniferum 140
Vitex agnus-castus 193

Sore gums
Mandragora autumnalis 167

Sore throats
Plantago major 146

Sores
Artemisia arborescens 54
Capparis decidua 40
Coriandrum sativum 180
Juniperus communis 79
Juniperus oxycedrus 79
Maerua crassifolia 42
Quercus coccifera 86
Salvadora persica 158
Senecio anteuphorbium 68
Vaccaria pyramidata 45

Spasmodic
Ruta chalepensis 158

Spasmodic conditions
Hyoscyamus albus 164
Hyoscyamus muticus 167

Spasmodic coughs
Hyoscyamus muticus 167

Spasmolytic
Pimpinella anisum 187

Spasms
Datura stramonium 164

Spermatogenic
Asparagus stipularis 130
Cyperus esculentus 80
Eryngium ilicifolium 183
Pinus halepensis 142

Spermatopoietic
Cyperus esculentus 80

Spermatorrhea
Tribulus terrestris 195

Spice
Cynomorium coccineum 80

Spleen
Salvadora persica 158

Spleen diseases
Ceterach officinarum 32

Spleen obstructions
Fumaria judaica 89

Spleen oedema
Tamarix aphylla 172

Spleen problems
Balanites aegyptiaca 35

Spleen troubles
Capparis spinosa 40

Sprains
Heliotropium bacciferum 37
Rosmarinus officinalis 110
Viscum cruciatum 131

Spreading sores
Rosmarinus officinalis 110

Sterility
Lepidium sativum 71
Thapsia garganica 187
Withania somnifera 168

Sternutatory
Anacyclus pyrethrum 52
Pulicaria crispa 67
Stachys officinalis 112

Stiffness
Zingiber officinale 193

Stimulant
Aceras anthropophorum 138
Ageratum conyzoides 52
Alliaria petiolata 70
Allium sativum 23
Ambrosia maritima 52
Ammi visnaga 175
Anacyclus pyrethrum 52
Anethum graveolens 175
Apium graveolens 175
Brassica nigra 70
Calendula officinalis 60
Cannabis sativa 40
Capparis spinosa 40
Capsicum annuum 164
Capsicum frutescens 164
Carum carvi 180
Chamaemelum nobile 60
Chamomilla recutita 60
Chenopodium ambrosioides 46
Cistus ladanifer 46
Cistus aurantium 155
Coriandrum sativum 180
Crithmum maritimum 183
Crocus sativus 97
Cuminum cyminum 183
Curcuma zedoaria 193
Cynara scolymus 64
Cyperus rotundus 82
Eruca sativa 71
Foeniculum vulgare 187
Galium odoratum 154
Geum urbanum 153
Hypericum perforatum 96
Juniperus oxycedrus 79
Lavandula angustifolia 101
Marrubium vulgare 101
Melissa officinalis 104
Myristica fragrans 135
Myrtus communis 135
Nasturtium officinale 71
Ocimum basilicum 109
Origanum vulgare subsp. *glandulosum* 109
Papaver somniferum 140
Paronychia arabica 45
Peganum harmala 195
Petroselinum crispum 187
Pimpinella anisum 187
Piper cubeba 142
Piper nigrum 142
Raphanus sativus 73
Salvia officinalis 110
Salvia sclarea 110
Santolina chamaecyparissus 67
Sisymbrium officinale 73
Solanum dulcamara 168
Stachys officinalis 112
Syzygium aromaticum 137
Teucrium polium 112
Thymus algeriensis 112
Trigonella foenum-graecum 128
Ulmus campestris 172
Verbena officinalis 191
Vitex agnus-castus 193
Zingiber officinale 193

Stimulate intelligence
Atropa bella-donna 162

Stomach cancer
Ricinus communis 86

Stomach conditions
Ocimum basilicum 109

Stomach fortifier
Salvadora persica 158

Stomach inflammations
Sesamum indicum 142

Stomach pains
Ajuga iva 98
Ammodaucus leucotrichus 175
Anethum graveolens 175
Citrus aurantium 155
Cotula cinerea 61
Pimpinella anisum 187
Rosa damascena 154
Ruta montana 158
Vicia faba 128

Stomach troubles
Marrubium vulgare 101
Ocimum basilicum 109
Origanum compactum 109
Teucrium polium 112

Stomach weakness
Zingiber officinale 193

Stomachache
Reseda luteola 151
Ricinus communis 86
Salvadora persica 158
Senecio anteuphorbium 68
Withania somnifera 168

Stomachic
Achillea fragrantissima 52
Achillea santolina 52
Aloe perryi 128
Aloysia triphylla 191
Ambrosia maritima 52
Ammi majus 175
Anethum graveolens 175
Apium graveolens 175
Artemisia absinthium 54
Artemisia herba-alba 57
Artemisia judaica 57
Asparagus stipularis 130
Berberis hispanica 35
Brassica nigra 70
Calotropis procera 27
Capsicum annuum 164
Capsicum frutescens 164
Carum carvi 180
Centaurea calcitrapa 60
Chamaemelum nobile 60
Chamomilla recutita 60
Chemopodium ambrosioides 46

Cichorium intybus 61
Citrus aurantium 155
Coriandrum sativum 180
Cotula cinerea 61
Cuminum cyminum 183
Ciscuta epithymum 70
Cymbopogon proximus 92
Cynara scolymus 64
Cyperus rotundus 82
Foeniculum vulgare 187
Fumaria officinalis 89
Juniperus communis 79
Laurus nobilis 116
Lavandula angustifolia 101
Lavandula stoechas 101
Melissa officinalis 104
Mentha spicata 104
Myrtus communis 135
Nasturtium officinale 71
Petroselinum crispum 187
Phragmites australis 96
Pimpinella anisum 187
Piper nigrum 142
Potentilla reptans 154
Raphanus sativus 73
Rosmarinus officinalis 110
Salvadora persica 158
Santolina chamaecyparissus 67
Solenostemma arghel 32
Stachys officinalis 112
Syzygium aromaticum 137
Thymus algeriensis 112
Verbena officinalis 191
Viola tricolor 193
Zingiber officinale 193

Stomachic tonic
Ocimum basilicum 109

Stomatitis
Geranium robertianum 92
Olea europaea 137

Strap broken limbs
Olea europaea 137

Strength restoration
Phoenix dactylifera 140

Strengthen the weak
Rosmarinus officinalis 110

Strengthening the body
Eleusine indica 94

Stupor
Ricinus communis 86

Sudorific
Ageratum conyzoides 52
Alliaria petiolata 70
Anchusa azurea 35
Borago officinalis 37
Buxus sempervirens 37
Calendula officinalis 60
Cuminum cyminum 183
Cupressus sempervirens 79
Cymbopogon schoenanthus 94
Cynodon dactylon 94
Echium plantagineum 37
Elymus repens 94
Eupatorium cannabinum 64
Hedera helix 27
Lactuca virosa 67
Laurus nobilis 116
Lavandula angustifolia 101
Origanum majorana 109
Peganum harmala 195
Petroselinum crispum 187
Ruscus aculeatus 155
Salvia officinalis 110
Sambucus ebulus 42
Sambucus nigra 42
Smilax aspera 162
Solanum dulcamara 168
Ulmus campestris 172
Viola odorata 193

Sunstroke
Calotropis procera 27
Inula viscosa 64
Otostegia fruticosa 110

Suppuration
Otostegia fruticosa 110

Sweetening agent
Glycyrrhiza foetida 123
Glycyrrhiza glabra 123

Swelling of spleen
Iris germanica 97
Trigonella foenum-graecum 128

Swellings
Borago officinalis 37
Capparis decidua 40
Heliotropium bacciferum 37
Inula viscosa 64
Polygonum maritimum 146
Ricinus communis 86
Ruta chalepensis 158

Swollen eyes
Ziziphus spina-christi 153

Sympathomimetic
Ephedra alata 82

Syphilis
Ageratum conyzoides 52
Asparagus stipularis 130
Balanites aegyptiaca 35
Buxus sempervirens 37
Lepidium sativum 71

Syphilitic cankers
Atractylis gummifera 57

Syphilitic lesions
Daphne gnidium 172

Syphilitic ulcers
Calotropis procera 27

Taenia
Dryopteris filix-mas 32
Santolina chamaecyparissus 67

Taenifuge
Santolina chamaecyparissus 67

Tapeworm
Otanthus maritimus 67

Teeth
Plumbago europaea 146

Teeth appearance in children
Hyphaene thebaica 138

Teeth cleansing
Juglans regia 98
Punica granatum 149

Teeth strengthener
Nirium oleander 25

Tenicide
Nigella sativa 150

Testes
Coriandrum sativum 180

Thinness
Thapsia garganica 187

Thirst
Phoenix dactylifera 140
Portulaca oleracea 149

Thirst-quenching
Portulaca oleracea 149

Throat
Tamarindus indica 126

Throat catarrhs
Lagenaria siceraria 75

Throat pains
Mandragora autumnalis 167
Nicotiana rustica 167

Throat troubles
Geranium robertianum 92
Glycyrrhiza glabra 123
Pistacia lentiscus 145
Thynus broussonettii 112

Tincture
Viola odorata 193

Tinea
Ballota nigra 101
Lupinus albus 123

Toes irritation
Lupinus albus 123

Tongue paralysis
Anacyclus pyrethrum 52

Tonic
Aceras anthropophorum 138
Ageratum conyzoides 52
Allium sativum 23
Aloe perryi 128
Ammi majus 175
Artemisia herba-alba 57
Avena sativa 92
Ballota nigra 101
Capparis spinosa 40
Capsicum annuum 164
Capsicum frutescens 164
Chamomilla recutita 60
Cichorium intybus 61
Cistanche phelypaea 138
Citrus aurantium 155
Corrigiola telephiifolia 42
Crocus sativus 97
Cynara scolymus 64
Cynomorium coccineum 80
Cyperus rotundus 82
Eucalyptus globulus 135
Eupatorium cannabinum 64
Euphorbia echinus 83
Ficus carica 134
Foeniculum vulgare 187
Fraxinus angustifolia 137
Galium odoratum 154
Geranium robertianum 92
Geum urbanum 153
Juglans regia 98
Juniperus communis 79
Lavandula stoechas 101
Lepidium sativum 71
Lythrum salicaria 131
Marrubium vulgare 101
Morus alba 135
Myristica fragrans 135
Myrtus communis 135
Origanum compactum 109
Origanum majorana 109
Otanthus maritimus 67
Phoenix dactylifera 140
Piper cubeba 142
Piper nigrum 142
Ranunculus sceleratus 151
Rubia peregrina 154
Rubia tinctorum 155
Ruscus aculeatus 155
Salix alba 158
Salvadora persica 158
Salvia officinalis 110
Salvia sclarea 110
Senecio anteuphorbium 68
Sesamum indicum 142
Silybum marianum 68
Stachys officinalis 112
Teucrium polium 112

Thymus capitatus 112
Tribulus terrestris 195
Trigonella foenum-graecum 128
Viola tricolor 193
Viscum cruciatum 131
Zingiber officinale 193
Ziziphus lotus 151

Tonic for arteriosclerosis
Capparis spinosa 40

Tonicardiac
Adonis annua 150
Crataegus monogyna 153
Syzygium aromaticum 137

Tonsillitis
Geranium robertianum 92
Trigonella foenum-graecum 128

Toothache
Achillea santolina 52
Ammi visnaga 175
Anacyclus pyrethrum 52
Asphodelus aestivus 130
Calotropis procera 27
Capparis decidua 40
Maerua crassifolia 42
Nicotiana rustica 167
Nigella sativa 150
Peganum harmala 195
Ricinus communis 86
Rosa damascena 154

Toothbrush
Atriplex halimus 45
Phoenix dactylifera 140
Salvadora persica 158

Toxic
Aloe perryi 128
Anagyris foetida 119
Androcymbium gramineum 128
Atractylis gummifera 57
Atropa bella-donna 162
Bryonia dioica 73
Colchicum autumnale 130
Coriaria myrtifolia 70
Daphne gnidium 172
Ecballium elaterium 75
Hyoscyamus faleslez 167
Retama raetam 126
Ricinus communis 86
Solanum nigrum 168
Spartium junceum 126
Urginea maritima 130
Withania somnifera 168

Tranquilizer
Ballota nigra 101

Trembling limbs
Lolium temulentum 96

Tuberculosis
Allium sativum 23
Inula viscosa 64
Lepidum sativum 71
Lycium intricatum 167

Tumors
Althaea officinalis 134
Anagyris foetida 119
Nerium oleander 25
Ocimum basilicum 109
Ricinus communis 86
Urginea maritima 130

Tumors of the eye
Ocimum basilicum 109

Typhoid
Allium sativum 23
Marrubium vulgare 101

Typhus
Marrubium vulgare 101

Ulcers
Ageratum conyzoides 52
Alkanna tinctoria 35
Anagyris foetida 119
Artemisia absinthium 54
Asphodelus aestivus 130
Borago officinalis 37
Capparis spinosa 40
Cynoglossum officinale 37
Globularia alypum 92
Pistacia lentiscus 145
Plantago afra 145
Plantago major 146
Punica granatum 149
Ranunculus sceleratus 151
Rosmarinus officinalis 110
Rubia tinctorum 155
Stellaria media 45
Urtica urens 191
Vaccaria pyramidata 45
Withania somnifera 168

Ulcers in animals
Nerium oleander 25

Ulcers of genital organs
Phoenix dactylifera 140

Ureter stones
Centaurium spicatum 89

Urinary affections
Plantago afra 145

Urinary ailments
Eryngium campestre 183

Urinary bladder
Physalis alkekengi 168

Urinary calculi
Daucus carota 183

Urinary diseases
Malva sylvestris 134

Urinary disorders
Ammi visnaga 175

Urinary incontinence
Globularia alypum 92

Urinary infections
Viola tricolor 193

Urinary inflammations
Plantago afra 145

Urinary system diseases
Inula viscosa 64
Zea mays 96

Urinary tract
Daucus carota 183
Juniperus communis 79
Ononis spinosa 126
Piper cubeba 142
Solenostemma arghel 32

Urinary tract dialator
Ononis spinosa 126

Urinary tract inflammations
Linum usitatissimum 131

Urinary tract stones
Juniperus phoenicea 79

Urinary troubles
Solenostemma arghel 32

Urine
Phoenix dactylifera 140

Urine contractions
Cynodon dactylon 94

Urine incontinence
Apium graveolens 175

Urine retention
Apium graveolens 175
Lavandula dentata 101
Leptadenia pyrotechnica 27
Narcissus tazetta 25
Zea mays 96

Urinogenital disorders
Piper cubeba 142

Uroliths expeller
Leptadenia pyrotechnica 27

Urticaria
Lavandula dentata 101

Uterine ailments
Helianthus annuus 64

Uterine haemorrhages
Eryngium campestre 183

Uterine infections
Daucus carota 183

Uterine muscles
Glycyrrhiza glabra 123

Uterine problems
Capsella bursa-pastoris 71

Uterine relaxant
Punica granatum 149

Uterus affections
Tamarix aphylla 172
Trigonella foenum-graecum 128

Uterus congestion
Trigonella foenum-graecum 128

Uterus contractions
Juniperus phoenicea 79
Juniperus thurifera 80

Uvula
Argania spinosa 162
Juniperus thurifera 80

Vaginal bleeding
Eleusine indica 94

Vaginal injection
Ruta montana 158
Solanum nigrum 168

Vaginal pessaries
Solanum nigrum 168

Varices
Phoenix dactylifera 140

Varicocele
Echinops spinosus 64

Varicose veins
Plantago major 146
Silybum marianum 68

Variola
Luffa cylindrica 79

Varix
Ruscus aculeatus 155

Vaso-constrictor
Capsella bursa-pastoris 71
Senecio vulgaris 68

Vasodilator
Echinops spinosus 64

Vemifuge
Senecio vulgaris 68

Venereal diseases
Daphne gnidium 172
Ricinus communis 86

Vermifuge
Ajuga iva 98
Alhagi graecorum 119
Alliaria petiolata 70
Allium sativum 23
Aloe perryi 128
Anagyris foetida 119
Artemisia absinthium 54
Artemisia atlantica 57
Artemisia herba-alba 57
Balanites aegyptiaca 35
Ballota nigra 101
Bryonia dioica 73
Calotropis procera 27
Carum carvi 180
Chamaemelum nobile 60
Chenopodium ambrosioides 46
Chrysanthemum coronarium 61
Crithmum maritimum 183
Cucumis melo 75
Cucurbita pepo 75
Curcuma zedoaria 193
Eupatorium cannabinum 64
Ferula communis 183
Foeniculum vulgare 187
Hypericum perforatum 96
Juniperus oxycedrus 79
Lavandula angustifolia 101
Lupinus albus 123
Nicotiana rustica 167
Nigella sativa 150
Physalis alkekengi 168
Portulaca oleracea 149
Punica granatum 149
Retama raetam 126
Rubia tinctorum 155
Santolina chamaecyparissus 67
Teucrium polium 112
Thymus broussonettii 112
Vitex agnus-castus 193

Vertebral pains
Zingiber officinale 193

Vertigo
Tribulus terrestris 195

Vesical calculus
Cynodon dactylon 94

Vesicant
Daphne gnidium 172
Plumbago europaea 146
Urginea maritima 130

Vesicatory
Clematis flammula 150
Euphorbia helioscopia 83

Veterinary medicine
Allium sativum 23
Artemisia herba-alba 57
Calotropis procera 27
Cedrus atlantica 142
Cuminum cyminum 183
Dryopteris filix-mas 32
Euphorbia resenifera 83
Heliotropium bacciferum 37
Tetraclinis articulata 80

Veterinary preparations
Citrullus colocynthis 73

Veterinary preparations for itch
Euphorbla balsamifera 83

Vitality
Fumaria parviflora 89

Vomiting
Coriandrum sativum 180
Cotula cinera 61
Haplophyllum tuberculatum 155
Ruta chalepensis 158

Vulnerary
Acanthus mollis 23
Agrimonia eupatoria 153
Ajuga iva 98
Ambrosia maritima 52
Anthyllis vulneraria 119
Artemisia absinthium 54
Avena sativa 92
Centaurea calcitrapa 60
Chamaemelum nobile 60
Chamomilla recutita 60
Convolvulus arvensis 68
Cynodon dactylon 94
Eupatorium cannabinum 64
Galium odoratum 154
Geranium robertianum 92
Hypericum perforatum 96
Lavandula stoechas 101
Lawsonia inermis 131
Lythrum salicaria 131
Melissa officinalis 104
Morus alba 135
Origanum majorana 109
Panicum turgidum 96
Plantago coronopus 146
Polygonum aviculare 146
Rosmarinus officinalis 110
Ruta chalepensis 58
Salix alba 158
Salvia officinalis 110
Sambucus nigra 42
Stachys officinalis 112
Teucrium chamaedrys 112
Teucrium polium 112
Vaccaria pyramidata 45
Verbena officinalis 191

War poison
Hyoscyamus faleslez 167

Warts
Euphorbia echinus 83

Weight adding
Hyoscyamus faleslez 167
Juglans regia 98
Lolium temulentum 96
Lycium intricatum 167
Mandragora autumnalis 167
Trigonella foenum-graecum 128
Vitex agnus-castus 193

White spots on the eye
Panicum turgidum 96

Whitening the teeth
Mandragora autumnalis 167

Whitlow
Lepidium sativum 71

Whooping cough
Thymus algeriensis 112
Viola odorata 193

Withering
Crocus sativus 97

Women's sterility
Withania somnifera 168

Worms
Allium sativum 23
Ocimum basilicum 109
Ricinus communis 86

Wound healing
Ocimum basilicum 109

Wound ulcers
Hedera helix 27

Wounds
Acacia raddiana 116
Ageratum conyzoides 52
Anthyllis vulneraria 119
Artemisia absinthium 54
Artemisia arborescens 54
Balanites aegyptiaca 35
Borago officinalis 37
Calendula officinalis 60
Capparis decidua 40
Centaurium spicatum 89
Cynoglossum officinale 37
Cyperus papyrus 82
Erodium cicutarium 92
Helianthus annuus 64
Juniperus communis 79
Juniperus oxycedrus 79
Lawsonia inermis 131
Maerua crassifolia 42
Nicotiana rustica 167
Pinus halepensis 142
Plantago coronopus 146
Plantago major 146
Plumbago europaea 146
Quercus coccifera 86
Retama raetam 126
Ricinus communis 86
Rosmarinus officinalis 110
Rubia tinctorum 155
Senecio anteuphorbium 68
Stellaria media 45
Typha domingensis 172
Urginea maritima 130
Urtica urens 191
Vaccaria pyramidata 45

Wounds of camels
Cymbopogon schoenanthus 94

COMMON NAMES INDEX

Aas 135
Aas barri 155
Abaoual 80
Abaqua 153
Abawal 142
'Abbad esh-shams 64
Abbouk 25
Abeb 168
Abelbel 57
Aben drag 149
Abernid 119
Abisga 162
Aboaun 128
Abolask 153
Abou en-noum 140
Aboubal 183
Abougboug 46
Aboujoulj 60
Aboushel-n-tekkouk 138
Abqouq 27
Abraham's balm 193
Abser 116
Absinth 54
Absinthe 54
Absinthe arborescente 54
Absinthe bâtarde 52
Absinthe de Judée 57
Absinthe menue 54
Absinthium 54
Abu khangar 71
Abur 75
Abushal 80
Abzac 116
Acacia d'Egypte 116
Acanthe molle 23
Aceb 60
Acham 183
Achdirt 154
Ache des marais 180
Achnef 71
Achtouan 149
Acrid lettuce 67
Ad-dahma 134
'Adam 82
Addad 57
Adder's tongue 92
Addou 25
Addoua 35
Adekkoush 140
Aderias 187
Adhan el-ghazal 37
Adhan el-thour 37
Adiante 23
Adil-ououchchn 164
Adjar 42
Adjem 42
Adjou 162
Adkhar 92
Admam 153
Adonide automnale 150
Adonide d'été 150
Adonide estivale 150
Adonis goutte de sang 150
Adras el-kelb 149, 195
Adroumam 80
Afahlehlé-n-aheddan 130
Afal 27
Afalehlé 167
Afdad 80
Afedjedad 67
'Afernan 83
Aferoug 40
Afersiou 32
Afezou 96
Affar 94
Affelajet 119
Affer 94
Afgous bourhioul 75
Afhrilal 175
Afioun 140
Afistinoun 70
Afiyyash 162
Afligou 104
Afnen 119
Afqous 75
'Afrar 116
Afsantin 54
Afsdad 126
Aftimoun 70
Aganat 128
Agargarha 52
Agérate 52
Agerger 119
Ageridd 42
Agesmir 94
Aggaya 197
'Aggour 75
Agjjuf 140
Agneau chaste 193
'Agoua 83
Agoucin bourioul 146
'Agoul 119
Agourim imeksawen 110
Agouzinir 94
Agrima 71
Agrimony 153
Agueridd 42
Aguerma 71
Ahades 116
Ahajjar 52
Ahates 116
Ahon-n-igoura 83
'Ai'afein 71
Aiazidh 183
Aifz 79
Aigremoine 153
Aiguille 92
Ail commun 23
Ail cultivé 23
Ailelé 137

'Ain el-arnab 128
'Ain el-bouma 150
'Ain el-hadjla 150
'Ain el-katkout 61
'Ain esh-shams 64
'Ain if 46
'Ain serdouk 25
Aioual 80
Airni 27
Aizara 35
Ajrourj 151
Akaioud 172
Akamen 175
Akaraba 70
'Akefa 123
Akhella 175
Akhendous 112
Akhilwan 42
Aklel 110
'Akoub 68
'Akreish 130
'Akresh 94
Akshout 70
Al-hilla 68
Alala 57
Alanoudrag 101
Alaterne 151
Alaternus 151
Alcanna 131
'Alda 82
'Alda el-dabbaghin 82
'Alda el-gemal 82
Aldhaz 119
Alelga 82
'Alenda 82
Aleppo pine 142
Aleppo rue 158
Alexander's foot 54
Alezzaz 172
Alfilaria 92
Alhagi des maures 119
Alili 25
Alisma plantain 23
Alisme 23
Alizari 155
'Alk 92, 116
'Alk el-anbat 145
Alkanet 35
Alkanna 35
Alkat 73
Alkekeng 168
Alkekenge 168
'Allaiq 154
Allgo 126
Alliare 70
Alliare officinale 70
Allison 71
Almande de terre 80
Almes 94
Alo 35
Aloe 128
Alouaich 68
Alougo 126
Aluine 54
Alvine 54
Alype 92
Alypo globe daisy 92
Alysse argentée 71
Alysse maritime 71
Alysson maritime 71
Amagelost 195
Amagraman 64
Amaracus 109
'Ambar ed-dor 97
Ambre végétal 46
Ambroisie 46, 52
Ambroisie du Mexique 46
Ambrosie 52
Amedjir 134
Amelzi 80,142
Ameo 67
Ameskelit 64
Amezzir 101
Amezzour 101
Amil 137
Amirbaris 35
Amizzour 40
Amkouk 80
Amlilis 151
Ammi commun 175
Ammi inodore 175
Ammi officinal 175
Amome des Indes 195
Amourgha 137
Amsa 187
Amseilih 40
Amwashar 137
Amzmem 151
'Anab ed-dib 168
Anagyre fétide 119
Anagyris 119
'Anbar 97
Anbarbaris 35
Andjira 191
Aneb ed-dib 130, 168
Anesfal 68
Anet 175
Aneth 175
Aneth doux 187
Angarf 193
Anini 25
Anis 187
Anis vert 187
Anise 187
Aniseed plant 187
Anisun 187
Anjjil 154
Annual mercury 86
'Ansara 150
Anschfel 68
Ansérine fétide 46
Anthémis noble 60
Anthyllide vulnéraire 119
Aoudmi 154
Aoukeraz 94
Aourizi 168
Aourma 158
Aourmela 60
Aourmi 158
Aoushket 126
Aoutem 32
Aouti 130
Aouzed 61
Apple of Sodom 27

Apple-bearing sage 110
'Aqerban 32
'Aqoul el-gabal 130
Aqoullab 96
'Ar'ar 79, 80
'Ar'ar berboush 80
'Ar'ar berhoush 80
'Ar'ar el-ibel 80
Arac 162
Araignée 150
'Araira 67
Arak 162
Aramès 46
Arami 98
Arams 46
Aranim 96
Arar tree 80
Arbre à gomme 119
Arbre à soie 27
Arbre au poivre 193
Arbre blanc 116
Ardj 153
Ardjan 162
Ardjaqnou 60
Arella 79
Arellachem 32
Arendj 155
'Areq sous 123
'Arfeg 67
Argan 162
Argan tree 162
Arganier 162
Argel 32
Argiqon 60
Argis 35
Arhbita 67
Arhdon 61
Arhilem 149
Arhilon 61
Arig 158
Ariouri 42
Ariri 25
Arkenu 42
Arkerma 42
Armoise 57
Armoise arborescente 54
Armoise blanche 57
Armoise de Judée 57
Armoise en arbre 54
Armoise rouge 57
Armoun 149
Armstrong 146
Arn tree 42
Aroubian 155
Aroumane 149
Arqat 27
'Arq safir 110
Arrête-boeuf 126
Arrhis 35
Arroche 46
Arssfa 101
Artichaut 61, 64
Artichaut sauvage 61, 68
Artichoke 64
Arum d 'italie 27
Arwari 42
Arzaq 142
Arzema 109
Arzoum 82
Asabi' hermes 130
Asad el-ard 57
Asafsaf 158
Asal 98
'Asa Musa 116
Asef 40
Asel 137
Asfaqs 110
Asfar 97, 151
Asfarar 37
Asfarfar 37
Ash-shawka al-haddah 153
Asharab 64
Ashasha 150
Ashabardou 68
Ashbarto 68
'Asheq esh-shams 64
Ashkhis 57
Ashreq 119
'Asi rebbo 138
'Asloudj 145
Asloudya 61
'Asluj 61
Asnan 183
Asperge 130
Aspérule odorante 154
Asphodèle 130
Assaaf 40
Assabay 27
'Assa er-ra 'i 146
Assay 46
Asseln 137
Assengar 96
Asslift 32
Atai 46
'Atana 52
Atemen 153
'Athaq 37
Atil 42
Atkizounn 155
Atlantic cedar 142
Atlantic pistacio 145
Atlas cedar 142
Atoua 67
Atoukelissa 135
Atrar 35
Atrope 164
Attasa 67
Attertag 126
Aubépine 153
Auli 183
Aunée visqueuse 67
Aurone 57
Aurone des champs 57
Aurone femelle 52, 67
Autumn adonis 150
Autumn crocus 130
Avens 154
Avoine 92
'Awarwar 75, 162
Awermi 158
Awrioun 86
'Awsaj 167
Ayate 89
'Aynun 92

Azalim 23
Azar 151
Azarem 151
Azarkur 151
Azart 134
Azawo 116
Azazzer 37
Azcar 183
Azdjmir 82
Azeboudj 137
Azekdon 191
Azekkoun 92
Azeli 98
Azemai 98
Azemmour 137
Azemnoun 27
Azenzou 150, 154
Azeroual 183
Azir 110
Azkhar 92
Azlen 137
Azlim 23
Azouiout 60
Azoukni 112
Azouri imouchene 168
Azar azidane 123
Azzou 130
Ba'athran 57
Baba adjina 153
Babnouj 61
Babnouz 61
Babounag 60, 61
Babounag rumi 60
Babounig 52, 61
Babul 162
Babuni 67
Babunig et-tuyur 68
Bacille 183
Badarendjabouya 104
Badhisqan 126
Bagdouness 187
Baglet'Aisha 71
Baguenaudier 123
Bakhbakh 23
Bakhis 134
Bakhr 128
Bakhran 128
Balah 140
Balah harara 35
Balanite d'Egypte 35
Balbal 195
Balia 46
Ballote fétide 101
Ballout el-hallouf 86
Ballutah 101
Balm-leaf 104
Bambous 75
Banafsag 193
Banewort 164
Baq 68
Baqela 128
Baqilla masri 123
Baqlet el-hamqa 149
Baqlet el-mubareka 149
Baqnin 168
Baqninou 168
Baqs 37, 158
Baranbakh 27
Barbaris 35
Barbe de chèvre 183
Barbede capucin 61
Barberry 35
Barbina 191
Barbotte 128
Barbousha 180
Bardaqoush 109
Bardi 82, 172
Barga 27
Barghoutha 71
Barren privet 151
Barru 138
Basal el-far 130
Basal el-kelb 130
Basal far 'on 130
Basbayedj 149
Basees 45
Basfayedj 149
Basil 109
Basilic 109
Baslim 23
Basoun 54
Bassal 23
Bassisa 45
Bastard agrimony 52
Basul 130
Battoum 145
Batuniqa 112
Bawwal 195
Baymut 191
Bazegzour 153
Bazezour 151
Be'eitheran 52
Bean-clover 119
Bear's breech 23
Bec de cigogne 92
Bec de grue 92
Bec de héron 92
Becid 130
Beebalm 104
Beglet el-berba 27
Begouga 25, 27
Beguoun 142
Behar 25
Beid el-ghoul 167
Beid el-ghul 75
Beiqa 123
Bekkem 151
Belachem 40
Belacheqine 71
Belaidour 164
Belesfendj 193
Belladone 164
Belle téte 112
Belle-dame 164
Bellehu 168
Bellout el-ard 112
Belna'aman 140
Belouza 130
Belozet el-'onsol 130
Belwaz 130
Ben en-na'aman 150
Ben memoun 82
Ben na'aman 140, 150
Ben nour 168

Ben nout 191
Ben tabis 154
Benderakesh 149
Benefsig 97
Benoite 154
Bent en-nar 191
Bentalis 154
Beqoul el-kelb 119
Berberry 35
Berchenoussane 32
Berdi 94, 172
Berdougala 149
Berengat 25
Berghousti 145
Bermuda grass 94
Berqam 52
Berraq 146
Berraya 197
Bersemoun 97
Bersiana 46
Bersil 187
Berslouna 97
Berwag 130
Berwaga 130
Besbas 187
Besbas harami 183
Besbasa 187
Beshna 96
Besillet iblis 128
Besla 23
Besliga 126
Besnikha 175
Bessat el-ard 45
Bessat el-melouk 45
Bessat el-qa'a 45
Bestana 79
Betina 167
Bétonie 112
Betony 112
Betoum 145
Bettikha 75
Beuqs 37
Bezer 145
Bigaradier 155
Bikhe shoukaran 180
Bilasan 42
Binesar 134
Bing 164
Bint En-Nebi 70
Bird pepper 164
Birhoum 162
Bisaille 128
Bishop's weed 175
Bishop's wort 112
Bishrin 52
Bitter apple 75
Bitter gourd 75
Bitter orange 155
Bitter-sweet 168
Bittikh 75
Bizr qotuna 145
Black bryony 82
Black cumin 150
Black horehound 101
Black maidenhair fern 32
Black mustard 70
Black nightshade 168
Black oak fern 32
Black pepper 142
Black poplar 158
Black spleenwort 32
Black-leaved mullein 162
Bladder herb 168
Bladder-senna tree 123
Bladderdock 149
Blah 140
Blé de Turquie 96
Bleibsha 149
Blépharie 23
Bliha 151
Blue gum tree 135
Bodweya 94
Bois pointu 155
Bois puant 119
Bokhour el-berber 42
Bokhour mourshka 42
Bokkar 96
Bontouma 131
Boon tree 42
Borgoman 52
Botoum 145
Bottle gourd 79
Bou 'adjel 183
Bou djenah 146
Bou dweys 94
Bou el-kazit 149
Bou en-noum 140
Bou ghans 158
Bou kahli 71
Bou khsas 191
Bou krish 37
Bou mekherri 153
Bou meknina 168
Bou mentem 193
Bou metin 193
Bou neffa' 187
Bou neggar 60
Bou qesas 27
Bou qini 164
Bou qnina 168
Bou rekba 96
Bou rendjouf 164
Bou sassal 37
Bou seman 35
Bou shenaf 37
Bou shweika 60
Bou soufa 154
Bou sreira 151
Bou tania 82
Bou teriowa 73
Bou tertakh 126
Bou tnia 73
Bou zenzir 86
Bou zeqdouf 191
Bou zerwal 68
Bou 'aggad 146
Boubezzit 89
Boudi 140
Bougraouna 150
Bouguel 149
Boundi 140
Bounerdjoul 164
Bourg-épine 151
Bourrache 37

Bourrache bâtarde 37
Bourrache officinale 37
Bourrwabes 42
Bourse à pasteur 71
Bourse de capucin 71
Boursette 71
Bous 96
Bousidan 168
Bousir 162
Bousir aswad-el-waraq 162
Bousira 162
Bout 172
Bouteille 79
Bouton noir 164
Box-holly 155
Bqula 134
Brabra 149
Branc ursine 23
Branke ursine 23
Brazilian tobacco 167
Bread-root 126
Brisemmou 149
Bristle fern 32
Broad bean 128
Bryone 73
Bryone couleuvrée 73
Bryone dioique 73
Bryone douce à fruit et racine noir 82
Bubal 183
Bubqini 164
Buck's-horn plantain 146
Bughlam 45
Bugle 98
Buglosse 37
Buis 37
Buis toujours vert 37
Bulbes de colchique 130
Buplèvre 45
Buqul as-sabiya 89
Burbeit 82
Burbit 97
Buseil 130
Busweifa 45
Butcher's broom 155
Cactus raquette 40
Cade 79
Cadier 79
Calabash cucumber 79
Calebasse 79
Calebasse d'Europe 79
Calibtus 135
Callitris 80
Calotrope 27
Caltrops 60, 195
Camamel 60
Camel thorn 119
Camel's hay 92, 94
Camomile 60
Camomille commune 61
Camomille du Sahara 61
Camomille odorante 60
Camomille romaine 60
Camphire 131
Canker flower 154
Caper-spurge 83
Capillaire 23
Capillaire de maraille 32
Capillaire de Montpellier 23
Capillaire noire 32
Capillaire rouge des officines 32
Câprier 40
Câprier commun 40
Câprier épineux 40
Capsicum 164
Capsique 164
Caraway 180
Carde 61
Cardon 61
Cardoon 61
Carique 134
Carob tree 123
Carotte sauvage 183
Caroubier 123
Carthame gummifère 57
Carvi 180
Carvi officinal 119
Casse à feuilles étroites 119
Casse trompeuse 119
Castor oil plant 86
Cat tail 172
Cat thyme 112
Cat's milk 83
Catapuce 83
Catherinette 83
Cèdre 142
Cèdre de l'Atlas 142
Céleri 180
Céleri cultivé 180
Celery 180
Celery-leaved crowfoot 151
Célestine 52
Centaurée 60
Centaurée acaule 60
Centaury 60, 89
Centinode 146
Cerfeuil 175
Cerfolium 175
Cerise de Juif 168
Cétérach officinal 32
Chaihata 52
Chaméléon blanc 57
Chamoeleon blanc des anciens 57
Chamomile 60
Champignon de Malte 80
Chanvre 40
Chanvre d'eau 64, 101
Chanvre indien 40
Chanvrine 64
Chardon à glu 57
Chardon argenté 68
Chardon étoilé 60
Chardon Marie 68
Chardon Notre Dame 68
Chardon roland 183
Chasse diable 97
Chasse fièvre 112
Chasse puce 104
Chaste tree 193
Chausse-trape 60
Cheat 96
Chellalah 42
Chêne cocciné 89
Chêne garouille 89
Chêne kermès 89

Chênette 112
Cheveux de paysan 61
Chick-pea 123
Chicorée 61
Chicorée amère 61
Chicorée sauvage 61
Chicotin 75
Chiendent 94
Chiendent commun 94
Chiendent d'Italie 94
Chiendent pied de poule 94
Chiendent rampant 94
Chilla 164
Chira 40
Chou noir 70
Chouaya 57
Christ's thorn 153
Chrysanthème à carène 61
Cicérole 123
Ciguë 180
Ciguë officinale 180
Ciguë tachée 180
Cinquefoil 154
Ciste à ladanum 46
Ciste blanc 46
Ciste d'Espagne 46
Ciste de Montpellier 52
Ciste ladanifère 46
Citronelle 104, 191
Citronnelle 94
Citrouille 75
Clary 110
Clématite 150
Clématite brûlante 150
Cléematite flammette 150
Clématite odorante 150
Cléome 52
Clous de girofle 137
Clove tree 137
Clover dodder 70
Cloves 137
Cockle bur 153
Colchicum 130
Colchique 130
Colchique d'automne 130
Colocynth 75
Coloquinte 75
Colutéa 123
Colutier 123
Common borago 37
Common box tree 37
Common bryony 73
Common caper-bush 40
Common caraway 180
Common chickweed 45
Common cistus 46
Common cultivated radish 73
Common eryngo 183
Common fennel 187
Common fennel flower 150
Common fig tree 134
Common flax 131
Common garden parsley 187
Common germander 112
Common ginger 193
Common groundsel 68
Common hedge mustard 73
Common ivy 27
Common lavender 101
Common lettuce 67
Common mallow 134
Common mint 109
Common polypody 149
Common reed 96
Common rosemary 110
Common sage 110
Common spleenwort 32
Common stork's-bill 92
Common strawberry 153
Common vetch 128
Common white horehound 104
Concombre d'âne 75
Concombre d'attrape 75
Concombre sauvage 75
Congourde 79
Conyze vulgaire 61
Coquelicot 140
Coqueret 168
Coqueret somnifère 168
Corail des jardins 164
Corbeille d'argent 71
Coriaire 70
Coriander 180
Coriandre 180
Corn bind 68
Corn de cerf 146
Corn lily 68
Corn poppy 140
Cornichon d'âne 75
Coronille 123
Coronope 146
Corroyère 70
Corroyère à feuilles de myrthe 70
Cotton weed 67
Couch grass 94
Courge torchon 79
Courgette 75
Cow-herb 45
Cresse 70
Cresse à feuille d'herniaire 70
Cresson alénois 71
Cresson de fontaine 71
Cresson des jardins 71
Cressonnette 71
Crève chien 168
Criste marine 183
Crithme 183
Crocus 97
Croix de Malte 195
Crotalaire 123
Crown daisy 61
Crown marigold 61
Cubeb pepper 142
Cubèbe 142
Cumin 183
Cumin à laine 175
Cumin des prés 180
Cumin du Sahara 175
Cumin laineux 175
Cumin noir 150
Curcuma zédoaire 193
Cure dents du Prophète 175
Cuscute 70
Cuscute de thym 70

Cynoglosse 37
Cynomoir écarlate 80
Cyprès 79
Cyprès commun 79
Cypress tree 79
Dabbab 104
Dactyle 94
Dadaifa 45
Daddès 154
Dadhi 97
Dadhi rumi 97
Dafla sahrawia 67
Dafs 175
Daghmus 83
Daikon 73
Dalia beida 73
Dall 151
Damask rose 154
Damdamun 42
Danaqah 96
Danewort 42
Danun 138
Danun el-gin 138
Daphné paniculé 172
Dar felfel 164
Dar sini 135
Dardar 137
Daret esh-shams 64
Darnel 96
Darrhis 35
Dars el-'agouz 195
Darw 145
Dasisah 54
Date palm 140
Dattier 140
Dattier du désert 35
Datura 164
Dauphinelle staphisaigre 150
Daurade 35
Deadly nightshade 164
Debsha 180
Defla 25
Degoufet 57
Dehada 101
Deil el-qott 94
Deis 94, 172
Delkmouch 131
Dellakal 32
Demamai 153
Demia 32
Demsisa 52
Dentelaire 146
Derhis 146
Derias 187
Deris 138
Dermous 86
Derw 145
Desert date 35
Devil's apple 164
Devil's trumpet 164
Deydahan 140
Dhaqn esh-sheikh 54
Dharirah 27
Dhou 145
Dohu el-keffin 149
Diabé 131
Dik 'aroum 195
Dill 175
Dill-seed 175
Dingel 73
Dirw 145
Dis 82
Ditch reed 96
Dj'eida 101
Dja'ad 112
Djabbar 96
Djaboub 96
Djahnama 164
Djamir 60
Djarna 92
Djashwan 61
Djei 101
Djelban 128
Djelbane 123
Djelif 94
Djell 158
Djemra 60
Djerdjir 71
Djerdjir el-maa 71
Djerir 180
Djerniz 57
Djertil 112
Djettiat 126
Djilla 128
Djimmar 61
Djimri 60
Djineda 79
Djir 134
Djirouad 75
Djolanar 149
Djouldjoulan 61
Djoumaira 60
Djoushshen 112
Djouz 98
Djouz er-ra'ian 146
Djouza matel 164
Djouzet er-ra'iane 172
Dodder of thyme 70
Dog briar 154
Dog rose 154
Dog's chamomile 61
Dog's orache 46
Dog's-toothgrass 94
Dokhan 167
Dokhan akhdar 167
Dokhan barri 167
Dokhan soufi 167
Domran 109
Dorade 35
Doradille 32
Doradille noire 32
Dorran 96
Douce-amère 168
Douhreig 128
Douilat 68
Doujnilourman 68
Doum 138
Doum d'Egypte 138
Doum oriental 138
Doum palm 138
Doumiat shouka 183
Dra 96
Dra shami 96
Draia 96

Drias plant 187
Drinn 96
Dubb'a 75
Dura shamiyah 96
Dutch rush 98
Dwale 164
Dwarf elder 42
Dwarf stinger 191
Dyer's bugloss 35
Dyer's madder 155
Dyer's rocket 151
Dyer's weed 151
Earth almond 80
Earth-gall 89
East Indian ginger 193
Ebora 35
Echinops ritron 64
Eclipte droite 64
Ecorce de garou commun 172
'Eddeis 128
Edgeish 142
Edible cyperus 80
Eglantier 154
Eglantine 154
Egyptian acacia 116
Egyptian balsam 35
Egyptian henbane 167
Egyptian lupin 126
Egyptian privet 131
Egyptian thorn 116
Egyptian towel gourd 79
Eimim 151
El-'attasa 67
El-'eteytesa 67
El-betbat 146
El-harra 73
El-hashal 138
El-henna 37
El-kemsha 70
El-kmisha 70
El-nakheil 140
El-sedab el-jebli 158
Elder tree 42
Elm 172
Emohi 134
'Enab ed-dib 168
'Enab el-haiya 73
'Enab et-ta'lab 168
Endjil 94
Endormie 164
English elm 172
English ivy 27
Entifa 154
Ephédra 82
Epiaire bétonie 112
Epine blanche 153
Epine de mai 153
Epine du Christ 153
Epine-vinette 35
Epithym 70
Eponge végétale 79
Epurge 83
Erbyan 61
Erg 158
Erigère 61
Erigéron 61
'Ern 25
Erode 92
Erodion cicutin 92
Erq el-share'e 45
'Erq et-tayyoun 64
Erqeita 27
Erynge 183
Erythrée centaurée 89
Erz 142
'Esh en-niml 128
Eshb el-malek 126
Eshba hamra 45
Eshbet el-ghorab 112
Eshbet el-kelb 104
Eshbet mariam 54
Eshbet netegerfa 112
Eshbet salema 68
Estakhoudes 101
Etel 172
'Etr 92
Eucalyptus 135
Eucalyptus officinal 135
Eupatoire 64, 153
Eupatoire chanvrine 64
Eupatoire d'Avicenne 64
Euphorbe 86
Euphorbe épurge 83
Euphorbe hélioscope 83
Euphorbe peplis 83
Euphorbe résinifère 86
Euphorbium 86
Euphorbium gum-plant 86
Evergreen cypress 79
Fachirchin 82
Fadhiss 145
Fafetone 27
Faggous el-hemar 75
Faghia 131
Faham 138
Faham d'Algérie 138
Falezlez 167
False daisy 64
Far'on 130
Farandal 131
Faraorao 168
Faraoun 138
Farfah 149
Farsh el-ard 45
Fashira 73
Fasoukh 183
Fausse sabine 79
Faux capillaire 32
Faux fenouil 187
Faux réséda de teinturiers 151
Faux séné 123
Faux turbith 187
Fawaniya 138
Feg'aa 64
Fegane 64
Feggous 75
Felfel ahmar 164
Felfel akhal 142
Felfel aswad 142
Felfel el-djebel 40
Felfel essudan 80
Felfel glib-el-ttir 164
Felfel haar 164
Felfel helw 164

Felfel merrakshi 164
Felfel rumi 164
Felfel torshi 164
Felfela 112
Felfila 164
Felgou 104
Feliet el-hami 67
Felon-wort 168
Femeterre 89
Fennel 187
Fenouil 187
Fenouil batard 175
Fenouil doux 187
Fenouil marin 183
Fenouil puant 175
Fénugrec 128
Fenugreek 128
Ferash el-qa'a 45
Ferasioun 101
Ferasioun aswad 101
Ferasioun mai 101
Ferbyoun 83
Ferkai 168
Férule 183
Fethies 145
Fève 128
Fève cultivée 128
Fève de loup 119
Fève de marais 128
Fèverolle 128
Feverwort 89
Feyyasha 162
Fezmir 151
Fidjel 158
Fidjla 158
Fidjla el-djebeli 158
Field eryngo 183
Field poppy 140
Figl 73
Figl el-gimal 73
Figuier 134
Figuier d'Inde 40
Figuier de barbarie 40
Figuier nopal 40
Fijel 155
Filaly 154
Five finger grass 154
Five leaf 154
Flambe 97
Flambe bâtarde 97
Flambe d-eau 97
Flambe des marais 97
Flea-wort 145
Fleabane 61
Fliet ghadir 52
Flilou 140
Fliou 104
Floss flower 52
Flowering flag 97
Flûteau 23
Foetid horehound 101
Foirole 86
Foqqish 168
Fouarek 68
Fouassier 134
Foudeoum 131
Fougat el-gamal 64
Fougère mâle 32
Fougga' el-djemel 183
Foul 128
Foul el-'arab 45
Foul hashadi 128
Foulet el-kalb 168
Fowwa 155
Fox geranium 92
Fragon 155
Fragon piquant 155
Fraisier 153
Fraisier des bois 153
Fraisier sauvage 153
Frasioun 104
Frasioun abiad 104
Frawlah 153
French cotton 27
French daffodil 25
French lavender 101
French mercury 86
Frêne de kabylie 137
Friar's cow 25
Fromageon 134
Ftozzer 73
Fudang 104
Fulayha 104
Fulayya 104
Fumeterre 89
Fumeterre officinale 89
Fumitere 89
Fumitory 89
Fustuq sharqi 145
Fuwwa 154
Fuwwa regiga 154
Fuwwat as-sabbaghin 155
Ga'ada 98
Gadwar 193
Gafit 64
Gafouli masri 96
Gairance 123
Galanga 193
Galanga mineur 193
Garance 154, 155
Garance des teinturiers 155
Garance voyageuse 154
Garde-robe 52
Garden chrysanthemum 61
Garden cress 71
Garden purslain 149
Garden sage 110
Gargir 71
Garlic 23
Garlic mustard 70
Garmoulya 153
Garnoun 61
Garou 172
Garrud 119
Garsa'na 183
Gatouf 145
Gattilier 193
Gaude 151
Gazar baladi 183
Gazar barri 183
Gazar esh-sheytan 175
Gazar shaytani 175
Gazon anglais 94
Gazoun 94

Gdari 25
Gemliya 61
Gendoul 126
Genêt d'Espagne 126
Genévrier 79
Genévrier commun 79
Genévrier de Phénicie 80
Genévrier oxycèdre 79
Genévrier rouge 79
Genévrier thurifère 80
Gengeit 164
Gengi 167
Genièvre 79
Genina 61
Gentaine centaurée 89
Genthus 54
Geranion 92
Geranium grass 94
Gerda 146
Gerga' 98
German iris 97
Germandrée 112
Germandrée officinale 112
Germandrée petit-chêne 112
Germandrée polium 112
Germandrée tomenteuse 112
Germi 27
Gern el-ail 146
Gertoufa 61
Gertufa 61
Gery 71
Gesoum 52
Gettiat 67
Ghab 96
Ghabsha 37
Ghafath 64
Ghafith 153
Ghalqa 32
Ghar 116, 193
Ghardeq 167
Gharfala 128
Gharghar 172
Ghassa 110
Ghassel 153
Ghazil 92
Gheshwa 151
Ghislah 92
Ghobbeira 52, 67
Ghobbeisha 52
Ghorara 70
Ghoreird 57
Ghorime 68
Ghoumran 46
Giant fennel 183
Gidar 89
Gihwana 61
Gingelly 142
Gingembre 195
Gingembre bâtard 193
Gingeolier 153
Ginger bread tree 138
Gingil 142
Gipsy flower 37
Gipsywort 101
Giraumon 75
Girofle 137
Giroflier 137
Gladdon 97
Gladwin 97
Glaieul des marais 97
Glaoua 154
Globulaire 92
Globulaire turbith 92
Globularia 92
Gmredj 60
Gnidium 172
Goat pepper 164
Goat weed 52
Golden flower of Peru 64
Golden locks 149
Gommier bleu 135
Gommier d'Egypte 116
Gommier de Tunisie 116
Gommier rouge 116
Goose-grass 94
Goudhim 145
Goudhoum 145
Gouët à capuchon 25
Gouët d'Italie 27
Gouffaz 52
Goulglam 149
Goumshi 96
Goungat 167
Gourd 75
Gourde 79
Gourt 126
Goushi 96
Goustt el-hayya 89
Goutiba 112
Goutte de sang 150
Gouz bouwa 135
Gouz et-tib 135
Gouzbir 180
Grand basilic 109
Grand iris 97
Grand plantain 146
Grand soleil 64
Grande absinthe 54
Grande ciguë 180
Grande mauve 134
Greater plantain 146
Grenadier 149
Grinouch 71
Gros chiendent 94
Ground cypress 67
Ground elder 42
Ground oak 112
Guebaba 180
Gueddain 145
Guengit 23
Guernech 71
Guessis 89
Gui 131
Gui rouge 131
Guigne de cote 164
Guimauve 134
Guimauve officinale 134
Guinea pepper 164
Gum-Arabic tree 116
Gurti 116
Guzmir 94
Hab el-kheraf 193
Hab er-rashad 71
Habaq 104, 109

Habaq el-ayalet 109
Habaq el-bahr 104
Habaq el-maya 104
Habb el-'arous 142
Habb el-'aziz 80
Habb el-foua 164
Habb el-kela 119
Habb el-lahw 168
Habb el-zalam 80
Habb er-ras 150
Habb er-reshad 71
Habb esh-shams 64
Habb geuzzoula 86
Habb ghar 116
Habb talaout 187
Habba helwa 187
Habba souda 150
habbeila 45
Habbet el-barakah 150
Habbet el-muluk 83
Habid 73
Habl el-masakin 27
Habriga 40
Hadaj 73
Hadaq 73
Hadd 46
Haddaq 70
Hade 96
Hadja 73
Hadriegs 187
Hafer el-mohar 130
Haffar 94
Hafina 64
Hagna 96
Hagueleg 35
Haguellet 73
Haida 112
Hairuari 42
Halama 37
Halbita 83
Halbub 86
Haldjamin 71
Half 71
Half barr 92
Halfa 94
Halfa mt'a kufra 94
Halfet makkah 94
Halhal 101
Halhal el-djebel 101
Halib de-diba 83
Halib el-ghazal 68
Halime 46
Haliyun 130
Hall 142
Hallaba 32
Halmoush 135
Halouk baladi 61
Hama 126
Hamahim 109
Hamaz 123
Hamella 131
Hammar tardjilel 92
Hamret er-ras 45
Hamriya 112
Hamsdir 101
Hamzousha 112
Hana 109
Hanbeit 149
Handal 73
Handaquq murr 126
Hanini 126
Haqq 61
Haras 116
Haraz 116
Hares 116
Hargel 32
Harif 73
Hariq amless 86
Harir igran 140
Hariret el-shami 96
Hariret el-za'atar 70
Harmal 195
Harmal el-djezair 180
Harmel 195
Harmel sahari 195
Harmola 145
Haroud tardjilel 92
Harouka 67
Harra el-berria 71
Harra el-gharin 71
Harriqa 71
Harrous 191
Harsha 37
Harshaf barri 68
Hart's-tongue fern 35
Hartaman 92
Hasak 195
Hasaka 195
Hasaknit 96
Haselra 92
Hasha 112
Hashish 40
Hashish el-awinet 52
Hashish el-faras 64, 94
Hashish el-fogara 40
Hashish el-gabal 61
Hashish el-line 86
Hashisha thawmiyah 70
Hashishat el-jourh 97
Hashishet as-sebyan 89
Hashishet ed-dabb 119
Hashishet ed-dahab 32
Hashishet el-'aqrab 89
Hashishet el-asnan 146
Hashishet el-baraghit 145
Hashishet el-kelb 104
Hashishet el-mabrouka 153
Hashishet el-mubarek 153
Hashishet el-qalb 97
Hashishet el-qizaz 45
Hashishet en-nahl 104
Hashishet er-rih 112
Hashma 94
Hasoub 68
Hassak 60, 89
Hassalban 110
Hatssa louban 110
Haut bois 42
Hawdja 145
Hawkal 80
Hawmanah 126
Hawmar 128
Hawthorn 153
Hayat 79

Hayat en-nefous 83
Hayshar 61
Hazdacht 140
Hdawa 96
Headed thyme 112
Heart's ease 193
Hebrew manna plant 119
Heddad 57
Hedej lehmar 73
Hedge mustard 73
Heglig 35
Heish 94
Heish moddeid 96
Helba 128
Helein 94
Helhal 101
Helianthe 64
Hemlock 180
Hemlock geranium 92
Hemp weed 64
Hen and chickens 60
Hendi 40
Henebane 167
Henna 131
Henna el-Ghula 35
Henné 131
Heprose 154
Herb ivy 98
Herb Louisa 191
Herb Robert 92
Herb trinity 193
Herb-bennet 154
Herba buena des espagnols 67
Herbe à cochon 146
Herbe à dorer 35
Herbe à la fièvre 89
Herbe à la rate 35
Herbe à Robert 92
Herbe au centaure 89
Herbe aux chantre 73
Herbe aux cure-dents 175
Herbe aux piqûres 97
Herbe aux plaies 110
Herbe aux poux 150
Herbe aux puces 61, 104, 145
Herbe aux sorcières 164
Herbe aux tanneurs 70
Herbe aux verrues 83
Herbe aux vers 54
Herbe blanche 67
Herbe de coronille 123
Herbe de la trinité 193
Herbe de Saint Jean 97
Herbe de Saint-Benoit 154
Herbe de Saint-Guiliaume 153
Herbe de Saint-Laurent 104
Herbe du bermudes 94
Herbe du citron 104
Herbe sacrée 110, 191
Herbe terrible 92
Herbe vierge 104
Herniare 45
Hidouret er-ra'ai 45
Hièble 42
Hierba buena 67
Hiermi 25
Hillou 167
Hirri 130
Hobeiq es-sedr 110
Hodengal 193
Holy herb 191
Hommad 149
Homme pendu 138
Hommos 123
Hommos el-hamir 195
Horf 71
Horf el-babln 73
Horf el-maa 71
Horreiq 191
Horse mint 104
Horse tongue 35
Hortania safra 96
Houbbail 164
Hound's tongue 37
Hound's-berry 168
Hour aswad 158
Houx frêlon 155
Hozouggart 151
Hridj 153
Hulba 128
Hulwa mura 168
Hulwort 112
Hummad el-arnab 70
Hurfa 149
Iazir 110
Ibeqqoula 134
Ibiqis 37
Ibitt 96
Iblez 142
Ibororhen 35
Ibret el-'agouz 92
Ibret er-raheb 92
Ibsel idam 131
Icha 71
Ichammen 183
Ichkil 131
Ichkis 57
Ichoumane 183
Idergis 138
Idgel 142
Idj 145
Idjened 25
Idkhir 94
Idmine 153
Ifelfel 164
Ifilkou 32
Ifsi 57
Ifzi 104
Igdil 142
Igengen 142
Iggiz 101
Iggt 145
Igigiz 101
Iglim 162
Ignens 54
Iguengen 142
Ihader 40
Iherriqet 191
Ijujer 89
Ikfilen 131
Ikidou 119
Ikiker 123
Iklil 110
Iklil el-gabal 110

Iklil el-malek 126
Ikshir 64
Ilès ougendouz 37
Ilili 96
'Ilk el-kelkh 183
Imejjir 134
Imelzi 94
Imereksin 191
Imezri 191
Imidek 145
Imzi 187
Imzir 101
'Inab at-ta'leb 168
'Inab ed-dib 168
'Inab el-ta'leb 168
Indian corn 96
Indian fig 40
Indian hemp 40
Indian jujube 153
Indian senna 119
Ingri 130
Inguel 142
Init 172
Inouthoun 119
Inzzriki 167
Iourzèz 71
Iqq 145
Irgel 52
Irhkri 80
Iris commun 97
Iris des marais 97
Iris faux acore 97
Iris fétide 97
Iris germanique 97
Iris gigot 97
Iris jaune 97
Irisa 97
Irni 25
Irz 80
Isfil 131
Isgaren 140
Ishhouane 149
Islel 137
Islène 137
Islih 151
Issel 158
Issin 158
Italian alkanet 37
Italian arum 27
Italian poplar 158
Ivary 96
Ivette musquée 98
Ivraie 96
Ivraie vivace 94
Ivy 97
Izmine 153
Izri 57
Ja'ada 112
Jack by the hedge 70
Jacob's sword 97
Jeljlan 142
Jenah en-nesr 61
Jerusalem pine 142
Jonc 98
Jonc aigu 98
Jonc aromatique 94
Jonc du Nil 82
Jonc odorant 94
Jonc piquant 98
Judean wormwood 57
Jujube tree 153
Jujubes 153
Jujubier 153
Jujubier des totophages 151
Jujubier sauvage 151
Juniper tree 79
Juniper-gum tree 80
Jusquiame 167
Jusquiame blanche 167
Jusquiame d'Egypte 167
Jusquiame du désert 167
Jusquiame flaeslez 167
Kababa hindiya 142
Kababa sini 142
Kababa tchini 142
Kababah 142
Kabar 40
Kabar abiad 73
Kabats 162
Kabbar 40
Kabéoualen 75
Kabouia 75
Kaddab el-durra 96
Kaf maryam 193
Kaff as-sabu' 151
Kaff ed-dabb 151
Kaff ed-dubb 110
Kaff El-'Adra 70
Kaff el-hirr 151
Kaff el-thour 37
Kaff en-nesr 35
Kaff es-sabbagh 97
Kaff Lella Fatma 70
Kaff Maryam 70
Kafur 135
Kahila 37
Kahla 35, 92
Kakang 168
Kakenedj 168
Kalenba 27
Kamaash 70
Kammoun el-djmel 101
Kammoun helw 187
Kammun aswad 150
Kammun el-akhal 150
Kammun karmani 195
Kanouri 27
Kar'a leghrab 94
Karafs 180
Karawiet el-djmel 101
Karawiya 180
Karaz el-quds 168
Karm 134
Karm barri 82
Karma beida 73
Karma souda 82
Karmouz en-nsara 40
Karmus 134
Karsun 71
Karsun mai 71
Kasba 98
Kashir 64

Kashout 70
Kbidet ed-dobb 83
Kebbaba 142
Kef ed-dib 183
Keff el-djerana 151
Kelkh 183
Kelkha 183
Kemmoun 183
Kemmoun abiad 187
Kemmoun bou-tofa 175
Kemmoun el-ibel 175
Kemmoun habashi 175
Kemmoun lemsewuf 175
Kemmoun soufi 175
Kemshe 70
Kemshet En-Nebi 70
Kera'a ed-djaja 61
Kerafess 180
Kerbaboush 83
Kerdwy 187
Kerefs el-maa 180
Kerkas 71
Kerkhash 89
Kerma 134
Kermes oak 89
Kerroush el-qermez 86
Kershoud 70
Kershout 128
Kesbour 180
Keshbur 183
Keshrt 86
Kessaba 126
Kettan 131
Kezber es-sakhr 32
Kezmir 94
Khabour 126
Khadd el-bint 64
Khafour 94
Khalis-n-imidkh 151
Khallachem 32
Khamal 130
Khaman 42
Khaman kabir 42
Khaman saghir 42
Khamira 130
Khanouf 67
Kharad 137
Khardal 70, 73
Khardal abiad 73
Khardal aswad 70
Kharma 162
Kharnah 110
Kharnub 119
Kharrara 83
Kharroub 119
Kharroub el-khinzir 119
Kharroub el-maiz 119
Kharroub tourshane 119
Kharrouba 119
Kharrub 116
Kharshaf barri 61
Kharshuf 64
Khashkhash aswad 140
Khass 67
Khass ez-zeit 67
Khathiri 145
Khayat el-djurhat 110
Khebab 175
Khelal 175
Khell 175
Khelwan 42
Khelwan saghir 42
Khenfdj el-hadjera 71
Khenfej 71
Khenounat el-wsif 97
Khenounat En-Nebi 25
Kherwa' 86, 193
Kheshkhash 140
Kheshkhash aswad 97
Kheyyat el-jrah 110
Khieta 112
Khilaf 158
Khilla 175
Khilla baladi 175
Khilla sheitani 175
Khisoum 57
Khitmi 134
Khiytah 73
Khizana 155
Khobaiza 134
Khobbeiza 134
Khobbeiza reziza 134
Khobz el-fara'na 175
Khokh barri 110
Khorshef 61, 64
Khorshef en-nasara 64
Khortan 92
Khou helhal 101
Khoudab 175
Khozama 151
Khulingan 193
Khurkum 193
Khurm el-ibrah 71
Khushkhash manthur 140
Khussa hermes 86
Khuzama 101
Khweitmah 123
Kidney-vetch 119
Kif 40
Kikout 130
Kis er-ra'i 71
KIzzen 27
Kmisa 70
Knee holly 155
Knot-grass 146
Knot-weed 146
Knotted marjoram 109
Kohheila 101
Korink 52
Korna 153
Kouaba 75
Koubbar 27
Kourras 61
Koussoms 40
Kouzrkoum 97
Krafsa 180
Kreisha 45
Krenka 27
Kronbeiza 40
Kruku 97
Ksila 35
Kufayfah 70
Kummel 180
Kurkum 193

Kusbara 180
Kusfarat el-himar 89
Kushuth rumi 54
Kuzama zarqa 101
Kuzbarat el-bir 23
Laban el-hamir 32
Lablab kebir 27
Lac sumach 25
Ladan 46
Ladanier 46
Ladanum de crête 46
Ladanum-resin tree 46
Ladies' seal 82
Lady's fingers 119
Lagmez 86
Lahlah 130
Lahu 168
Lahw 168
Laichour 96
Laitue cultivée 67
Laitue d'huile 67
Laitue sauvage 67
Laitue scariole 67
Laitue vireuse 67
Lakor 119
Laktounia 86
Lalle 131
Lamedij 134
Lance du Christ 101
Land caltrops 195
Langue de boeuf 37
Langue de cerf 35
Langue de chien 37
Laqttine 75
Lareng 155
Large cuckoo-pint 27
Larisq 142
Lassaf 40
Lattilel 175
Laurel 116
Laurier 116
Laurier commun 116
Laurier d'Apollon 116
Laurier des poètes 116
Laurier franc 116
Laurier-rose 25
Laurier sauce 116
Lavande 101
Lavande officinale 101
Lavande stoechas 101
Lavande vraie 101
Lavender cotton 52, 67
Lawn-grass 94
Lead-wort 146
Lebalig 37
Lebbein 67
Lebena 68
Leblab 27
Lebsal 23
Lebsan el-khil 71
Leddad 57
Left azouggar 73
Lehbaliya 37
Lehshash 75
Lekhlakh 68
Lekshash 75
Lellousha 60
Lembetha 83
Lemkheinza 52
Lemmad 94
Lemmam 109
Lemon verbena 191
Lemon-balm 104
Lemsous 187
Lendj 154
Lenjbar 131
Lentisk 145
Lentisque 145
Leqq 25
Lerz 142
Lesan el'asfour 137
Lesan el-aiyel 35
Lesan el-kheil 35
Lesan et-teir 137
Lesser bindweed 68
Lesser dodder 70
Lesser galangal 193
Lezzaz 172
Lfernan 83
Lggt 145
Liazir 101
Libdan 70
Libsan 70
Libyan strawberry tree 82
Lierre 27
Lierre grimpant 27
Liez-ou-illeg 145
Lifsan 70
Lihha el-ghul 32
Lin 131
Lints 128
Liqamt 109
Liquorice plant 123
Liroun 151
Lirriaq 86
Lis bleu 97
Lis sauvage 97
Lisan ed-dib 37
Lisan el-hamal 35, 145, 146
Lisan el-kalb 37
Lisan el-qitt 35
Lisan el-thour 35, 37
Lisan hamad 146
Liseron de Provence 68
Liseron des champs 68
Liseron épineux 162
Liseron fausse-guimauve 68
Lishlish 68
Liverwort 153
Lmeshasha 146
Lobsol bouchen 131
Locust tree 123
Lofut 128
Lolium 96
Loof 25, 27
Lotus des anciens 151
Lotus jujube 151
Lotus tree 151
Louas 32
Loueg 68
Louiza 104
Loul 96
Lousewort 150
Louz el-berber 162

Louzga 68
Lowwaya 73
Lsan el-bergi 146
Lsan el-hamal 146
Lubanah maghrabi 83
Luf 79
Lufa 79
Lufa el-djin 167
Luf ga'd 27
Lufah 167
Luffa d'Egypte 79
Lupin 126
Lupin d'Egypte 126
Luwwaya 68
Lwiza 191
Lyciet 167
Lycope 101
Lycope des marais 101
Lyebzar 142
Lysimachie rouge 134
Lysimaque rouge 134
Ma'adnous 187
Ma'as 149
Maddad 68
Madder 155
Magnuna 52
Magraman 64
Mahareb 94
Maidenhair 23
Main de Fathma 70
Maîs 96
Maize 96
Makir 45
Male fern 32
Male polypody 32
Malfouf el-kelb 86
Malherbe 146
Mallow bindweed 68
Maltese mushroom 80
Maluh 45
Mamejjirt 134
Mandeliya 61
Mandragore 167
Mandrake 82
Mandrée en capitule 112
Maqdunis rumi 187
Maraget Musa 116
Maraq es-sedra 151
Mardaddoush 109
Mardaqoush 109
Marguerite 61
Marguerite des champs 61
Marhoum 73
Marijuana 40
Marjolaine 109
Majrolaine à coquille 109
Markh 27
Marmid 126
Marriout 104
Marriout el-kelb 104
Marrochemin 104
Marrube 104
Marrube aquatique 101
Marrube blanc 104
Marrube d'eau 101
Marrube noir 101
Marrube puant 101
Marsh crowfoot 151
Marsh mallow 134
Marsh parsley 180
Marshoush 80
Maryamyah 110
Masrur 80
Massas 23
Massasah 146
Massette 172
Massette à feuliile étroites 172
Massette des étangs 172
Mastic tree 145
Matak 123
Matricaire 61
Matricaire camomille 61
Mauve 134
Mauve sauvage 134
May-bush 153
Mazahr 155
Mazrour 80
Meadow saffron 130
Mechtehiya 73
Meddad 137, 142
Medeb 37
Medicinal squill 131
Medja el-abiad 134
Medjir 134
Meghnenou 168
Meharga 101
Mejennena 195
Mejennin 155
Mejjir 134
Melfouf el-kalb 46
Melifa 70
Meliles 151
Melilot 126
Mélisse 104
Mélisse officinale 104
Melliha 70
Melon 75
Menash ed-dibban 89
Menthe 109
Menthe douce 109
Menthe pouliot 104
Menthe sauvage 104
Menthe silvestre 104
Menthe verte 109
Mércuriale annuelle 86
Merraret el-sekhour 73
Merriwa 104
Mersag 61
Mersin 135
Mersit 64, 109
Mersita 109
Merwash 145
Merzizou 104
Merzizua 104
Mesaisa 146
Mesalem 67
Mesenzer mazir 146
Meshit 45
Mesiouka 67
Mesistrou 109
Meskeh 98
Meslah 162

Mesmoum 97
Mesran lehwar 68
Messekra 164
Messharwan 137
Messila 168
Mesuak 162
Methnan 172
Methnan akhdar 172
Metnan 172
Meule 134
Meurdjel 155
Mexican goose-foot 46
Mexican tea 46
Mezouqesh 112
Mezri 191
Mekhlet er-ra'i 71
Milk thistle 68
Millepertuis 97
Mioukou 96
Miseyka 98
Misk el-gin 112
Mizmar er-rai 23
Mkheinza 46
Mledor 164
Mlila 151
Mloul 109
Moddad 94
Moddeid 68, 137
Mofassa 110
Molène 162
Molene noire 162
Momordique 75
Monk's tree 193
Mordjan 42
Morelle furieuse 164
Morelle grimpante 168
Morelle noire 168
Morgan 168
Morgeline 45
Morrar 60, 68
Mort aux poules 167
Mother's heart 71
Mouchita 92
Mouker 45
Mountain germander 112
Mountain rue 158
Mourara 61
Mourkeba 86
Mouron blanc 45
Mouron des oiseau 45
Moursal 104
Mouse-thorn 60
Mousowrar 80
Moutarde blanche 73
Moutarde noire 70
Mrennebo 110
Mstoura 96
Mu-qnina 168
Mudar plant 27
Mufassiha 110
Mugwet 154
Muntinah 46
Muql makki 138
Muraya 68
Mûrier 135
Mûrier blanc 135
Murier des haies 154
Murrar 60
Murraret el-hanash 89
Muscadier 135
Mushraf 60
Musk melon 75
Musky bugle 98
Muslih al-andar 162
Myrte 135
Myrtle 135
Myrtle spurge 83
Myrtle-leaved sumach 70
Myrtle-leaved tanner's tree 70
Mzertrioud 42
Mzouchen 45
Na'ad 82
Na'ama 110
Na'na 52d
N'na' 109
Na'na' akhdar 109
Na'na' et-teroundj 104
Na'oudh 104
Nab el-djemel 150
Nab el-kelb 154
Nabca 153
Nabk tree 153
Nabq 151, 153
Nabta 175
Nadjir 94
Nadwa 70
Nafa 187
Nafal 126
Nagour 60
Nahari 109
Najem 94
Naked ladies 130
Nakhl 140
Nanoukha 175
Nar berd 150
Narcisse 25
Narcisse tazette 25
Nard 183
Nardjes 25
Narendj 155
Nargis 25
Nashash ed-dibban 89
Natash 123
Natna 46
Navet du diable 73
Ndjil 94
Nebat en-nar 191
Nedjem 94
Nedjil 94
Nefel 128
Nefir 164
Negil 94
Neiret 67
Nekhal 140
Nemdar 104, 109
Neshem 172
Nesri 154
Nettin 150
Ngeyi 27
Nigelle 150
Negil 94
Nile papyrus 82

Niriche 25
Nisrin 154
Noble épine 153
Nounkha 175
Nowar bellaremj 60
Nowar el-mdilla 151
Nowar zouawa 25
Nowara hindia 40
Nowaret el-karmouz 40
Noyer 98
Noyer commun 98
Nusay 94
Nut-grass 82
Nutmeg 135
Oak of Cappadocia 52
Oats 92
Odessir 57
Oeil de bouc 54
Oeil de perdrix 150
Oftazzen 73
Oignon 23
Oignon marin 131
Oil lettuce 67
'Okna 130
Old woman 54
Oleander 25
Oleandre 25
Olive tree 137
Olivier 137
Olivier sauvage 137
Onion 23
'Onsal 130
'Onseil 130
'Onsel 130
'Onsol 130
'Onsul 130
'Onsul bahari 131
Ophrys homme 138
Opium poppy 140
Oqhowan 61
Orairyia 52
Orangier amer 155
Orangier de sévile 155
Orcanette 35
Origan 110
Origan du Maroc 109
Orizia 168
Orme 172
Orme campêtre 172
Orme pyramidale 172
Ornoba 149
'Oronfel 25
'Oroug sabbaghin 155
Ortie 191
Ortie bâtarde 86
Ortie brulante 191
Ortie grieche 191
Ortie romaine 191
Ortie rude 191
Orvale 110
Oseille d'Amérique 149
Oseille sauvage 149
'Oshar 27
Osier blanc 158
Ossis 167
Ouabejjir 134
Ouailoulou 40
Oualbarda 92
Ouari 151
Ouazouri 142
Ouberka 42
'Oud al-'anbar 97
'Oud el-'attas 52
'Oud el-kheir 151
'Oud el-maa 158
'Oud en-nuwwar 137
Ouden el-'anz 23
Ouden el-arnab 37
Ouden el-fil 25, 27
Ouden el-hallouf 151
Ouden el-homar 162
Ouden esh-shah 37
'Oud es-salib 138
Ouerga 60
Oufadia 75
Oufni 119
Ouheireche 191
Ouisd 158
Oulmou 172
Oumana 75
Ouowi 75
Ouqil boulrhoun 150
Ourdj 153
'Ourouq homor 155
Ourzima 45
Ousmiche 35
Ouzag 60
Ouzbir 110
Oxycèdre 79
Oyok 52
Ozomaine 191
Paille de la mecque 94
Palma Christi 86
Palmier doum 138
Palmier-dattier 140
Panias 183
Panicant 183
Panicaut 183
Pansayh 193
Pansy 193
Pantine 138
Paper reed 82
Papier du Nil 82
Papyrus 82
Pariètaire d'Espagne 54
Parsley 187
Parsnip 183
Pasquier 128
Passe-pierre 183
Passerage cultivée 71
Passerine 172
Pastende 183
Pavot 140
Pavot des moissons 140
Pellitory 54
Pellitory of Spain 54
Pennyroyal 104
Pensée 193
Perce pierre 183
Père de la santé 187
Perfoliate St. John's wort 97
Persil 187
Persil cultivé 187
Peter's cress 183

Petit chêne 112
Petit chiendent 94
Petit cyprès 67
Petit houx 155
Petit liseron 68
Petit muguet 154
Petit poivre 193
Petit sureau 42
Petite centaurée 89
Petit cuscute 70
Petite ortie 191
Pétron 79
Peuplier franc 158
Peuplier noir 158
Peuplier suisse 158
Pheasant's eye 150
Phoenician juniper 79
Pick-needle 92
Pick-tooth 175
Pied de loup 101
Pigeon's grass 191
Piment 164
Piment cultivé 164
Piment d'oiseau 164
Piment de cayenne 164
Piment des jardins 164
Piment enragé 164
Pin blanc 142
Pin d'Alep 142
Pin de Jérusalem 142
Pin-grass 92
Pipperidge 35
Pistachier de l'Atlas 145
Pivoine 138
Plantain 146
Plantain corne de cerf 146
Plantain d'eau 23
Plantain des oiseaux 146
Plantain majeur 146
Plante au beurre 73
Plombagine 146
Pois chiche 123
Poison-hemlock 180
Poivre 142
Poivre à queue 142
Poivre cubèbe 142
Poivre d'Inde 164
Poivre de Guinée 164
Poivre noir 142
Poivrier commun 142
Poivrier long 164
Poivron 164
Polium 112
Polygale de Syrie 45
Polypode 149
Polypode de chêne 149
Polypody wall fern 149
Polystic fougère mâle 32
Polytric des officines 32
Pomegranate 149
Pomme de prairie 126
Pomme de sauge 110
Pomme de sodome 27
Polle du diable 164
Pomme épineuse 164
Ponceau 140
Poppy 140
Porcelet 167
Pot marigold 60
Potentille rampante 154
Potiron 75
Pouliot 104
Pouliot de montagne 112
Pourcellaine 149
Pourpie potager 149
Pourpier 149
Pourpier de mer 46
Prickly artichoke 61
Prickly cedar 79
Prickly ivy 162
Prickly lettuce 67
Prickly pear 40
Psoralier 126
Psyllium 145
Pucière 145
Pudding grass 104
Pumpkin 75
Purple crocus 130
Purple loosestrife 134
Purple viper's-bugloss 37
Purslane 149
Pyrèthre 54
Pyrèthre d'Afrique 54
Pyrèthre salivaire 54
Qalb el-djadj 183
Qallab 94
Qamis bent-el-malek 150
Qantarioun 89
Qantarioun saghir 89
Qar'a 75
Qar'a aslawiya 75
Qar'a dubb'a 75
Qar'a duruf 75
Qar'a hamra 75
Qar'a maghrabi 75
Qar'a rumi 75
Qar'a tawil 75
Qarad 116
Qarqahan 60
Qasab el-bardi 82
Qasba 96
Qased 151
Qasuris 97
Qatab 64
Qataf 45
Qataf bahari 45
Qatel el-kelb 130
Qattayah 126
Qawleh 96
Qawoun 75
Qawqhan 60
Qaysoum 52
Qaysun 52
Qaysun 67
Qazzah 187
Qbala 96
Qebaboush 140
Qebad 70
Qehaniya 46
Qelilou 89
Qelouta 123
Qennarya 64

Qenneb 40
Qer'aa 75
Qer'aa beida 75
Qer'aa el-leben 75
Qer'aa gardousi 75
Qer'aa medwen 75
Qerfa 71
Qeriou'aa 73
Qersa'na 183
Qesas el-lesan 27
Qesbir el-bir 32
Qessous 27
Qezaza 45
Qinawa 175
Qistus 46
Qittaa barri 75
Qittat en-na'am 73
Qoddab 146
Qorissa 149
Qoronfel 137
Qoronfel abiad 137
Qorreis 191
Qors begra 123
Qort 52, 126
Qotaiba 89
Qozzah 187
Qrei'a 75
Qseiba 175
Qtout 45
Qttania 96
Quatre épice 150
Quereillet 101
Quintefeuille 154
Quitch grass 94
Quittaa el-hemar 75
Qurras 60, 61
Qurrat el-'ayn 71
Qushet el-hayya 89
Qwaleh 96
Rabal 67
Rabd 67
Raboul 67
Racine de chiendent 94
Racine giroflée 154
Racine vierge 82
Radis cultivé 73
Radjoudjte 98
Rag gourd 79
Rafia 94
Rajraf 23
Ramberge 86
Ramram 45
Rand 116
Raqma 134
Raqmiya 134
Rashad 71, 149
Ratam 126
Rattle-box 123
Rawq 71
Ray-grass 94
Rayhan 109
Rahyan dawoud 109
Rebba 112
Rebruba 61
Rechig 96
Red darnel 94
Red pepper 164
Red sand-wort 45
Reda'a 83
Redjel el-wa'al 123
Redoul 70
Redoul commun 70
Redradj 155
Reed-mace 172
Réglisse 123
Réglisse glabre 123
Réglisse officinale 123
Regma 92
Reine des bois 154
Reiniche 25
Rejeguenu 60
Rejla 149
Remth 46
Rennet 168
Renoncule 151
Renoncule scélérate 151
Renouée des oiseaux 146
Renouée maritime 146
Reqraq 126
Requemaya 92
Reshad 71
Retem 126
Retem behan 126
Réveille-matin 83
Rezaima 61
Rhanni 131
Ribba 119
Ribyan 54, 61
Ricin 86
Rigl el-ghorab 175
Rigl el-hamam 35, 191
Rigla 149
Rihan 135
Rihanet el-maa 131
Rjel el-ghorab 146
Rjel leghrab 94
Roast-beef plant 97
Robita 61
Rock samphire 183
Rocket 71
Roghata 45
Rokheima 45
Roman chamomile 60
Roman laurel 116
Roman nettle 191
Roman pellitory 54
Romarin 110
Romman 149
Ronce 154
Roquette 71
Roquette épineuse 73
Roquette vraie 71
Rose de Damas 154
Rose de jéricho 70
Rose de quatre saisons 154
Rose of jericho 70
Rose sauvage 154
Roseau 96, 172
Roseau balais 96
Roseau commun 96
Roseau de maris 96
Rosemary 110

Rosier des chiens 154
Rosier sauvage 154
Rosin weed 70
Rotrayt 195
Roubia 104
Rough bindweed 162
Rouida 70
Rouk 32
Rouka 71
Roum 96
Rourawa 42
Rue 158
Rue d'Alep 158
Rue des montagnes 158
Rue des murailles 32
Rue sauvage 158, 195
Rummadah 83
Rush broom 126
Rush-nut 80
Rusty-back 32
Ruta 158
Rutsa 158
Rye-grass 94, 96
Sa'ad 82
Sa'ad el-homar 82
Sa'ada 83
Sa'adan 195
Sa'aet el-naqa 64
Sa'ed 79
Saal 82
Sabad 67
Sabat 96
Sabine a gros fruit 80
Sabine thurifère 80
Sabir suqutri 128
Sabline rouge 45
Saboun el-'arais 37
Sabounia 23
Sabun el-'aris 131
Sadhab 158
Sadhab el-barr 158
Dadhab el-djebeli 158
Safar 96
Saffron 97
Safira 104
Safirous 75
Safran 97
Safran batard 130
Safran cultivé 97
Safran d'automne 130
Safran des prés 130
Safran vrai 97
Safsaf 158
Safsaf abiad 158
Safsag 64
Sagadon 75
Sage apple 110
Sahbakou 42
Sahtor 35
Sain-bois 172
Sainfoin agul 119
Saint-bois 172
Sakaran 167
Salad mustard 73
Salicaire 134
Salicaire commune 134
Salima 110
Salma 110
Salmiah 46
Salmiya 110
Salsepareille 162
Salsepareille indigène 162
Salsepareille d'Italie 162
Sam el-far 131
Samar 98
Samar baladi 98
Samar murr 98
Samma 96
Sammah 94
Sammarah 73
Samphire 183
Samseyk 98
Sanawbar 142
Sand spurrey 45
Sandarach tree 80
Sandarus 80
Sanguinaire 45
Sanina 80
Sanoubar 142
Sanoudj 150
Sant 116
Santé du corps 71
Santoline 52, 67
Santoline blanche 67
Sanug 175
Saponaire 45
Saq el-akhal 23
Sarah 42
Saraqtoun 101
Sarghine 42
Sarha 42
Sarkh 42
Sarkhas 32
Sarkhas el-ballut 32
Sarsor 64
Sarw 79
Sarw gabali 79
Satarag 89
Sauge 110
Sauge écarlate 110
Sauge officinale 110
Sauge sclarée 110
Saule blanc 158
Sawsan asfar 97
Sawsan azraq 97
Sayal 116
Sbott 96
Scale fern 32
Scaly spleenwort 32
Scarlet oak 89.
Scarlet synomorium 80
Sceau de Notre Dame 82
Scenanth 94
Scented trefoil 126
Schoenanthe 94
Schoenanthe officinal 94
Scille 131
Scille maritime 131
Sclarée 110
Scolopendre 35
Scurfy pea 126
Scutch-grass 94

Se'd 82
Sea ambrosia 52
Sea bugloss 37
Sea cud-weed 67
Sea fennel 183
Sea onion 131
Sea purslane 46
Sea rush 98
Seaorache 46
Sebbarh 172
Sebbit 96
Sebenq 150
Sebet 94
Sebhora 25
Seboulet el-far 94
Sedira 35
Sedjra tenshama 37
Sedra 151
Seif el-ghorab 67
Seif el-maa 23, 146
Sekigigeren 168
Sekkin ed-dib 97
Sekkoum 130
Sekoura 154
Sekran 61, 168
Selarwa 119
Selattet el-bahr 183
Selikh 23
Sell 137
Sella 137
Sellaha 32
Sellata 180
Sellbou 98
Sellouf 32
Selmia 110
Semm el-far 164, 168
Semm el-firakh 168
Semmana 73
Semouma 23
Senbouqa 42
Séné 119
Séné bâtard 123
Séné d'Alep 119
Séné de Syrie 119
Séné du Sénégal 119
Séné du Soudan 119
Séné sauvage 92
Sénegrain 128
Senelles 153
Senesaq 155
Sénevé blanc 73
Sénevé noir 70
Senna 119
Senna barri 123
Senna beldi 92
Senna ghanami 119
Senna haram 119
Senna hindi 119
Senna mekki 119
Senna sa'eidi 119
Sennairya 175
Senné 119
Senoụber 142
Serghina 42
Serient 42
Seris 61
Serr 130
Serwal 79
Sésame 142
Sésame de l'Inde 142
Setwall 193
Seurti 40
Seville orange 155
Seyal 116
Sga'a 37
Sha'al 57
Sha'ar el-'agouz 191
Sha'ar el-ard 23
Sha'ar el-dra 96
Sha'ar el-ghul 23, 32
Sha'ar el-khanzir 23
Sha'ret et-trab 94
Shabat el-gabal 187
Shabrom 73
Shadjret mariam 54
Shagar el-mastika 145
Shagaret ed-damm 35
Shagaret el-ghazal 155
Shagaret el-hayat 79, 80
Shagaret el-muql 138
Shagaret er-rih 155
Shagaret es-sous 123
Shagaret Mariam 54
Shagaret wahhsh 52
Shagret Mriam 70
Shahtarag 89
Shahtredj 89
Shajaret et-talq 70
Shakuta 70
Shalem 40
Shalmun 135
Shamar 175, 187
Shamar bahariya 183
Shammam 75
Shamshad 37
Shandgoura 98
Shandjar 35
Shaqaqil 183
Shaqwas 46
Sharam 110
Shareka 52
Sharir 104
Sharma 168
Sharp cedar 79
Sharp grass 94
Sharp rush 98
Shatra 112
Shatreg 89
Shawashi el-dura 96
Shawk ed-dab'a 23
Shawk ed-dabb 23
Shawk ed-deeb 46
Shawk ed-dib 23
Shawk el-'elk 57
Shawk el-himir 61
Shawka yahoudiya 183
Shawka zarga 183
Shawkaran 180
Shawla beyda 86
Shay gabali 110
Shay gebeli 67
Shaybet el-ajouz 54
Shaylam 96
Shbarto 68

Shebet 175
Shebrog 130
Shedjeret el-aden 46
Shedjret el-janna 164
Shedjret el-jemel 164
Sheikh el-boukoul 35
Sheikh el-rabi 68
Shelgha 92
Shemouga 86
Shemsia 64
Shenaf 71
Shendgura 112
Shendjar 35
Shepherd's purse 71
Sherifa 45
Shge'a 128
Shge'at el-arneb 128
Shiba 54, 67
Shibit 175
Shibreq 68
Shibrim 68
Shih 57
Shihan 57
Shikaw 64
Shikouria 61
Shiltam 71
Shini 67
Shiria 61
Shirsh 126
Shitaradj 146
Shittah tree 119
Shittim wood 119
Shizi 79
Shlayk 153
Shmary 82
Shobroq 68
Shoka masrya 116
Shoka qibttya 116
Shoubbetan 150
Shoubroq 73
Shouk 130
Shouk boulti 68
Shouk el-abiod 183
Shouk el-diman 68
Shouk el-gamal 64
Shouk el-gemal 68
Shouk el-ghazal 96
Shouk el-gimal 119
Shouk el-yahoudi 23
Shouk en-nasara 68
Shouk sinnari 68
Shoukail 175
Shouket el-beida 68
Shtiwal 149
Shufan 92
Shuqaf 23
Shurrabet el-dura 96
Shurrabet er-ra'i 155
Shurud 32
Shush 96
Shwika yahoudiya 183
Shwikhia 61
Shwilia 61
Shwwiket Ibrahim 183
Sianama 46
Siba 54
Sidr 151, 153
Sidr barri 151
Sif ed-dib 97
Sif el-dib 97
Sifsfa 110
Sigarsou 162
Sikra 96
Sikran 164, 180
Silla 73, 94, 130
Silt 94
Simreeb 45
Simsim 142
Sindiyan el-ard 101
Sirr 73
Sisana 97
Sise 73
Sitt Khadigah 126
Siwak 162
Siyaf 97
Skengbir 193
Skoura 154
Small bulrush 172
Small nettle 191
Smallage 180
Smilax rude 162
Smooth thapsia 187
Snake bryony 73
Snei'ah 25
Snouber 142
Soapberry bush 35
Sobbaira 40
Sobhane khallaku 155
Socotra aloe 128
Soqqait 80
Soqqait barari 80
Sorr 64
Sorrel 149
Soubeirette 153
Soubou 138
Souchet à papier 82
Souchet comestible 80
Souchet rond 82
Souci 60
Souci des jardins 60
Souci officinal 60
Soufrat el-molouk 150
Sour orange 155
Sourendjan 130
Sous 123
Sowai 130
Sowak 98
Sowak En-Nebi 110
Spanish broom 126
Spanish chamomile 54
Spanish pellitory 54
Spartier genêt 126
Spearmint 109
Spider flower 52
Spindle wort 57
Spur pepper 164
Spurge flax 172
Squill 131
Squirting cucumber 75
St. John's-bread 123
St. Mary's flower 70
St. Mary's thistle 68

Staphysaigre 150
Star of the earth 146
Star thistle 60
Stavesacre 150
Stellaire 45
Stinking goose-foot 46
Stinking iris 97
Stinking wood 119
Stoechas 101
Stramoine 164
Succory 61
Sudaniya 164
Sulion 42
Sumac vernis 25
Summer adonis 150
Summer pheasant's eye 150
Sun spurge 83
Sunflower 64
Sureau 42
Sureau commun 42
Sureau hièble 42
Sureau noir 96
Suwal 96
Suweid 64
Swak En-Nebi 175
Swak er-ra-ian 146
Swallow-tailed willow 158
Sweet alison 71
Sweet basil 109
Sweet cumin 187
Sweet grass 154
Sweet marjoram 109
Sweet violet 193
Sweet virgin's-bower 150
Sweet woodruff 154
Sweet-bay 116
Sylphium 187
Syrian rue 158, 195
Taaferd 154
Taba 167
Tabac 167
Tabac du Brézil 167
Tabac rustique 167
Tabakat 151
Takakath 153
Tabel 180
Tabellaout 175
Tabellout igilef 89
Tabenenna 167
Tabera 167
Tabga 154, 167
Taboraq 35
Tabounekkart 57
Tabouret 71
Tabourzigt 164
Taboushisht 137
Tabrakat 172
Tabuda 172
Taburzigt 131
Tachkal 32
Tadist 145
Tadjdjart 116
Tadjellet 73
Tadjibout 140
Tadjilban 128
Tadjira 140
Tadjnouft 195
Tadoumkheit 25
Tadrisa 195
Tafeqeloujla 75
Taferzizt 73
Taffa 71
Tafinaout 140
Tafiyyasht 162
Tafouri 83
Tafrha 154
Tafrira 23
Tafrita 149
Tafrut 97
Taga 64, 79
Tagamait 94
Taganasu 67
Tagart 42
Tagasiba 96
Tagga 79
Taggult 183
Tagha 61
Tagouft 57
Tagoug 57
Tagruft 195
Taguerourt 134
Tahammak 25
Taharadjt 35
Taheli 172
Tahindest 104
Tahouet 46
Tahsoult 60
Tai el-'areb 45
Taicest 94
Taida 142
Tailoula 73
Tailoulout 40
Tairart 67
Taka 79
Takaout 172
Takert 86
Takhsaît 75
Takka 80
Takkilt 61
Takout 86
Talah 92
Talakh 119
Taleggit 98
Talewort 37
Talezzast amellal 158
Talh 116
Tall adonis 150
Tall rest-harrow 126
Taloubat 140
Talout 96
Talsatt 45
Tamarin 128
Tamarind tree 128
Tamarix à galle 172
Tamarnier 128
Tamart 32
Tamat 116
Tamazate 134
Tamazout 52
Tamechttibt 52
Tamehit 134
Tament 37
Tamenunnait 167
Tamenzirt 92

Tamerbout 79
Tamessaout 187
Tamezlagelt 195
Tamiah 45
Tamier 82
Taminier 82
Tamk 175
Tamkelt 70
Tammam 96
Tamoshalet 137
Tamr 140
Tamr hindi 128
Tanaglet 134
Tanahot 86
Tanahout 83
Tanakfail 71
Tanar'ant 86
Tanater 67
Tanekht 140
Tanesfalt 68, 162
Tannoun 52
Taoualt 80
Taoucatt 45
Taoulouaza 183
Taoulzit 61
Taoumiah 45
Taourza 25
Tara 82
Tara bouchehen 73
Taratir el-dura 96
Tarbush el-ghorab 68
Tardiut 61
Tare 128
Tareda 126
Tarhi 96
Tarihant 135
Tariouba 154, 155
Tarka Ir'en 79
Tarmiga 45
Tarmint 149
Taroubent 155
Taroubia 155
Taroumant 149
Tarout 80
Tarrhsimte 75
Tartaqah 83
Tartous 80
Tartout 80
Tartout el-beni-edem 80
Tartut 138
Tartut el-kelb 138
Taryala 167
Taselbou 82
Taselgha 92
Tasemmumt 149
Taset 116
Tasetta Meriem 54
Tashtiwan 149
Taskarat 64
Taskrunt 92
Taslent 137
Tasmas 23
Tassergint 42
Tassouflal 27
Tastiwan 149
Tataoura 68
Tatil 42
Tatoutet 135
Tatura 164
Tawalment 146
Taybult 40
Taynanast 150
Tayniyut 140
Tazait 138
Tazbboujt 137
Tazdait 140
Tazenzena 80
Tazert 134
Tazgemmut 162
Tazgouart 35
Taziout 130
Tazmait 98
Tazouggert 151
Tazoura 151
Tazout 80
Tazzawt 130
Tazzourt 110
Tebbaq 64
Tebs 175
Tecemlall 145
Techeredjili 57
Tefchoune 151
Tefel el-djouza 146
Teffah 110
Tefi 116
Tefrat el-kheil 60
Tefshoun 151
Tegtag 126
Teif ed-dib 25
Teisset 35
Teka 79
Telbaout 151
Telfa-giddaoun 138
Telh lebiad 116
Telit 126
Tellak 83
Tellakh 32
Tellemt izimer 151
Telmoumi 73
Temahaq 116
Temarsa 104
Temzelit 138
Teqmezoutin 112
Teqout 130
Terbuna 73
Tereri 42
Terfaq 153
Terhala 64
Termes 123
Terrehla 64
Terroumt 168
Tertag 126
Tertakh 126
Terzous 80
Tesker 164
Teskera 64
Tezzount 191
Thala 119
Thalilen 175
Thapsia 187
Thapsie 187
Thaqib el-hajar 149

Thatimt 137
Thé arabe 45
Thé de France 104
Thé de Grèce 110
Thé du Mexique 46
Therilal 175
Thil 94
Thirsty thorn 119
Thorfel 71
Thorn tree 35
Thorn-apple 164
Thoum 23
Three-lobed sage 110
Thuia à la sandaraque 80
Thuia articulé 80
Thulthulan 168
Thuya 80
Thym 112
Thym de Crète 112
Thym des steppes 57
Tibb 134
Tiberrimt 94
Tibinsert 134
Tibisrennit 134
Tibn Makkah 94
Tibsal 23
Tichmougin 52
Tiddi 79
Tidekst 145
Tidekt 145
Tidilla 164
Tidjat 162
Tidmamai 68
Tieredjeli 57
Tif es-sabounya 45
Tifersit 73
Tifert 40, 131
Tifest 40
Tifidas 128
Tifizza 80
Tifrhout 64
Tifroua 57
Tigenthast 52
Tigigesht 45
Tiglish 130
Tigourma 154
Tihendit 40
Tijujar 89
Tikammin 150
Tikelmout 27
Tikheloulin En-Nebi 25
Tikherroubt 123
Tikida 119
Tikidat 119
Tikiout 86
Tikiut 83
Tikoukt 89
Tilfaf 61
Tilidout 140
Tililsen 57
Timaiart 82
Timegsin 71
Timeriout 104
Timermenna 42
Timersat 104, 109
Timersidi 109
Timersitine 109
Timerzat 101
Timerzouga 61
Timeskine 71
Timetfest 67
Timezrit 191
Timgelest 195
Timijja 109, 110
Timizagt 61
Timmuma 167
Timtshish 112
Timzi 191
Timzourin 112
Tin shawki 40
Tine 134
Tinjara 61
Tinnevelly senna plant 119
Tiougda 25
Tiouinet 89
Tiouli 96
Tiourmi 168
Tiqqi 79
Tir'ad guisri 89
Tiranimine 96
Tiranrat 80
Tirarar 80
Tirhounam 35
Tiriresht 45
Tirki 79
Tisermt ouakal 92
Tisernas 92
Tiskert 23
Tisliwha 119
Tissendjelt 96
Tisseraw 162
Tissert 23
Tit-n-tacekourt 150
Titarek 27
Tiyni 140
Tizizoua 37
Tizizwit 104
Tizmit 94
Tiznint 162
Tlirin 67
Tobbana 68
Toffa 73
Tohar 46
Tongue-grass 71
Tooth pick 175
Tooth-brush tree 162
Toothwort 146
Torcha 27
Torchon 79
Tortelle 73
Touchanina 168
Touchanine 86
Toudari 73
Toufalt 183, 187
Touffelt 162
Toufi 138
Toulloult 96
Toum 23
Toundoub 40
Toungane 94
Tournesol 64
Touroudjan 104

Tourwagat 42
Tourza 27
Toushna 112
Tousslat 60
Tout 135
Tout abyad 135
Tout el-ard 153
Tout el-harir 135
Tout el-khela 154
Tout el-qa'a 153
Tout en-nasara 153
Tout helw 135
Touta 135
Toute bonne 110
Toute épice 150
Touzala 110
Touzimt 150
Touzla guizgaren 60
Touzzal 110
Touzzala 46
Touzzalt 46
Touzzelt 137
Tra'a 96
Trainasse 146
Tree wormwood 54
Trèfle des sables 119
Trèfle jaune des sables 119
Trèfle musqué 126
Tribule terrestre 195
Triolet jaune 119
Troumoucht 40
Tsaboun ghett 83
Tsailaloul 40
Tsalal el-antar 162
Tsalina 61
Tseffa 71
Tselgoust 126
Tsil 94
Tsminoun 82
Tosouik 98
Ttmer 140
Tubbaq 64
Tudharig 73
Tue chien 130
Tuffah el-muzzah 153
Tuftolba 98
Tugga 35
Turbad 92
Turbith 92
Turbith blanc 92
Turfas 138
Turkey wheat 96
Turkia 96
Tuzelt 52
Twitch grass 94
Tzetta 137
Tzndjan 104
Ubruzi 75
'Ud er-rihh 35
Ugin 172
Uhri 94
'Ulleiq 68
'Ulliq 162
Umm aliya 46, 52
Umm djeladjel 52
Umm ed-driga 175
Umm el-laban 32
Umm el-lbina 83
Umm ghfara 96
Umm kalb 119
Umm re-roubia 104
Umm rekba 96
Umm rwis 145
'Unnab 153
'Unnab barri 155
'Uqdah 35
'Uqruban 35
'Ushba 162
'Ushba maghrabiya 162
'Ushba rumiya 162
Uzeina 146
Vaccaire 45
Vegetable sponge 79
Velar 73
Velar officinal 73
Venus's hair 23
Vernix 80
Vervain 191
Verveine 191
Verveine citronelle 191
Verveine odorante 191
Verveine officinale 191
Vesce 128
Vigne de judée 168
Vigne noir 82
Vinettier 35
Violet 193
Violette 193
Violette odorante 193
Vipérine 37
Vrillée 68
Vulnéraire 119
Vulvaire 46
Wahhsh 52
Wairurud 42
Walnut 98
Ward 154
Wrd barri 154
Ward djouri 154
Ward el-homar 25
Ward es-sini 154
Ward es-siyag 154
Ward ez-zawan 134, 138
Ward ez-zeroub 154
Warraq saboun 146
Wartwort 83
Water celery 151
Water cress 71
Water grass 71, 83
Water hemp agrimony 64
Water horehound 101
Water plantain 23
Waybread 146
Weden el-djedd 146
Weld 151
Werd 46
West African black pepper 142
White acacia 116
White chameleon 57
White henbane 167
White mallow 134
White mulberry 135

White mustard 73
White thorn 153
White wild vine 73
White willow 158
Whorled mint 109
Wideina 146
Wild carrot 183
Wild celery 180
Wild chamomile 61
Wild chicory 61
Wild jujube 151
Wild lettuce 67
Wild mint 104
Wild olive 137
Wild rue 158
Wild tea 67
Wild tobacco 167
Willow weed 134
Winter cherry 168
Wire-grass 94
Wood avens 154
Woody nightshade 168
Wormseed 46
Wormwood 54, 57
Wound-wort 112, 119
Xyris puant 97
Yabruh 167
Yansum 187
Yaqtin 75
Yasmin el-khela 168
Yedd Fatma 70
Yellow iris 97
Yellow water flag 97
Yellow weed 151
Za'atar 112
Za'atar barri 112
Za'atar el-hmir 112
Za'atar el-mediya 112
Za'atar farsi 112
Za'ater 109, 110
Za'atar hindi 109
Za'faran 97
Za'rour 25
Za'rur al-awdiyah 153
Zabak 94
Zachum oil tree 35
Zafrin 151
Zafwa 168
Zaghalanta 151
Zaghlil 140, 150, 151
Zaita 146
Zakouk 187
Zalim 23
Zamechttibt 52
Zanbag azraq 97
Zandjir 86
Zaqqoum 35
Zaqqum 83
Zarqottouna 145
Zaytun 137
Zaz 68
Zbib barri 150
Zbib el-jbel 150
Zbib el-laidour 164
Ze'itra 112
Zebboudj 137
Zebbour 137
Zedoaire 193
Zedoary 193
Zefzouf 153
Zeggoum 84
Zegzeg 153
Zeita 32
Zekmuna 162
Zeku 23
Zekza 101
Zellechem 32
Zenina 119
Zenjabil 193
Zent 158
Zeqresh 162
Zerara 150
Zerga 92
Zeri 57
Zerreiga 92
Zerzira 60, 71
Zezzeri 57
Zfeizef 153
Zfenari el-ma'iz 175
Zgallem 138
Zglem 138
Zgougou 142
Ziata 180
Zibl el-far 61, 67
Zibl el-ma'iz 82
Zilla 73
Zimeba 79
Zimzellil 138
Zingar 193
Zirr el-ward 154
Ziwan 92
Zizanie 96
Zob ed-dib 138
Zob el qa'a 138
Zob el-ard 138
Zob en-nasrani 138
Zob er-roumi 138
Zobb el-ard 80
Zobb el-ghaba 80
Zobb el-qa'a 80
Zobb el-tourki 80
Zobeida 60
Zorbeih 46
Zouhmouk 70
Zouzzalt 46
Zoweitna 92
Zreiga 183
Zriga 92
Zughaf 23
Zummeir 92
Zu'rur 153
Zuwan 94, 96
Zzit 137

INDEX TO SPECIES

Page numbers in boldface denote illustrations.

Acacia albida 116
Acacia arabica var. *nilotica* 199
Acacia nilotica **115**, 116, 199
Acacia raddiana 116, **117**, 199
Acacia seyal 116
Acacia tortilis subsp. *raddiana* 199
Acanthus mollis 23
Aceras anthropophorum 138
Achillea fragrantissima **49**, 52
Achillea santolina **50**, 52
Adiantum capillus-veneris **22**, 23
Adonis aestivalis 150
Adonis annua 150, 200
Adonis autumnalis 200
Ageratum conyzoides 52
Agrimonia eupatoria 152
Agropyron repens 199
Ajuga iva 98, **99**
Alhagi graecorum **118**, 119, 199
Alhagi mannifera 199
Alhagi maurorum 199
Alisma plantago-aquatica 23
Alkanna tinctoria **34**, 35
Alliaria officinalis 198
Alliaria petiolata 70, 198
Allium cepa 23
Allium sativum 23
Aloe perryi 128
Aloysia citriodora 200
Aloysia triphylla 191, 200
Alpinia officinarum 193
Althaea officinalis 134
Alyssum maritimum 199
Ambrosia maritima **51**, 52, 94
Ammi majus 175
Ammi visnaga **173**, 175
Ammodaucus leucotrichus 175
Ammoides pusilla **174**, 175, 200
Ammoides verticillata 200
Anacyclus pyrethrum 52
Anagyris foetida 119
Anastatica hierochuntica **69**, 70
Anchusa azurea 35, 198
Anchusa italica 198
Androcymbium gramineum 128, 199
Androcymbium punctatum 199
Andropogon laniger 199
Andropogon schoenanthus 199
Anethum graveolens 175, **176**
Anthemis nobilis 198
Anthemis pseudocotula **53**, 54
Anthyllis vulneraria 119
Apium graveolens 175, **177**
Arbutus pavari 82
Argania spinosa **160**, 162
Arisarum vulgare **24**, 25
Aristida pungens 199
Artemisia absinthium 54, 57
Artemisia arborescens 54
Artemisia atlantica 57
Artemisia campestris 57
Artemisia herba-alba **55**, 57, 198
Artemisia inculta 198
Artemisia judaica **56**, 57
Artemisia judaica subsp. *sahariensis* 57
Arum italicum 27
Asparagus horridus 199
Asparagus stipularis **129**, 130, 199
Asperula odorata 200
Asphodelus aestivus 130, 199
Asphodelus microcarpus 199
Asplenium adiantum-nigrum 32
Asplenium scolopendrium 198
Asplenium trichomanes 32
Atraclylis gummifera 57
Atriplex halimus 45
Atropa bella-donna 162
Avena sativa 92
Balanites aegyptiaca **33**, 35
Ballota nigra 101
Berberis hispanica 35
Betonica officinalis 199
Blepharis ciliaris 23, 198
Blepharis edulis 198
Boerhavia repens 137, 200
Borago officinalis **36**, 37
Brassica nigra 70, 199
Brocchia cinerea 198
Bryonia dioica 73
Buxus sempervirens 37
Calendula officinalis 60
Callitris articulata 199
Callitris quadrivalvis 199
Calotropis procera **26**, 27
Cannabis sativa 40
Capparis decidua **38**, 40, 198
Capparis sodada 198
Capparis spinosa **39**, 40, 198
Capparis spinosa var. *aegyptia* 198
Capparis spinosa var. *rupestris* 198
Capsella bursa-pastoris 71
Capsicum annuum 164
Capsicum frutescens 164
Carum ammoides 200
Carum carvi 155, **178**, 180
Caryophyllus aromaticus 200
Cassia acutifolia 199
Cassia angustifolia 199
Cassia aschrek 199
Cassia italica 119, **120**, 199
Cassia obovata 199
Cassia senna 119, **121**, 199
Cedrus atlantica 142
Centaurea acaulis 60

Centaurea alexandrina **58**, 60
Centaurea calcitrapa **59**, 60
Centaurium erythraea **88**, 89, 199
Centaurium spicatum 89, **90**
Centaurium umbellatum 199
Ceratonia siliqua 119
Ceterach officinarum **31**, 32
Chamaemelum nobile 60, 198
Chamomilla recutita 60, 198
Chenopodium ambrosioides **44**, 46
Chenopodium vulvaria 46
Chrysanthemum coronarium 61
Cicer arietinum 123
Cichorium intybus 61
Cistanche phelypaea 138, 200
Cistanche tinctoria 200
Cistus albidus 46
Cistus ladanifer 46
Cistus monspeliensis **47**, 52
Citrullus colocynthis **72**, 73
Citrus aurantium 155, 200
Citrus bigaradia 200
Clematis flammula 150
Cleome amblyocarpa **48**, 52
Colchicum autumnale 130
Colocynthis vulgaris 199
Colutea arborescens 123
Conium maculatum 80
Convolvlus althaeoides 68
Convolvulus arvensis 68
Convolvulus hystrix 68
Conyza ambigua 198
Conyza bonariensis 61, 198
Coriandrum sativum **179**, 180
Coriaria myrtifolia 70
Cornulaca monacantha 46
Coronilla scorpioides 123
Corrigiola telephiifolia 42
Cotula cinerea 61, 198
Cotula coronopifolia 61
Crataegus monogyna 153, 200
Crataegus oxyacantha 200
Cressa cretica 68
Crithmum maritimum 183
Crocus sativus 97
Crotalaria aegyptiaca **122**, 123
Cucumis melo 75
Cucurbita pepo 75
Cuminum cyminum 140, **181**, 183
Cupressus sempervirens 79
Curcuma pallida 200
Curcuma zedoaria 193, 200
Cuscuta epithymum 70
Cuscuta planiflora 70
Cymbopogon proximus 92, **93**, 199
Cymbopogon schoenanthus 94, 199
Cymbopogon schoenanthus subsp. *proximus* 199
Cynara cardunculus 61
Cynara humilis 64
Cynara scolymus 64
Cynodon dactylon 94
Cynoglossum officinale 37
Cynomorium coccineum **78**, 80
Cyperus esculentus 80, **81**
Cyperus papyrus 82
Cyperus rotundus **81**, 82
Daemia cordata 198
Daphne gnidium **170**, 172
Datura stramonium **163**, 164
Daucus carota var. *boissieri* **182**, 183
Delphinium staphisagria 150
Diotis candidissima 198
Diotis maritima 198
Dittrichia viscosa 198
Dryopteris filix-mas 32
Ecballium elaterium **74**, 75
Echinops spinosus 64
Echium maritimum 198
Echium plantagineum 37, 198
Eclipta alba 198
Eclipta prostrata **62**, 64, 198
Eleusine indica 94
Elymus repens 94, 199
Elytrigia repens 199
Eminium spiculatum 27
Ephedra alata 82
Erigeron crispus 198
Erodium cicutarium 92
Eruca sativa 71
Eryngium campestre 183
Eryngium ilicifolium 183
Erysimum officinale 199
Erythraea centaurium 199
Erythraea spicata 199
Erythrostictus punctatus 199
Eucalyptus camaldulensis 135
Eucalyptus globulus 135
Eucalyptus rostrata 135
Eugenia aromatica 200
Eugenia caryophyllata 200
Eupatorium cannabinum 64
Euphorbia balsamifera var. *sepium* 83
Euphorbia echinus 83
Euphorbia falcata 83
Euphorbia granulata 83
Euphorbia helioscopia 83
Euphorbia lathyrus 83
Euphorbia peplis 83
Euphorbia resenifera 83
Ferula cummunis 183
Ficus carica 134
Foeniculum vulgare **184**, 187
Fragaria vesca 152
Francoeuria crispa 198
Fraxinus angustifolia 137, 200
Fraxinus oxycarpa 200
Fumaria judaica **87**, 89
Fumaria officinalis 89
Fumaria parviflora 89
Galium odoratum 154, 200
Geranium robertianum 92
Geum urbanum 152
Globularia alypum **91**, 92

Glycyrrhiza foetida 123
Glycyrrhiza glabra 123
Haloxylon scoparium 46
Haplophyllum tuberculatum 155
Hedera helix 27
Helianthus annuus 64
Heliotropium bacciferum 37, 198
Heliotropium undulatum 198
Herniaria hirsuta 45
Hyoscyamus albus 164, **165**
Hyoscyamus faleslez 167, 200
Hyoscyamus muticus **166,** 167
Hyoscyamus muticus subsp. *faleslez* 200
Hypericum perforatum 96
Hyphaene thebaica 138
Imperata cylindrica 94
Inula viscosa **63,** 64, 198
Iris foetidissima 97
Iris germanica 97
Iris pseudacorus 97
Juglans regia 98
Juncus acutus 98
Juncus maritimus 98
Juniperus communis 79
Juniperus oxycedrus 79
Juniperus phoenicea **77,** 79
Juniperus thurifera 80
Kleinia pteroneura 198
Koniga maritima 199
Lactuca sativa 67
Lactuca scariola 198
Lactuca serriola 67, 198
Lactuca virosa 67
Lagenaria siceraria 75, 199
Lagenaria vulgaris 199
Laurus nobilis 116
Lavandula angustifolia 101, 140, 199
Lavandula dentata 101
Lavandula multifida 101
Lavandula officinalis 199
Lavandula stoechas **100,** 101
Lavandula vera 199
Lawsonia alba 200
Lawsonia inermis 42, 135, 154
Lepidium sativum 71
Leptadenia pyrotechnica 27, **28**
Linum usitatissimum 131
Lippia citriodora 200
Lithospermum callosum 198
Lobularia maritima 71, 199
Lolium perenne 94, **95**
Lolium temulentum 96
Lolium temulentum var. *leptochaeton* **95**
Lolium temulentum var. *macrochaeton* **95**
Luffa aegyptiaca 199
Luffa cylindrica **76,** 79, 199
Lupinus albus 123, **124,** 199
Lupinus termis 199
Lycium intricatum 167
Lycopus europaeus 101
Lythrum salicaria 131
Maerua crassifolia **41,** 42
Malva parviflora **132,** 134
Malva sylvestris **133,** 134
Mandragora autumnalis 167
Marrubium vulgare 101, **102**
Matricaria chamomilla 198
Matricaria recutita 198
Melilotus indica 126
Melissa officinalls 104
Mentha longifolia subsp. *typhoides* **103,** 104 199
Mentha pulegium 104, **105,** 140
Mentha rotundifolia 199
Mentha spicata 104, **106,** 199
Mentha spicata x *Mentha suaveolens* 199
Mentha suaveolens **107,** 109, 199
Mentha sylvestris 199
Mentha x *villosa* 107, 109, 199
Mentha viridis 199
Mercurialis annua **84,** 86
Moltkia callosa 198
Moltkia ciliata 198
Moltkiopsis ciliata 37, 198
Morus alba 135
Myristica fragrans 135, 200
Myristica moschata 200
Myrtus communis 135, **136,** 154
Narcissus tazetta 25
Nasturtium officinale 71
Nerium oleander 25
Nicotiana rustica 167
Nigella sativa 150
Ocimum basilicum 109
Olea europaea 137
Olea europaea var. *sylvestris* 137
Ononis antiquorum 199
Ononis pungens 199
Ononis spinosa 126, 199
Ononis tournefortii **125,** 126
Opuntia ficus-indica 40, 96
Origanum compactum **108,** 109
Origanum glandulosum 199
Origanum majorana 109
Origanum vulgare subsp. *glandulosum* 109, 199
Otanthus maritimus **65,** 67, 198
Otostegia fruticosa 110
Paeonia coriacea 138, 200
Paeonia corralina var. *coriacea* 200
Panicum turgidum 96
Papaver dubium **139,** 140
Papaver rhoeas 140
Papaver somniferum 140
Paronychia arabica 45
Paronychia argentea **43,** 45
Peganum harmala **194,** 195
Pergularia tomentosa **29,** 32, 198
Periploca laevigata 32
Petroselinum crispum **185,** 187, 200
Petroselinum sativum 200
Phelypaea lutea 200
Phelypaea tinctoria 200
Phoenix dactylifera 140

Phragmites australis 96, 199
Phragmites communis 199
Phyllitis scolopendrium 35, 198
Physalis alkekengi 168
Pimpinella anisum 187
Pinus halepensis 142
Piper cubeba 142
Piper nigrum 142
Pistacia atlantica 145
Pistacia lentiscus **143,** 145
Pituranthos tortuosus **186,** 187
Plantago afra 145, 200
Plantago coronopus 146
Plantago major **144,** 146
Plantago psyllium 200
Plumbago europaea 146
Polygonum aviculare 146
Polygonum maritimum 146
Polypodium vulgare 149
Populus nigra 158
Portulaca oleracea **147,** 149
Potentilla reptans 154
Psoralea plicata 126
Ptychotis ammoides 200
Pulicaria desertorum 198
Pulicaria crispa 67, 198
Pulicaria incisa **66,** 67, 198
Pulicaria undulata 198
Punica granatum **148,** 149
Quercus coccifera 86
Ranunculus lanuginosus 200
Ranunculus macrophyllus 151, 200
Ranunculus sceleratus 151
Raphanus sativus 73
Reseda luteola 151
Retama raetam 126
Rhamnus alaternus 151
Rhamnus zizyphus 200
Rhus tripartita 25
Ricinus communis **85,** 86
Rosa canina 154
Rosa damascena 154
Rosmarinus officonalis 110
Rubia peregrina 154
Rubia tinctorum 155
Rubus ulmifolius 154
Rumex roseus 200
Rumex vesicarius 149, 200
Ruscus aculeatus 155
Ruta chalepensis **156,** 158
Ruta montana **157,** 158
Salix alba 158
Salvadora persica 158, **159**
Salvia fruticosa 110, 199
Salvia libanotica 199
Salvia officinalis 110
Salvia sclarea 110
Salvia triloba 199
Sambucus ebulus 42
Sambucus nigra 42
Santolina chamaecyparissus 67
Saponaria vaccaria 198
Scilla maritima 199
Scolopendrium officinale 198
Scolopendrium vulgare 198
Senecio anteuphorbium 68, 198
Senecio vulgaris 68
Sesamum indicum **141,** 142, 200
Sesamum orientale 200
Silybum marianum 68
Sinapis alba 73
Sinapis nigra 199
Sisymbrium alliaria 198
Sisymbrium officinale 73, 199
Smilax aspera 162
Sodada decidua 198
Solanum dulcamara 168
Solanum nigrum 168
Solenostemma arghel **30,** 32. 198
Solenostemma oleifolium 198
Spartium junceum 126
Spergularia campestris 198
Spergularia marginata 198
Spergularia media 45, 198
Spergularia rubra 45, 198
Stachys officinalis 112, 199
Stellaria media 45
Stipagrostis pungens 96, 199
Syzygium aromaticum 137, 200
Tamarindus indica 126
Tamarix aphylla 172, 200
Tamarix articulata 200
Tamus communis 82
Tetraclinis articulata 80, 199
Teucrium chamaedrys 112
Teucrium polium **111,** 112
Thapsia garganica 187, **188**
Thymelaea hirsuta **171,** 172
Thymus algeriensis 112, 199
Thymus broussonettii 112, **113**
Thymus capitatus 112, **114**
Thymus ciliatus 116
Thymus maroccanus 116
Thymus serpyllum 116
Thymus vulgaris 116
Thyumus zattarellus 199
Thymus zygis 116
Tribulus terrestris 195
Trigonella foenum-graecum **127,** 128
Triticum repens 199
Typha angustata 200
Typha angustifolia 200
Typha australis 200
Typha domingensis 172, 200
Ulmus campestris 172
Urginea maritima 130, 199
Urginea scilla 199
Urtica pilulifera **189,** 191
Urtica urens **190,** 191
Vaccaria pyramidata 45, 198
Vaccaria segetalis 198
Vaccaria vulgaris 198

Verbascum sinuatum **161**, 162
Verbena citriodora 200
Verbena officinalis 191, **192**
Verbena triphylla 200
Vicia faba 128
Vicia sativa 128
Viola odorata 193
Viola tricolor 193
Viscum cruciatum 131
Vitex agnus-castus 193
Withania somnifera 168, **169**
Zea mays 96
Zilla macroptera 199
Zilla spinosa 73, 199
Zingiber officinale 193
Ziziphus jujuba 200
Ziziphus lotus 151, **152**
Ziziphus sativa 200
Ziziphus spina-christi **152**, 153
Ziziphus vulgaris 200
Ziziphus zizyphus 92, 152, 200
Zygophyllum coccineum 195, **196**
Zygophyllum gaetulum 197

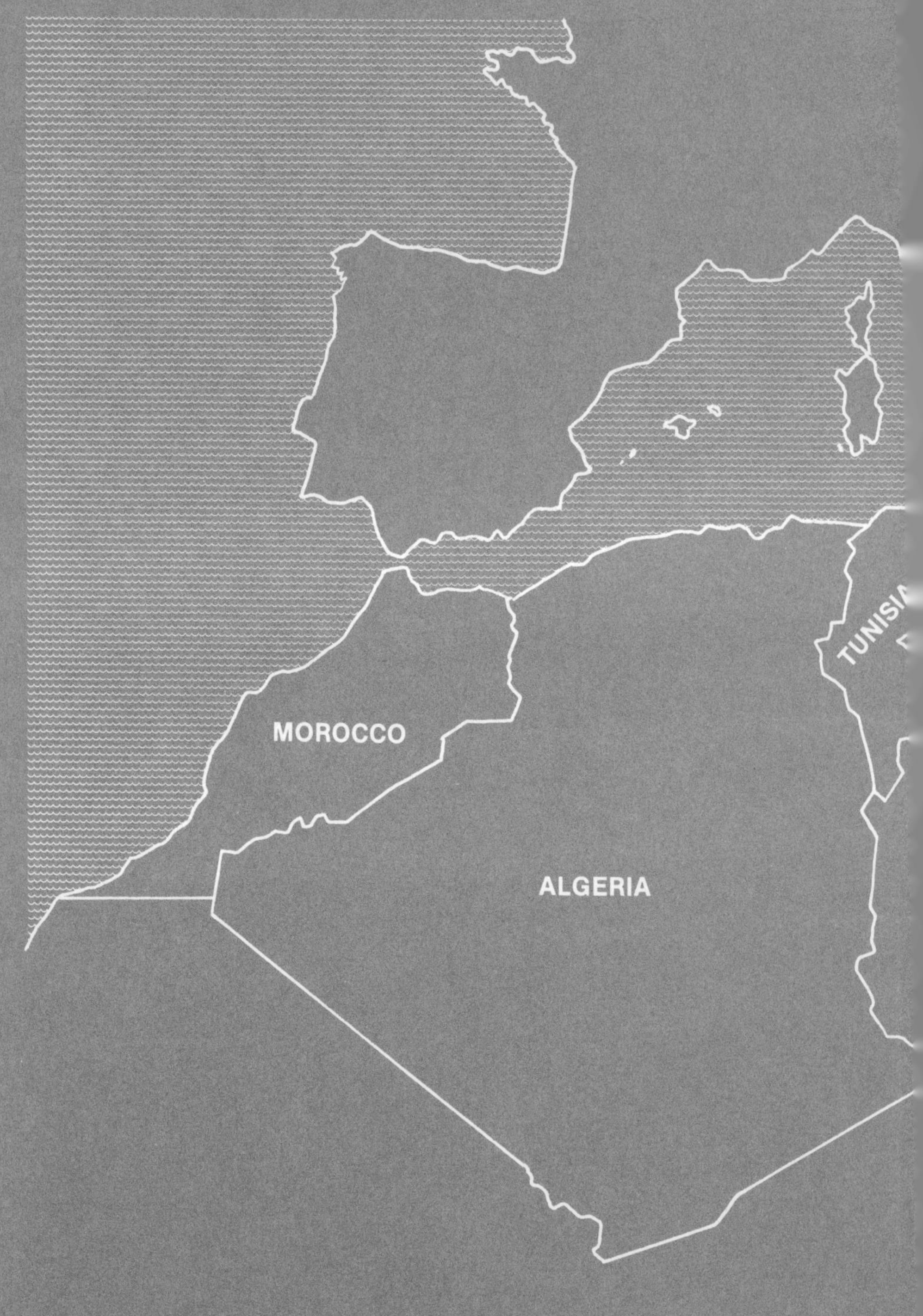

This map, which illustrates the area covered in this work, does not represent any political opinion concerning the boundaries between the countries of North Africa.